Medicine, Sport and the Law

EDITED BY

SIMON D. W. PAYNE

MB, BS, FRCS (Ed. and Eng.)
The Medical Protection Society
London;
Department of General Surgery
Central Middlesex Hospital
London

EDITORIAL CONSULTANTS

EDWARD GRAYSON

MA (Oxon)
of the Middle Temple and
of the South Eastern Circuit,
Barrister

SIR JOHN ELLIS

KBE, MA, MD, FRCP
Past President
The Medical Protection Society
London

JOHN DAVIES

MRCS, LRCP, DPhysMed
Medical Director
Harley Street Sports Clinic
London

BERNARD KNIGHT

MD (Wales), MRCP, FRCPath, DMJ (Path),
Barrister;
Professor of Forensic Pathology
University of Wales
College of Medicine
Cardiff

FOREWORD BY

HRH THE PRINCESS ROYAL

BLACKWELL SCIENTIFIC PUBLICATIONS

OXFORD LONDON

EDINBURGH BOSTON MELBOURNE

To Ailsa, Thomas and Jet

© 1990 by
Blackwell Scientific Publications
Editorial Offices:
Osney Mead, Oxford OX2 0EL
25 John Street, London WC1N 2BL
23 Ainslie Place, Edinburgh EH3 6AJ
3 Cambridge Center, Suite 208
  Cambridge, Massachusetts 02142, USA
107 Barry Street, Carlton
  Victoria 3053, Australia

First published 1990

Set by Best-set Typesetter Ltd,
Hong Kong
Printed and bound in Great Britain
by Hartnolls Ltd,
Bodmin, Cornwall

DISTRIBUTORS

Marston Book Services Ltd
PO Box 87
Oxford OX2 0DT
(*Orders:* Tel: 0865 791155
         Fax: 0865 791927
         Telex: 837515)

USA
Year Book Medical Publishers
200 North LaSalle Street
Chicago, Illinois 60601
(*Orders:* Tel: (312) 726−9733)

Canada
The C. V. Mosby Company
5240 Finch Avenue East
Scarborough, Ontario
(*Orders:* Tel: (416) 298-1588)

Australia
Blackwell Scientific Publications
(Australia) Pty Ltd
107 Barry Street
Carlton, Victoria 3053
(*Orders:* Tel: (03) 347-0300)

British Library
Cataloguing in Publication Data

Medicine, sport and the law.
  1. Sports & games. Medical aspects
  I. Payne, Simon D. W.
  617.1027

ISBN 0−632−02439−9

Contents

v

Part II: Specific Sports

List of contributors

L. M. ADAMS BSc, MB, ChB, PhD
Lecturer, Department of Anatomy, University of Leeds, Leeds LS2 9JT; Honorary Member of the Medical Commission of the Amateur Boxing Association of England

M. ALLEN MB, ChB, DMRD
Jockey Club Medical Consultant, The Jockey Club, 42 Portman Square, London W1H 0EN

T. J. ANSTISS BM, MEd
Research Assistant, Charing Cross Hospital; Honorary Registrar, Ealing Health Authority, Ealing Hospital, Southall, Middlesex UB1 3EU; past international athlete

I. S. BENJAMIN BSc, MD, FRCS
Senior Lecturer, Royal Postgraduate Medical School; Honorary Consultant Surgeon, Hammersmith Hospital, Du Cane Road, London W12 0NS

J. C. BETTS MB, BS LRCP, MRCS, MRCGP
General Practitioner, 82A Roman Road, London E2 0PG; Vice President of the British Sub Aqua Club

M. BOTTOMLEY MB, ChB, DObstRCOG
Medical Officer, Bath University Medical Centre, Claverton Down, Bath BA2 7AY; Medical Officer to the British athletes team

J. F. BUCHAN
Sleepers Hill Lane, Cocking Causeway, Midhurst, Sussex GU29 9QQ

J. M. CAMERON MD, PhD, FRCS(Glas.), FRCPath, DMJ
Professor of Forensic Medicine, Department of Forensic Medicine, The London Hospital Medical School, Turner Street, Whitechapel, London E1 2AD; Medical Officer to the British and Olympic swimming teams

J. C. CHAWLA MD, FRCS
Senior Lecturer in Rehabilitation, Demonstration AIDS Centre, Spinal/ Rehabilitation Unit, Rockwood Hospital, Llandaff, Cardiff CF5 2YN

J. CRANE MB, ChB
General Practitioner, Aylesbury Health Centre, Thurlow Street, London SE17 2UN; Team Physician to Arsenal Football Club and the England football team

A. R. CRAWFURD MA, MRCP
General Practitioner, Ivy Court Surgery, Tenterden, Kent TN30 6RB; Honorary Medical Officer to the Amateur Fencing Association and corresponding member of the Medical Commission of the Fédération Internationale d'Escrimé

J. DAVIES MRCP, LRCP, DPhysMed
Medical Director, Harley Street Sports Clinic, 110 Harley Street, London W1N 1AF; Consultant in Physical Medicine and Rehabilitation, The Devonshire Rehabilitation Hospital, Devonshire Street, London W1N 1RF; Honorary Physician to the Welsh Rugby Union; member of the International Rugby Board Medical Advisory Committee; Medical Officer to the British Lions

E. GRAYSON MA(Oxon)
Of the Middle Temple and of the South Eastern Circuit, Barrister, 4 Paper Buildings, Temple, London EC4 7EX

P. J. A. GRIFFIN FRCs
Associate Specialist, Renal Transplant Unit, Cardiff Royal Infirmary, Newport Road, Cardiff CF2 1FZ; Medical Officer to the British Transplant Games team

F. T. HORAN MSc, FRCS
Consultant Orthopaedic Surgeon, Cuckfield Hospital, Hayward Heath, West Sussex RH17 5HQ; Medical Officer to the MCC

R. W. KENDRICK MB, FDS, FFD
Consultant Oral and Maxillofacial Surgeon, Northern Ireland Plastic and Maxillofacial Service, The Royal Victoria Hospital, Grosvenor Road, Belfast BT12 6BA; International Board and World Cup hockey referee

K. W. KENNEDY MB, BCh, DPhysMed
Consultant in Orthopaedic Medicine, 30 Harley Street, London W1N 1AB; past Irish international rugby player

B. KNIGHT MD(Wales), MRCP, FRCPath, DMJ(Path), Barrister
Professor of Forensic Pathology, Institute of Pathology, University of Wales College of Medicine, Cardiff Royal Infirmary, Newport Road, Cardiff CF2 1FZ

C. LOVEDAY MB, BS, MIBiol, PhD
Lecturer in Virology, Department of Virology, University College Hospital, London

D. A. D. MACLEOD MB, ChB, FRCS(Ed.)
Consultant Surgeon, Lothian Health Board, West Lothian Unit, St John's Hospital at Howden, Howden Road, West Livingstone, West Lothian EH54 6PP; Honorary Medical Adviser to the Scottish Rugby Union

G. R. McLATCHIE MB, ChB, FRCS
Consultant Surgeon, The General Hospital, Hartlepool, Cleveland TS24 9AH;

*Former Chairman of the Medical Control Commission of the World Union of Karate
Organisations*

F. NEWTON MRCS, LRCP, DA
*Sports Physician, Grafton Leys, 39 Cattle End, Silverstone, Northamptonshire NN12
8UX; Medical Officer to the Admirals Cup team*

R. N. PALMER Llb, MB, MRCS
Secretary, The Medical Protection Society, 50 Hallam Street, London W1N 6DE

G. RADHAKRISHNAN MB, MRCPsych
*Lecturer, Department of Psychological Medicine, University of Wales College of
Medicine; Honorary Registrar, Academic Unit, Ely Hospital, Ely, Cardiff CF5 5XE*

P. G. RICHARDS FRCS
*Consultant Neurosurgeon, Regional Neurosciences Centre, Charing Cross Hospital,
Fulham Palace Road, London W6 8RF; Medical Officer for Brands Hatch*

R. R. H. SHIPWAY
*Partner, Le Brasseur and Monier-Williams, 71 Lincoln's Inn Fields, London WC2A
3JF*

J. C. TAYLOR MRCS, LRCP, DObstRCOG, MRCPsych
*Consultant Forensic Psychiatrist, Northeast Thames Region Health Authority,
Friern Hospital, Friern Barnet Road, London N11 3BP*

P. L. THOMAS MB, BS
*General Practitioner, Reading Clinic, 10 Eldon Road, Reading, Berkshire RG1 4DH;
past British Olympic oarsman; Honorary Secretary to the British Association of
Sport and Medicine*

A. L. WHITESON MB, BS, MRCS, LRCP
*General Practitioner, 58A Wimpole Street, London W1M 7DE; Medical Officer to the
British Boxing Board of Control*

J. G. P. WILLIAMS MD, MSc, FRCS, FRCP
*Consultant in Rehabilitation Medicine, Wexham Park Hospital, Slough, Berkshire
SO2 4HL; Medical Adviser to the Squash Rackets Association*

J. P. R. WILLIAMS MBE, MB, BS(Lond.), MRCS, LRCP, FRCS(Ed.)
*Consultant Orthopaedic Surgeon, Princess of Wales Hospital, Coity Road, Bridgend
CF13 1RQ; Junior Wimbledon Champion; past Welsh international rugby player*

P. J. WREN MB, ChB, MD, FRCGP, MIBiol
*Monksgate, Hardacre Lane, Wittle-Le-Woods, Chorley, Lancashire PR6 7PQ;
Chairman of the Medical Commission of the Amateur Boxing Association of
England*

MEDICINE, SPORT AND THE LAW

FOREWORD - HRH THE PRINCESS ROYAL

Organised sport forms an important part of the heritage of the people of the United Kingdom. Many of the games that are now enjoyed throughout the world have their origins in these isles, and the development of their rules of play and codes of conduct owe much to British influence in standards of civilisation and fair play. The United Kingdom is still in a position to influence those standards and this book could be a major factor in respect to medicine, sport and the law.

It is extremely important for the continued integrity of our society that the diverse activities enjoyed by so many, both as spectators and as participants, are seen to attempt to maintain a high reputation in terms of safety and standards of conduct. Unfortunately, in the same way that sport can be effective both in promoting health and causing injury, ever increasing standards of competitiveness and of professionalism, can likewise bring about progressively higher levels of excellence in conjunction with dubious standards of conduct. Our athletes continue to break world records but some will stoop to base levels and unfair methods in the attempt. The so called "professional foul" is now unfortunately only too well known in the context of competitive sport.

Sport can prevent its own destruction by appropriate action from its respective governing bodies. They will, however, need all the help they can muster and consequently it may be timely to enlist the assistance that medicine and the law may offer. It could also be argued that medicine and the law have already been enlisted - unfortunately for some of the wrong reasons - to research and prescribe undetectable drugs and arguments to avoid the rules of sport. The general conduct of sport at all levels will not improve if doctors and lawyers drive "four in hands" (coach and horses) through the spirit of the law.

However, when medical knowledge and research into the mechanism of injury is combined with relevant legal considerations, the results could offer sports legislators an excellent basis for sound reform of their rules with a view to increasing safety and eliminating undesirable practices.

The authors of this pioneering work have provided a much needed benchmark which may materially assist those involved in the assault on the problems which beset modern sport.

This book outlines the common medical and legal problems, and discusses some of the moral issues with which doctors attending sports men and women may be faced. By describing how these situations should be handled for the benefit and safety of sports men and women, this work has made a significant contribution to sports medical literature.

Anne

Preface

This book offers definitive, practical and authentic advice on the legal, ethical and professional problems with which any doctor concerned with a medical sporting issue may be faced. It is hoped that sports administrators of the relevant governing bodies, and the athletes themselves, in addition to medical practitioners of all disciplines, will benefit from the advice contained herein, for the future well-being of all sports enthusiasts and of sport itself.

'No gain without pain' is a concept known well to athletes of all disciplines. It may be more completely understood, however, when reflected in their achievements on the field of play against the clock, or in overcoming the adversity of disablement or disease; in the experience of most competitive sports men and women the contrasting sensations of pleasure and pain meet on the dark side of the same moon.

Sport may defy complete definition but few can doubt its role in promoting health and fulfilment in those taking part. The capacity of sport to forge bonds between competitors locked in friendly rivalry, or between nations participating in international games, is a manifestation of its nature as a true international language.

Such formidable potential requires appropriate and careful handling if it is to be harnessed to the best effect. Morever, this common understanding amongst nations may be subject to abuse if it is not adequately protected from those who would seek its exploitation for their own political or commercial ends.

At the Central Council for Physical Recreation's annual conference in November 1986, John Wheatley, the then Director-General of the Sports Council, highlighted the importance of sport as a national pastime: 'Participation in United Kingdom sport and recreation involves about 22 million people in all, on at least one occasion per month . . . it embraces all generations from the cradle to the grave.'

Although complete statistics are inevitably unavailable because of the diverse nature of sporting endeavour, it has been calculated that 1.5 million sporting injuries occur annually in the UK (*Daily Telegraph* 24 September 1984). This produces two major consequences: the sufferers are unable to continue with their respective sports and 10% of injuries cause absence from work.

The healthy human body exists as a self-regulating machine for a remarkable period of time. As William Boyd in his textbook of pathology notes, 'strange that a harp with so many strings should stay in tune so long'. Many studies have shown that regular physical activity contributes significantly towards health, well-being and longevity in the individual. The capacity of physical recreation to promote health, however, must be recognised alongside its capability to cause injury, producing a spectrum of damage ranging from trivial self-limiting disablement to death.

Doctors who are trained to treat 'disease' may be incompletely aware of the benefits and hazards to health that sport can provide. Increasing numbers of sports men and women who present as 'patients' will include the capability to resume sport as an important ingredient in the quality of their existence and therefore also as a criterion for 'cure'. Thus it may be necessary for doctors, who may not immediately realise or recognise the true value of sport to their patient and also to the community, to extend their concept of disease to include the situation in which the athlete/patient is unable to practise or compete. Although the bulk of the population engaged in sport will regard the capability to take part simply as a source of enrichment of their quality of life, for a specialist minority this activity will also represent their major means of income.

Both ordinary and élite participants will look to medicine to assist in their preparation, enhance their performances and treat their ills. A significant legal liability will exist for doctors who attend such patients in ignorance of their needs. The speciality which describes these obligations is sports medicine. Relatively few texts exist to describe the standards of care required of the doctor generally and none so far as we are aware in relation to sports medicine itself. It is therefore hoped that this contribution to the literature, written primarily to advise doctors and other health professionals, may help by raising the level of consciousness of medical men and women to the responsibilities that they face in various sporting contexts. It is anticipated that the need for this knowledge will continue to increase.

In the UK the administration of sport of various types is entrusted with approximately 390 governing bodies. This is a necessary and prudent arrangement for the proper running of the individual disciplines and sensible updating of playing rules. It is as well to remember however that certain games, and especially those involving physical contact, aggression or speed, are from time to time subject to a degree of lobbying by pressure groups who seek to restrict the sport in question or abolish it altogether, allegedly on the grounds of safety. The governing bodies do indeed already have an ethical duty — and also, more significantly, a legal duty — to ensure that the sport over which they preside is reasonably safe for its participants and spectators.

Alterations in the playing laws brought about as a result of research in sports medicine have already occurred and have helped to effect demonstrable reductions in casualties in such sports as boxing, rugby football, motor-racing, horse-racing, American football and hockey, to name but a few. The role of the doctor in this regard must be to explain and maintain the pressure of medical evidence presented to the governing bodies in order that continuing beneficial amendments to the laws of the game are made, so that the game itself may be protected from the sometimes warranted attacks on its safety record.

Recourse to law is available to injured parties to settle disputes in situations of conflicting interests. Where sport is involved, the playing, administrative and organisational laws that have been created are all subordinate to national laws, although this fact may come as a surprise to some. An increasing number of examples exist where the common law and Parliamentary influence have been brought into play, and perhaps this is a sign that the pressures of competition and public interest in certain activities have caused these games to outgrow their administrative and playing rules, a situation that in itself demands reform, or at least a critical reappraisal of existing playing laws and regulations of the sport in question.

That part of medical decision-making which lies beyond the boundaries that the law may control occurs within the territory governed by ethical considerations. Such factors are of no less importance to the doctor than the law itself. The fall of the Canadian athlete, Ben Johnson, from 'hero to zero' at the Seoul Olympics in 1988 exemplifies the charged moral climate surrounding the issue of drug-abuse in sport. In the same vein, the use of violent foul play demonstrates a further illustration of the malaise which affects modern competitive endeavour. It is essential that doctors should be appraised of the issues and facts of life involved in the use of outlawed performance-enhancing substances and in over-zealous activity in competition, in order that their patients and they themselves do not suffer in this ethical and medico-legal minefield.

HIV disease and consent for participation in sport by the mentally handicapped are further areas which require ethical exploration and guidance for the medical practitioner, and debate on these subjects is provided in these pages.

The Corinthian ideal of sport is summed up in the phrase *mens sana in corpore sano* — a healthy mind in a healthy body. Since the modern Olympic Games were resurrected by Baron de Couberin in 1896 sport has progressed considerably. A totally new dimension has been introduced in the emergence of professional codes, aided and abetted by the attention of media coverage. Sport is now big business that projects powerful images that may be used well or abused by their promoters and other vested interests.

The medical profession must ensure that it is adequately protected from the twin perils of damage to the sport which the practitioner him- or herself may enjoy, and professional liability which may be incurred by practising inappropriate or inadequate standards of care, remembering that the categories of negligence are never closed.

Sport is the problem child of the late twentieth century and the law alone is unable to control it. The law ultimately will be the final arbiter of conduct, but medical men and women have a golden opportunity to influence its development and this is a chance which none of the interested parties concerned can afford to miss.

Simon Payne
London W3
September 1989

Acknowledgements

A production of this size and complexity would only ever be undertaken by an individual who at the time of starting had no real grasp of the magnitude of the problems to be encountered. It could only ever be completed by someone who had the serendipitous good fortune to enjoy unreserved support and assistance from colleagues, friends and relations.

The editor is indebted to many in this regard, but in particular to Dr John Barker, Acting Deputy Secretary of the Medical Protection Society, and to Dr Oscar Craig of its Council, both of whose wisdom, counsel and support have helped to keep the editor going at times when the going got tough.

The contributing authors have observed a commendable punctuality in production of their manuscripts and any delays that have occurred are essentially the fault of the editor for completely misjudging the number of hours in a day, misreading the number of days in a week, and miscalculating the number of weeks in a year.

Accurate collation and presentation of detailed information from multiple sources requires efficient and dedicated secretarial application. The production of this work owes much to the conscientiousness of Miss Frances Azque-Bright, whose considerable secretarial talents proved indispensible in the preparation of the manuscript throughout numerous amended versions. Additional supporting secretarial assistance has been ably supplied by Miss Janice Thompson, and the editor is most grateful to these ladies for their devotion to the project.

The contribution made by the consultant editorial board is more fully acknowledged elsewhere, but any tribute would be incomplete without recording our thanks to Mr Huw Knight, who, as a skilled linguist, cast an expert eye over the manuscript to modify construction in places and to improve grammar in general!

On points of law, further technical advice is gratefully acknowledged from Mr Colin Brown who is a senior litigation partner with the solicitors, Le Brasseurs and Monier-Williams.

Dr Heather Payne and Dr Norman Doe comprised the proof-reading support team, by kind permission of Rachel and Elizabeth Doe, and my sincere thanks are due to them as well as to my mother and father for their encouragement and Sunday luncheons.

The appearance of a work such as this within the same general epoch as the projected date of publication seems to rely as much on the understanding of the publishers as it does on the co-operation

of the authors. For this the editor has to thank Peter Saugman and
Julian Grover of Blackwell Scientific Publications, and must acknowledge the kindness, courtesy and understanding of the whole
of their production team.

Finally recognition and heartfelt thanks are owed for many
months of privation, accepted without complaint by Ailsa and
Thomas and also by Jet who never seemed to mind.

Simon Payne
London W3
September 1989

Part I: General Issues

Sports medicine and the law

1

EDWARD GRAYSON

'The Law fills gaps which the world of sport can never reach'

Prologue

The law linked collectively to medicine and sport was the last thought in my mind as a law student, after the Second World War had just ended, when the gross mistreatment of a simple fibula fracture from a mistimed tackle in the Oxford University soccer trials ended my active participation forever in the game, as a player. It led indirectly to a love for the law blending with a lifelong enthusiasm for all sports and thinking, writing and ultimately practising law as applied to sport.

Initial thoughts in that direction were developed with topics which the medical world in a sporting context may never need to contemplate. They were fired by dining in the Hall of Exeter College (where Britain's first organised Athletic Meeting and Club were formed in 1850 and nearly a century later Sir Roger Bannister dreamed of breaking the four-minute mile barrier), beneath a portrait of Mr Justice Eve. He had pioneered the concept of sporting educational charities with a High Court judgment delivered during the First World War. It confirmed a former schoolmaster's bequests to Aldenham School for the purpose of building Eton fives courts or squash rackets courts and an annual athletics school sports prize. In *re Mariette* [1915] 2 Ch. 284 was a landmark decision which the House of Lords unanimously endorsed 65 years later in the Football Association's Youth Trust Deed decision of *Inland Revenue Commissioners* v. *McMullen* [1981] AC 1.

Ch: Chancery (Law Reports)

AC: Appeal Cases

That inspiration for sporting–legal thoughts led to published explanations after commencing practice at the Bar in the *FA Bulletin* and *Rating and Income Tax* during 1953 on the taxation anomalies between professional cricketers' tax-free benefits from public subscriptions and those of professional footballers which were then contractually based and thereby liable to income tax. They were followed by an abortive attempt to argue the now well-established restraint of trade principle in a county court case on behalf of Ralph Banks who had played against the immortal Stanley Matthews in the celebrated Coronation Year FA Cup Final of 1953 when Blackpool beat Bolton Wanderers 4–3 (*Aldershot Football Club* v. *Banks* (1955) *Aldershot News* 4, 25 November 1955).

Medical issues never surfaced at all during that period, although the personal suffering from that self-inflicted soccer injury was a classic case of *volenti non fit injuria* (he who voluntarily consents to lawful injury risks cannot claim compensation damages for it). It is correctly qualified by my co-editor Professor Bernard Knight's contribution on p. 72. Deliberate criminal and civilly actionable breaches of playing law nullify it. My broken fibula, when my foot stabbed the hard Iffley Road ground, tackling for a ball already whisked away by my opponent, illustrates it perfectly. Subsequent negligent hospital treatment, which created a legal liability, was sufficiently remedied elsewhere by specialist skills to deflect parental thoughts from the available compensation claim against the local hospital authorities.

Yet four decades later, when Butterworths' *Sport and the Law* (with 15 chapters and 10 appendices) took shape in the later 1980s, the chapter headed 'Sports medicine and the law' was the first to be written because its subject matter was then uppermost in my own and the general public's minds. It has contributed to the structure of the pages which follow. For the intervening years have developed this area of the application of the law to medicine within sport into the most important for sport in particular and society in general. It affects all sections of the community from the cradle to the grave as the national concept of sport for all becomes synonymous with health for all.

As a member of the editorial board I have had the opportunity and privilege to obtain an overview of all contributions to these pages, and thus to identify a pattern which emerges that is common to all the differing sporting disciplines where legal involvement cannot be ignored. They can be conveniently summarised as follows:

1 Any medical or paramedical practitioner in this growth area, as evidenced by our contributors, clearly has, or should have, an enthusiasm for his or her particular sports discipline.

2 Different sporting categories demand different levels of medical experiences and awareness and action, often in an international context. Yet as Dr F. Netwon says at the end of his chapter, 'Medical hazards of water sports — and how to avoid them', in respect of the profile of the team doctor, with words of general application, it 'is much that of the old-fashioned family doctor.'

3 The medical adviser must always keep in mind the overriding duty to the individual performer as an individual patient.

4 Conflicts of duty between responsibility to the athlete patient and any governing or managing body should be recognised, identified and resolved in favour of the overriding professional duty to the patient, and liaison should be established, if required, with the patient's more permanent GP. This position is comparable to the in-house industrial and commercial practitioner's relationship with employees (while being alert to the potential differences created between ambitious athletic achievers and/or their administrators desiring and, indeed, perhaps demanding, for competitive or individual participation, a medical opinion for fitness which conflicts with the patient's individual welfare).

5   There is a necessity for medical advisers to administrative governing, managerial, organisational or promotional bodies to:
(a) understand, identify and, if necessary, record their own legal relationships and areas of legal control and responsibility as contractors or agents;
(b) where appropriate, advise on suitable facilities and equipment, including communication with associated or back-up services for supplying appropriate medical action for every occasion; and
(c) recognise and act upon an entitlement to withdraw from any commitment if such advice is not pursued effectively, thereby placing such advice at risk for potential legal liability.

6   A requirement for keeping or logging adequate records for future reference in case of disputes over diagnosis and treatment may appear to be self-evident, but in circumstances of sporting medical emergencies this benefit to both patient and doctor may be overlooked.

7   There is a general across-the-board absence of adequate statistical information for assessing the extent of sporting injuries and levels of seriousness in order to gauge the problems which require the most immediate remedial action.

8   A precise definition of relationships and responsibilities and cross communication is essential, if time permits in writing, between all parties concerned in respect of the sports doctor's appointment to act for an individual, team or governing body, for the purpose of accepting or avoiding a duty of confidentiality to an individual athlete or participant.

These common denominators emerge as the most apparent features which bind all the different sporting medical requirements in a common interest. Furthermore, the number of additional examples and citations which have been specifically identified in my own text here as having been incorporated while these pages were being prepared for the printers during the autumn and early winter of 1989, after its earlier structure based on the Butterworths' *Sport and the Law* publication in January 1988, demonstrates beyond doubt the rapid development of a growth area. It is illustrated almost daily, and indeed, inevitably, as the sporting world expands its horizons internationally to every corner of the world. Against this background, what follows here is an attempt to explain, within the limitations of space as comprehensively as possible, how the law and medicine can combine to benefit not only sport and its personnel in general, but also society, which all three disciplines should seek to serve. The laws are stated as at Remembrance Sunday, 12 November 1989.

Introduction and issues

The role of sport within the international community was described by Professor Sir Ludwig Guttman in 'Reflections on sport in general' in his *Textbook of Sport for the Disabled*, published in 1976, with words which are as true now as they were when he wrote, 'Today sport plays an ever-increasing part in the life of the individual, as it does in the life of nations, and represents as much a positive element in the culture of our modern life as it did in the culture of ancient nations.'

The survival of sport on the public stage through sponsorship caused one of Britain's best known and experienced commentators, Ron Pickering, to address British sport's governing bodies at the Central Council of Physical Recreation's (CCPR's) annual conference at Bournemouth in 1985 with the following citation from the *Observer*'s leading sports writer, Peter Corrigan: 'Sport took its soul to the pawnbrokers so long ago that finding the redemption ticket is not going to be easy.'

Four years later, in early 1989, that redemption ticket emerged at an international medical congress on injuries in rugby and other contact sports, organised by the South Africa Sports Medicine Association, within a heartbeat of where Dr Christiaan Barnard pioneered the internationally acclaimed first successful heart transplant operation at Cape Town's Groot Schur Memorial Hospital. For if medicine and music spell out an international language known to all peoples of the world, which transcends or should transcend all known barriers, so, too, does sport, and the injuries and damage to health that it can cause.

In two crucial areas, violence and drugs (sport's own VD problem), medical services and their associated disciplines such as physiotherapy, pharmacology and biochemistry can alone identify the causes for which the law, in and out of sport, should be able to provide the remedy. Correspondingly, if medicine and its ancillary services err, the law provides areas for redress, particularly in the field of negligence and even, in the most extreme circumstances, through criminal liability.

Within the drugs scenario, doctors, pharmacologists and biochemists and laboratory staff have uncorked the bottles from which have poured the disagreeable evidence of cheating and attempted cheating by artificial stimulants. No less disagreeable, and of equal actual and potential consequence, is the other form of sporting injury to health: violent foul play. Curiously, and for reasons connected with long-established sporting mores and customs, linked to the macho image of robust play, any notion of cheating by physical injury has hitherto been underplayed, if not ignored: with increasing frequency throughout the world an offender or an offending team gains an unfair advantage over and against the victim through breaches of playing laws. This can also create breaches of national civil and criminal laws which merit intervention by traditional legal processes, in addition to sporting institutions and governing bodies' disciplinary tribunals.

Thus sports medicine involves not only traditional treatment and availability of facilities, it is also a guide and reflection on the state of play according to sporting rules and laws or breaches of them. This was evidenced as long ago as 1978 when two crucial sporting medical contributions to the *British Medical Journal* (December 1978) identified medical evidence which crystallised respectively the injurious consequences of existing playing laws which required amendment and the civil and criminally liable consequences of undoubtedly violent foul play in breach of existing playing laws. J. P. R. Williams, surgical registrar, and Professor B. McKibbin, in the Department of Traumatic and Orthopaedic Surgery at Cardiff Royal Infirmary, warned in an article entitled 'Cervical spine injuries in Rugby Union football': 'Referees and coaches should be aware of the dangers of scrum collapses, especially as it seems to be an increasingly popular tactic to bring about this purposefully.' J. E. Davies, Research Registrar, and T. Gibson, Consultant Physician, recorded in an article entitled 'Injuries in Rugby Union football': 'in a prospective study of 185 players attached to 10 British rugby clubs . . . foul play might have caused as many as 47 (31%) of all reported injuries. Complete eradication of deliberately dangerous play would considerably reduce the high incidence of injuries in this sport.'

These two complementary examples of a common denominator for health hazards illuminate ideally the relationship between sports medicine and the law. They would also appear to reflect to this particular non-medical editor and contributor one of the factors which influenced the first Lord Horder in his early days at Bart's at the turn of the century, as explained in the memoir by his son entitled *The Little Genius* (1966): 'that preoccupation with the post-mortem room . . . and an examination of the body after death was often, as it sometimes still is, the only way to arrive at the truth about a particular case, to confirm or upset a diagnosis, and to push forward the frontiers of knowledge in general. There is no arguing with the corpse on the slab.' A corollary to this appears in the current and 13th edition (1973) of *Glaister's Medical Jurisprudence and Toxicology*. Written initially by successive holders of the Regius Chair of Forensic Medicine in the University of Glasgow, John Glaister, Sr., and his son John Glaister, Jr., kinsmen of the BBC producer, Gerard Glaister, of such authentic television programmes as *Colditz* and *Howard's Way*, the Conclusions to the chapter entitled 'The medico-legal aspects of wounds' advise at p. 256 '. . . the examiner should direct his attention to the reconstruction of the cause of the injuries. He should first decide the instrument, then the degree of violence, the possibility of accident, the direction of the wound, and the relative position of the parties'. For sporting injuries caused by violent foul play this formula cannot be improved, and leads logically to the next citation from six years later.

In June 1979, after the British Medical Journal for 1978 cited above, P. N. Sperryn, in a paper to the British Association of Sports Medicine symposium, published in the *British Journal of Sports Medicine* (vol. 14, nos 2 & 3, August 1980, pp. 84−9), reaffirmed: 'It has recently become evident that deliberate foul play in certain sports is directly responsible for many sports injuries. It could be argued that the medical profession, on becoming aware of such trends in the style of play in sport, should be among the first to initiate the political changes which should lead to elimination of dangerous unfair play.'

No magic or new dimension exists for either medicine or the law in their application to sport. The law applies recognised criteria and principles to an area where it was traditionally recognised as a needless intruder until the complexities of modern administration and the intensity of modern competition demanded its arrival on a scene which conventional sporting sources were unable to regulate and control. The necessity for compulsory purchase orders and planning consents were as essential for the preservation and development of sporting premises as the necessity for courts of law to compensate victims and punish offenders of violent foul play.

More recently the nexus was highlighted in the sustained and extensive publicity in relation to the Sheffield Wednesday Football Club's Hillsborough Stadium disaster. At the time of writing in autumn 1989, in between Lord Justice Taylor's interim report (CM 765), published in August 1989, and his final report, due to be published early in 1990, the recommendations, under the separate headings of 'Co-ordination of emergency services' and 'First aid, medical facilities and ambulances', are sufficiently comprehensive and relevant, in principle, not only to the tragic events which gave rise to this particular judicial inquiry, but also to all sports activities generally. Accordingly they are reproduced in Appendix 1.1. For the boundaries of sports medicine and the law are clearly not limited to playing areas.

So long as sport, leisure and recreational activities are capable of self-regulation, or careful or responsible control by sporting governing bodies or institutions or promotional organisations, without injurious or potentially injurious consequences, traditional legal sources are rarely required to intervene. When health and safety are at risk, the general legal system alone cannot protect the community which obtains its pleasures within the conventional sporting spheres. It not only needs evidence from the medical world, whether with regard to drugs, violence or maladministration, to prove specific breaches of regulations and of the rule of law with consequential health hazards. It also needs an awareness of the ethical and moral climate in which it operates.

Medicine as well as sport is caught up in the whirlwind of changing attitudes and scientific developments which demand decisions on many contentious ethical issues outside the sporting arena. Yet, as long ago as 1979, Sir Roger Bannister, from his standpoint as the first four-minute mile record-holder and neurologist before becoming Master of Pembroke College, Oxford, wrote in his foreword to Professor Peter McIntosh's book *Fair Play: Ethics in Sport and Education*: 'It is an increasingly popular notion among many young people that we can throw off ethical and moral principles in more and more spheres of life ... The fact of the matter is that we are faced with moral choices many times a day and if we do not notice them it must be that our intelligence or sensitivity is becoming blunted. Sport, which occupies the professional time of a few and the spare time of many, is a fit study for ethics.'

That study is beyond the scope of this chapter and of this book. Yet, as Bernard Crick, from his standpoint as Professor of Politics at Birkbeck College in the University of London, wrote in his preface to *Law and Morality*, edited by Louis Blom-Cooper and Gavin Drewry, in 1976: 'The structure of ethical arguments is hardly something to be determined *a priori* ... Both the fascination and the general problem today of the relation of law to morality — Does the law rest upon morality? Should the law concern itself with private morals? — arise because we no longer live in a society in which there is a clear moral code (whatever its basis) or in which there is consensus in the Ciceronian sense of common agreement as to right and interest.'

Nature nevertheless creates its own norm from the cradle to the grave. Medical remedies for healing and preservation of life have progressed down the years with new frontiers identified in succeeding centuries and generations: from Simpson with chloroform, Madame Curie with radiology, Pasteur with immunology, down to our own times with Banting, Best and Macleod with insulin and Chain, Florey and Fleming with penicillin. Yet, for the world of sport and its own capacity to operate as a mirror of and for society generally, medicine is the sole continuing area which can create a standard of awareness and recognition within the widest possible public for assessing tolerable or unacceptable conduct and attitudes. Within the context of this particular chapter, definitions and terms of reference to identify the areas affected are essential. Accordingly, attention will be focused on:

1 Definitions and terms of reference: sport, medicine and the law.
2 Violence and drugs (sport's own VD problem).

3   Medical intervention for women in sport and the law.
4   Medical standards and medical negligence.
5   Sport's future needs for medicine and the law.

1. Definitions and terms of reference: sport, medicine and the law

Sport

In Butterworths' *Sport and the Law* (1988) I cited two authoritative sources who independently arrived at the same conclusion from different points of the sporting compass. One was Sir Denis Follows, a wise and courageous administrator with three renowned sporting bodies: the British Olympic Association, the Central Council of Physical Recreation and the Football Association. In 1980 as Chairman of the British Olympic Association he effectively opposed Mrs Thatcher's embargo on the participation by British athletes in the Moscow Olympics staged shortly after Russia's invasion of Afghanistan. The other was the Director-General for many years of the Government-funded Sports Council, John Wheatley.

Before Follows died of cancer in 1983 he explained in a memorable Philip Noël-Baker Memorial Lecture at Loughborough College, 'I have reached the conclusion, after many years of trying, that sport defies definition. The Sports Council tried it and gave it up as a bad job.'

Two years later in 1985 during the course of a written Sports Council Memorandum to the House of Commons Environment Committee, which reported to the House of Commons in February 1986, based on the Council's conclusions under the title of 'Financing of sport in the United Kingdom', Wheatley stated: 'A study of the financing of sport produces a problem of definition. There is no single list of activities which would meet with universal agreement. Many years ago sport was felt by some to encompass hunting, shooting and fishing. A much wider view is now taken by many people.'

Indeed, with the television coverage of such diverse activities as darts, snooker and motor-racing, the time may well have come for a reassessment and re-evaluation of what constitutes sport, and particularly what sport is in relation to health and medicine. The *Concise Oxford Dictionary* traces its meaning derivatively to be an abbreviated form of the Middle English (1200–1500) 'disport' with various meanings, including 'frolic, gamble, enjoy oneself'. The celebrated Joseph Strutt in his book *Sports and Pastimes of the People of England, including Rural and Domestic Recreation from the Earliest Period to the Present Time* (1801) began his text with the classic claim, 'In order to form a just estimation of any particular people, it is absolutely necessary to investigate the Sports and Pastimes most generally prevalent among them.'

Nearer our own time during an address to the CCPR's annual

conference in Bournemouth during November 1986, John Wheatley explained that, in the UK, participation in sport and recreation involved about 22 million in all 'on at least one occasion a month'. He added that 'Many of these, however, clearly do not see the need to join the governing bodies of sport, though their interests are affected by these governing bodies [which he numbered at approximately 390], which exercise some measure of control or guidance in the four countries of the UK.'

A great jurist, Lord Bryce, in his *Studies in History and Jurisprudence* (vol. 11, p. 181), observed that 'there are some conceptions which it is safer to describe than to attempt to define'. Sport is one of them. Hence Professor Sir Ludwig Guttman, in his *Textbook of Sport for the Disabled*, included among others this attempt by Unesco: 'Any physical activity which has the character of play and involves a struggle with oneself or with others, or a confrontation with natural elements, is sport. If this activity involves competition it must be performed with a spirit of sportsmanship. There can be no true sport without fair play. All rules must be observed with this in mind.' Within this context it is at least arguable that sport's function must include elements of health and education and risks within a self- or externally disciplined control; and those elements of control are essential to the manner in which the law and rules of play must apply to sport.

Legal

In the opening chapter to Butterworths' *Sport and the Law*, I have explained how *Britain: 1987*, an official handbook prepared by the Central Office of Information, explains at the beginning of Section 24, entitled 'Sport and recreation': 'The British invented and codified the rules of many of the sports and games which are now played all over the world', and within the sporting context they can be identified and categorised at four separate levels.

1 Playing laws: for players and participants to play. These are, in general, facilitative.
2 Penal playing laws: for referees and umpire to control and discipline play. These are, in general, restrictive.
3 Administrative laws: for fair and sensible organisation and control.
4 National laws: the overriding control for justice and fair play at all the above three levels.

They are extended by the international dimension in modern sport to two more widely embracing areas:
5 International governing body.
6 Overseas national laws.

I also illustrated their interaction by explaining that when a Welsh international rugby player in the autumn of 1985 punched a defenceless opponent during the course of a club rugby match without being seen by the referee:

1 There was a clear breach of rugby playing laws.

2 The player concerned was not disciplined by the referee in control.

3 The incident was ignored by club administrators.

Therefore as a last resort the national criminal law was invoked to the extent that a prosecution was launched for a criminal assault, which resulted in a conviction following a guilty plea. During the preliminary committal court proceedings, the chairman of Abercarn, Gwent, South Wales, magistrates' court on 13 May 1986 explained, 'It is difficult to decide where the rough and tumble of sport ends, and where criminality begins to appear in the game of rugby football. We therefore think the case would be more properly dealt with by a Crown Court.'

At the Crown Court, on a plea of guilty to common assault, David Bishop was sentenced to a custodial period of one month. A Court of Appeal reduced this to a suspended sentence for the same period. A month later, when this precedent was pleaded by counsel for an appellant who was a police officer who had been convicted of the offence of inflicting grievous bodily harm with intent (contrary to Section 18 of the Offences Against the Person Act 1861), and sentenced to six months' imprisonment for having bitten an opponent's ear when the two players were in close proximity immediately after a rugby tackle, Lord Lane, the Lord Chief Justice, commented that Bishop 'may consider himself lucky to have been treated so leniently.'

A few months earlier, in April 1985, a Court of Appeal in the Civil Division of the High Court affirmed an earlier County Court judge's award of £4000 damages to the victim of a foul soccer tackle in an amateur soccer match, resulting in a broken leg. The claim was couched in both negligence and trespass to the person, a civil assault, but the award was based on 'an obvious breach of the defendant's duty of care towards the plaintiff' (*Condon* v. *Basi* [1985] 2 AER 453).

In both illustrations the law of each game had been broken. The damage to the victim invoked the national law, too: in Bishop's case the criminal code, in Basi's case the civil code. On each occasion the complainant was a victim of a crime of violence, confirmed by medical evidence. Thus does medicine partner the law in illustrating Sir Ludwig Guttman's citation from Unesco, 'There can be no true sport without fair play.'

Sports medicine

An international publication, originating from Sweden in 1983 and first published in the UK in 1986 with the title of *Sports Injuries*

— *Their Prevention and Treatment*, defined sports medicine as encompassing 'the following elements: preparation and training, prevention of injuries and illness, diagnosis and treatment of injuries and illness rehabilitation and return to active participation in sport. This definition relates to the athlete, the sport, sporting equipment and diagnostic instrumentation.' Each element in this area creates a potential legal issue and the definition must be regarded as incomplete unless the elements of administrative arrangements and provisions for their control and organisation, i.e. the responsibilities of promoters and employers, are included within or added to the final categories of 'sporting equipment and diagnostic instrumentation.'

One example has already been mentioned above: the recommendations for adequate medical services in the Sheffield Wednesday Hillsborough report, for which potential permutations of legal liabilities will be considered below (pp. 39–40). Another is illustrated by a vicarious liability which arose when Canadian courts awarded substantial damages against an employing club and doctors for rejecting complaints of serious sporting injurious consequences by a professional ice-hockey player suffered during the course of a game, explained in detail below on p. 37 (*Robitaille* v. *Vancouver Ice Hockey Club Ltd* [1981], 3 DLR 288). DLR: Dominion Law Report (Canada)

The strictly medical elements must be governed by the traditional and conventional legal sanctions within medical practice and its ancillary associations. Non-playing aspects such as sports equipment and diagnostic instrumentation are regulated by the general legal framework, which many people inside sport itself appear to be unaware can apply to the sporting scene equally as it does to the general community. Violent breaches of sporting laws and rules of play, condoned or inadequately disciplined by over-tolerant administrations, coaches, managers and referees, have created a misconception that sport could be a legal 'no-go' area on the basis that the law of the land stops at the touch-line or the boundary. How this is not the case is emphasised by medical evidence and clarified by the definitive manner in which the rule of law operates within a sporting context.

2. Violence and drugs

Each of these areas creates a cheating-at-sport situation. Violence is more clear-cut and identifiable. The issues of drugs in sport and how to deal with them can create confusion and injustice because of the overlap and, often, lack of communication between doctor, patient, administrator and lawyer. For violence there is no possibility of confusion. The only legal issue that arises is under what legal label violent misconduct in sport can be identified. Because of its comparative simplicity when contrasted with the complex administrative and medical drug scene, it may conveniently be dealt with first.

Violent sporting misconduct: the anatomy of foul play

This creates not only criminal and civil liabilities, but also claims for compensation from the Government-funded Criminal Injuries Compensation Board. It can also create ancillary contractual consequences, which, although not directly associated with medical issues, are nevertheless illustrative of violent misconduct. Thus in 1933 the Civil Court of Appeal in London reversed a trial judge's decision to reject a claim by an 18-year-old Irish heavyweight boxer, Jack Doyle, against the proprietors of the now demolished White City Stadium. He had forfeited his £3000 purse under the small print of the fight contract after the referee had disqualified Doyle for foul fighting in a contest for the heavyweight championship of Great Britain against Jack Petersen, now President of the British Boxing Board of Control. His lawyers had argued, because of their client's legal status as an infant, that the forfeiture was a legal penalty which was contractually disadvantageous and thereby not beneficial to their client. The test then, as now, under the Infant's Relief Act 1874, had been that an infant's contracts must be for beneficial necessaries. Lord Hanworth, one of Lord Denning's predecessors as Master of the Rolls, adjudicated, 'It is as much in the interest of the plaintiff himself as of any other contestant that there should be rules for clean fighting and that he should be protected against his adversary's misconduct in hitting below the belt or doing anything of the sort' (*Doyle* v. *White City Stadium Ltd* [1935] 1 KB 110).

The more directly actionable legal principles which have stood the test of time for over a century to outlaw violent sporting misconduct were reaffirmed as relatively recently as 1975 when the Court of Appeal Criminal Division in *R.* v. *Venna* [1975] 3 All ER 788 (p. 793 f–g) explained, '*R.* v. *Bradshaw* [1878] 14 Cox CC 83 can be read as supporting the view that unlawful physical force applied recklessly constitutes a criminal assault.'

In the Bradshaw case a jury acquitted a footballer who had been prosecuted for manslaughter after causing injuries during a friendly football match, no doubt because evidence was produced, from one of the two umpires in charge of the game, that no unfair play occurred. During prosecuting counsel's opening speech to the jury, Bramwell LJ interrupted a reference to the game's rules to say (p. 84), 'Whether within the rules or not, the prisoner would be guilty of manslaughter if while committing an unlawful act he caused the death of the deceased.'

The summing-up to the jury before its 'not guilty' verdict included these words, which with their references to intention and recklessness contain the key to both criminal and civil liability: 'If a man is playing according to the rules and practice of the game and not going beyond it, it may be reasonable to infer that he is not actuated by any malicious motive or intention, and that he is not acting in a manner which he knows will be likely to be productive of death or injury. But, independent of the rules, if the prisoner intended to cause serious hurt to the deceased, or if he knew that in charging as he did, he might produce serious injury and was indifferent and reckless as to whether he would produce serious injury or not, then the act would be unlawful. In either case he would be guilty of a criminal act and you must find him guilty, if you are of a contrary opinion you will acquit him.

Twenty years later, in *R. v. Moore* (1898) 14 TLR 229, the evidence had a stronger flavour with a stronger result. The accused offending footballer

1   jumped violently with his knees against an opponent's back;
2   threw the victim violently against a knee of the goalkeeper;
3   caused internal injuries resulting ultimately in death a few days afterwards.

The summing-up on this occasion to the jury by Hawkins J (pp. 229–30) explained: 'The rules of the game were quite immaterial ... it did not matter whether the prisoner broke the rules or not. Football was a lawful game, but it was a rough one and persons who played it must be careful to restrain themselves so as not to do bodily harm to any other person. No one had a right to use force which was likely to injure another, and if he did use such force and death resulted, the crime of manslaughter had been committed.... If a blow were struck recklessly which caused a man to fall, and if in falling he struck against something and was injured and died, the person who struck the blow was guilty of manslaughter, even though the blow itself would not have caused injury.'

After that verdict in 1898 no record of serious reported sporting violence from competitive as distinct from playground play has been traced for nearly 70 years until 1968. Then the crime explosion in society generally spilled over on to sporting fields, illustrated by the medical evidence provided ten years later by Davies and Gibson in the citation above (p. 7) from the *British Medical Journal* in December 1978 and subsequently by the Criminal Injuries Compensation Board. It was illuminated and high-lighted for all the world to see, as it can still see on telerecording films, as chronicled by one of the most renowned international athletes, the Brazilian soccer star, Pelé. In *My Life and the Beautiful Game* (1977) he has explained with Robert L. Fish, as I have narrated in Butterworths' *Sport and the Law* (pp. 205–206) citing Pelé and Fish at pp. 144–155, when identifying his experiences during the 1966 World Cup competition in Britain, '... against Bulgaria ... I had been the target of merciless attacks from Zechev of Bulgaria throughout the

TLR: Times Law Reports (as distinct from *The Times* reports)

*NB Jack Rollin,
football's leading
statistician and author
of the *Guinness Book
of Soccer Records*,
in his *World Cup
Triumph 1986* records
the referee as Herr
Tschenscher of West
Germany . Pelé's text
is as cited here.

entire game. Zechev did everything he could physically to cripple me, and the referee, Jim Finney* gave neither me nor any of the others on our team the protection we had a right to expect from an official in a game.'

'Morais, of Portugal, had a field day fouling me; eventually putting me out of the game. He tripped me, and when I was stumbling to the ground he leaped at me, feet first, and cut me down completely. It wasn't until I actually saw the films of the game that I realised what a terribly vicious double-foul it was. The stands came to their feet screaming at the foul, but the English referee, George McCabe allowed Morais to remain on the field, although again, even in the most inexperienced league in the world, he would have been thrown out for either of the two fouls, let alone both. Dr Gosling and Mario Americo came to help me from the field, and Brazil went on to play with ten men and ended up eliminated from the tournament.'

Those impressions of what the films showed for Pelé have been confirmed by my own viewing at least seven times of the nationally marketed official film of the 1966 World Cup Competition, *Goal*, by its scriptwriter and the *Sunday Times* football correspondent, Brian Glanville, and also by *The Times*' senior sportswriter, David Miller. The consequences legally are independently and interdependently the sixfold as set out at p. 11 above.

They were all repeated 14 years later during the semi-final of the 1982 World Cup competition in Spain. The West German goalkeeper Schumacher assaulted the French defender Battiston in a manner condemned internationally by the sporting press. Yet as David Miller recorded in his book on the 1966 World Cup, *The Boys of '66: England's Lost Glory* at p. 21, 'Any dignified sport would have suspended for life the West German goalkeeper for his atrocious foul in the 1982 semi-final, which shamefully handicapped the French. From FIFA there was no more than a murmur.'

Battiston's 1982 experience against West Germany and Pelé's experience against Portugal and Bulgaria in the 1966 World Cup created a classic combination of circumstances which *could* and *should* have demonstrated — but did not — how all six legal layers acted upon and with each other in an effective policy because the fouls merited the following sanctions:

1 Sending off from field punishment.
2 In breach of Law 12 — violent conduct or serious foul play.
3 Suspension or dismissal from competition in the manner suffered 12 years after Pelé by Scotland's star winger sent home from the 1978 World Cup in Argentina following a positive drugs test in breach of FIFA rules but lawfully prescribed under Parliament's Misuse of Drugs Act 1971 (see p. 27–28).
4 National prosecution for assault occasioning actual bodily harm.
5 International governing body as in (2) above with censure upon

referees and FIFA noted by David Miller for abdicating responsibilities.

6   Overseas national as in (3) above, with the precedents from other violent visitors or criminal offenders to visiting shores.

Nothing at all in fact ever happened. The offenders escaped back to their native lands without any effective punishment for their respective and undoubted criminality. The reluctance of the prosecuting authorities in the Liverpool area (covering Goodison Park where the Pelé assaults occurred) to take action could conceivably have resulted from diplomatic sensitivities. Since then, in the next World Cup, at Mexico City in 1970, England's captain, Bobby Moore, was intimidated by a false charge of alleged theft in the Colombian capital of Bogota; and as the world knows, 20 years later, the South Wales prosecuting authority charged the Welsh international amateur rugby footballer David Bishop with the offence identified and suffered by Pelé. It might well save rugby football from following the same slippery path to self-destruction taken by violent players and abject administrators at domestic and international levels. To those who supinely and irresponsibly say 'It's all part of the game', Pelé's beautiful game and that of others — the game of ballet without music — there is one question to be answered. What should happen to any member of a dance routine chorus whipping the feet from under the legs of Fred Astaire and Ginger Rogers? Punishment or condonement?

By 1980 the Criminal Injuries Compensation Board felt constrained to record in its paragraph 30: 'While there is now considerable public awareness of the existence and extent of football violence, we doubt whether the public is aware of the catastrophic effects which result from such criminal acts. The Board frequently deals with cases of people scarred for life, sometimes with cases of people seriously and permanently maimed and occasionally with people who are killed. We welcome the efforts which the courts, the police and many sporting organisations are making to attempt to lessen the number of such crimes.'

Seven years later, in 1987, the Board was still reporting (paragraph 37, p. 14): 'In the last few years, the Board has received an increasing number of applications arising from violence among players, particularly during rugby or football matches ... We consider that it is in the interests of everyone that people who commit criminal offences on playing fields should be prosecuted. Anyone who considers that an injury upon him was caused by a criminal offence should draw the attention of the police to it. If he does not do so, he is unlikely to receive compensation from the Board.'

This last caveat identifies paragraph 6(a) of the Board's Compensation Scheme, which provides for withholding or reducing compensation for delay, non-disclosure to the police and other inhibitory factors. The criminal and civil pattern which has emerged is summarised below (Table 1.1). The sample recorded represents only the tip of an ever-growing iceberg, the extent of which can never be fully known because of the absence of any means of collecting accurate data to gauge the range of the problem. This situation is well illustrated by a chance discussion while these pages were being prepared, with a former President of the Medico-Legal Society, Judge John A. Baker DL (a friend since our Oxford days) during a lull in court business at Kingston upon Thames. He enquired casually whether a judgment he had delivered in the Epsom County Court a few years ago for a soccer injury would be of interest and assistance. The response was positive, and the consequence now is that, to the list extracted below from Butterworths' *Sport and the Law* (and subsequent occurrences since its publication in January 1988), should be added the example which was unreported and embedded in the Epsom County Court archives until disclosed by this generous thought from the Circuit Judiciary with a very strong medico-legal association: disclosed in 1989, but relating to events in 1981, and heard at Epsom County Court in 1983. Because it emphasises this unknown and uncharted area of sporting injuries, it is placed out of chronological context near the head of Table 1.1.

While these pages were in preparation for the printers a chance meeting in the Temple with another practising barrister, Oliver Wise, produced yet another unreported case. This related to events at Basingstoke County Court in October 1989, in which he had been instructed before His Honour Judge Galpin, which precedes Judge John A. Baker's citation in the table below. Oliver Wise commented that his case which had been pleaded as a civil assault based on the tort of trespass to the person did not contribute to jurisprudence. Yet with Judge John A. Baker's precedent they each reflect a trend which was unheard of during our post Second World War Oxford days, but regrettably is being reproduced regularly in criminal courts at all levels as well as in the County Courts and High Courts to a degree which is unknown but cannot be ignored. Because they are the most recent to come to my notice they are designedly placed at the commencement of the Table 1.1.

In most of the examples in Table 1.1 the offences breached Rugby Law 26 or Soccer Law 12, which prohibits violent foul play, in addition to the civil and/or criminal law of the land. They are merely recorded examples of countless other less formally recorded examples throughout the world. Thus in 1985 a woman footballer who broke an opponent's jaw in a women's friendly (*sic*) soccer match on May Day was convicted of assault and ordered to pay £250 compensation by Clacton magistrates in Essex (*Baker* v. *Bridger* (1985) *Daily Express*, 1 May). And in 1986 from the USA an assault was reported which could have been prosecuted in the UK, arising from a fight between two women jockeys. One bit the arm of the

Table 1.1 A summary of Court cases resulting from sports injuries.

Date	Injury	Issue	Court	Case
1989	Kick during course of play to opponent causing two nights in hospital adjudicated to have been deliberate on spur of moment	Civil assault (trespass to the person) damages claim: £400 general damages; but claim for aggravated damages refused	Basingstoke County Court	*Vermont* v. *Green* (provided by Mr Oliver Wise, Barrister)
1983	Head butt causing broken nose and black eyes to 38 years old local player in local league match	Civil assault (trespass to the person) damages claim: £400 general damages and £5.80 special damages and costs	Kingston County Court	*Hewish* v. *Smailes* (provided from court archives by H. H. Judge John A. Baker, DL)
1968	Fatal blow causing death during niggling dispute in local league Essex soccer match	Criminal manslaughter prosecution. Convicted. Sentence: conditional discharge	Maidstone Assizes (transferred from Essex Assizes)	*R.* v. *Southby* (1969) *Police Review*, 7 February, p. 10
1969–70	Broken leg from foul tackle in local league Sussex soccer match	Civil assault (trespass to the person) damages claim: £4000 damages award and costs	Lewes Assizes and High Court, London for damages award	*Lewis* v. *Brookshaw* (1970) 120 NLJ 413
1977	Broken leg from foul tackle in local league Cornwall soccer match	Civil assault (trespass to the person) damages claim: £4000 damages award and costs	Bodmin Crown Court	*Grundy* v. *Gilbert* (1977) *Sunday Telegraph*, 31 July
1978	Fractured jaw in two places from off-the-ball punch in club Rugby Union match in South Wales	Inflicting grievous bodily harm contrary to s. 20 Offences against the Person Act, 1861. Convicted. Nine months' suspended sentence	Newport Crown Court	*R.* v. *Billinghurst* [1978] CLR 553

(1978 *British Medical Journal*, December, contributions: J. P. R. Williams and B. McKibbin, J. E. Davies and T. Gibson (see p. 7))

Date	Injury	Issue	Court	Case
1980	Fractured jaw, nose, cheekbone during 'friendly' rugby game	Inflicting grievous bodily harm contrary to s. 20 Offences against the Person Act, 1861. Plea: Guilty. Six months' custodial imprisonment (reduced without reasons on appeal to two months' custody)	Croydon Crown Court and Court of Appeal	*R.* v. *Gingell* [1980] CLR 661
1984–5	Broken leg from foul tackle in local league Leamington Spa soccer match	Negligence claim based on 'reckless disregard of plaintiff's safety which fell far below the standards which might reasonably be expected in anyone pursuing the game'. £4000 damages awarded and confirmed on appeal	Warwick County Court and Court of Appeal	*Condon* v. *Basi* [1985] 2 All ER 453
1985–6	Concussion from punch in off-the-ball Rugby Union incident	Guilty plea to common assault. Sentence: One month's custodial imprisonment reduced without reasons to one month's suspended imprisonment	Newport Crown court and Court of Appeal	*R.* v. *Bishop* (1986) *Times*, 12 October

Table 1.1 (Continued)

Date	Injury	Issue	Court	Case
1986	Ear bite after tackle in police Rugby Union match	Inflicting grievous bodily harm with intent contrary to s. 18 Offences against the Person Act, 1861. Convicted. Six months' custodial imprisonment. Confirmed on appeal	Cardiff Crown Court	R. v. *Johnson* [1986] 8 CAR (S) 343
1988	Broken jaw by professional soccer player in tunnel after match	Guilty plea. Inflicting grievous bodily harm contrary to s. 20 Offences against the Person Act 1861. £1200 fine £250 compensation and costs	Swindon Magistrates' Court	R. v. *Kamara* (1988) *The Times*, 15 April
1988	Broken cheekbone caused by amateur rugby player in club match kicking opponent on ground during course of play	Conviction: grievous bodily harm 18 months' imprisonment	Bristol Crown Court	R. v. *Lloyd* (1988) *The Times*, 15 September
1988	Broken jaw by amateur soccer player in 'friendly' match	Actual bodily harm	Wood Green Crown Court	R. v. *Birkin* (1988) *Enfield Gazette*, 7 April
1988	Damaged ligaments to professional footballer	Negligence claim based on illegal tackle. Agreed damages £130 000	High Court London	*Thomas* v. *Maguire and Queen's Park Rangers* (1989) *Daily Mirror*, 17 February
1989	Broken thigh and back injuries in fall caused by horse crossing in front of two other runners under guidance of jockey	Civil assault and negligence claim resulting in damages of $A121 490	Australian Supreme Court (Mr Justice Finlay)	*Frazer* v. *Jonst* (1989) *Racing Post*, 19 May, 26 May
1989	Concussion from kick on head to player on ground by soccer opponent	Grievous bodily harm. Eighteen months' custodial sentence. Confirmed on appeal	St Albans Crown Court and Court of Appeal	R. v. *Chapman* (Court of Appeal Criminal Division transcripts)

All ER: All England Reports. CAR: Criminal Appeal Reports. CLR: Criminal Law Review. NLJ: New Law Journal.

other, who needed a tetanus injection. The stewards imposed a $30 fine for 'causing a disturbance in the jockeys' quarters', a TV room (Calder Race Course, Miami, *Daily Express*, 1 July 1986).

The wider British Commonwealth, however, from Canada and Australia has entered two areas yet to be pursued in the UK, vicarious liability for sports field injuries against *non-players*, as in the Canadian case of a claim against Vancouver Ice Hockey Club Ltd and its doctors (see p. 37). In another Canadian case, this time from British Columbia, and in a case from New South Wales, Australia, victims of broken neck injuries sustained in rugby scrums are suing respectively:

1 the opposing club, and, in the Australian case, the coach too;
2 the opposing/controlling Rugby Union;

3 the controlling referees' association;
4 the referee;

on the basis that they were vicariously responsible for the victim's injury through negligent control and administration. This litigation at both ends of the Commonwealth is continuing at the time of writing.

Yet nearer home in the UK, the Scottish Football Association has disciplined two of its senior referees and downgraded the level of games which they can control because of alleged ineffective action against two fouling footballers, i.e. not dismissing them from the field of play: on one occasion when serious ligament injury resulted from an illegal tackle, and on another occasion for persistent dissent.

One frequent and insidious complaint about the national law entering into the realm of playing field illegalities is that sporting governing bodies can take care of it all. This, however, is not the case. For, separate and apart from inconsistencies in sentencing, they cannot, or at least do not, attempt to compensate a victim. Thus, when the Arsenal defender Paul Davis broke the jaw of the Southampton player Glenn Cockerill in full view of millions of television spectators during 1988 he was disciplined by an FA Commission which suspended him from playing in nine future games and imposed a £3000 fine. No one ever suggested by either inference or from facts that any money was paid to the victim. Yet two years earlier, when a Sussex County League player head-butted a referee, who was knocked unconscious, after the referee had penalised the offender, the victim consulted his local solicitor, Robert Rogers, who represents Sussex RFU on the RFU at Twickenham. The wise legal advice was to operate the Criminal Injuries Compensation Board's recommendations and place the matter in the hands of the police. A prosecution resulted. The charge of assault occasioning actual bodily harm was committed by local lay justices to Chichester Crown Court in West Sussex. The offender pleaded guilty. He was sentenced to 28 days' custodial imprisonment and ordered to pay £400 compensation to the victim. What sporting governing body would dare to order compensation to the victim? What sporting governing body would dare to arrogate to itself such powers, recognising its legal vulnerability in doing so, or, indeed, feel itself equipped to adjudicate and assess the level of compensation satisfactorily?

Those who whinge about the national law's involvement with sporting violence would best serve their own sport's discipline by reminding themselves that so far, to date, no known case can be traced for vicarious criminal provocation against an administrator, coach, manager or other official. Logic and the spiralling developments tabulated above, however, point inexorably in that direction if offenders do not desist from erroneously regarding bodily contact sports and other games as a licence to commit crime. If the upward pattern of unlawful, as distinct from accidental injurious conduct does not cease, then one day a criminal prosecution will be brought for aiding and abetting, counselling and producing such an offence against someone other than the offending player himself. If this sounds remote and beyond belief, it will be salutary for potential offenders to observe the words of Lord Goddard when Lord Chief Justice, a former Oxford University athletics half-blue and subsequently adjudicator in the inter-varsity Oxford–Cambridge athletics matches during his period of office in the 1950s at the now demolished White City Stadium in London. In 1951, with two other eminent judges, Humphreys J and Lord Devlin (as Devlin J) sitting in the King's Bench Divisional Court, they dismissed an appeal against conviction by a magazine proprietor of *Jazz Illustrated*, who had been convicted by Bow Street Magistrates' Court in London under Article 18(2) of the Aliens Order 1920 of aiding and abetting a breach of condition of entry into the UK of a greatly admired US citizen and musician, the jazz saxophonist, Coleman Hawkins. The basis for the conviction and its affirmation was that the offender had encouraged the breach by supporting a performance on stage. Lord Goddard emphasised that 'if he knew the offending proprietor had booed, it might have been some evidence that he was not aiding and abetting' (*Wilcox* v. *Jeffery* [1951] 1 All ER 464).

One of the generally unseen consequences of violent misconduct in the soccer scene was recorded in the *Guardian* on 18 November 1988 by its experienced football correspondent, David Lacey. He explained how 'Referees who officiate at football's lower levels are leaving the game in droves because of the rising number of assaults by players. The problem has become sufficiently serious for the FA to set up a special sub-committee to look into it ... There are 41 000 clubs in England, but only about 25 000 referees. Verbal abuse is bad enough but attacks on referees are running at more than 200 a session and the figure is rising.

After 230 assaults had been reported for the 1986–87 season the FA launched a referees recruitment drive but now, following prompting by the county FAs and the Referee's Association, they are going to give the matter a thorough investigation.'

Since those words were cited and while these pages were being prepared for the printers towards the end of 1989, Rugby Union referees have been reported requiring police protection publicly at renowned Rugby Union grounds after undoubted criminal assaults on referees; and thus the spiral of violence, especially against sources of authority, never diminishes. Many will recall the despair of the distinguished Metropolitan Police Chief Superintendant and referee, George Crawford, who felt obliged to walk off from refereeing what became fighting between two famous Rugby Union clubs during the mid-1980s. He now contents himself with adjudicating for school matches, where innocence can be protected if not corrupted by evil examples of public performers abusing great games as a vehicle and licence for criminal misconduct.

Before passing to the poisonous climate of the sporting drug scene, two final areas of sporting injuries require special attention. One has been confirmed by the London Court of Appeal since these pages were first formulated; schools sporting injuries, particularly for rugby, and insurance. The other is boxing and has been covered comprehensively in its medical and ethical context by the representative contributors from the amateur and professional disciplines (Chapters 18 and 19), and the Supervising Editor's note on the medical–moral arguments against the sport, particularly at professional level. The legal position of boxing has never been defined with certainty and finality for mainly historical reasons, and, as we shall see it is still developing. Parliamentary legislation in Australia, Canada and South Africa has attempted to regulate it. In Britain its only overall control is through the courts. The reported cases for over a century have moved from validating limited sparring as lawful (*R. v. Young* [1866] 10 Cox CC 370), via prize fighting until defeat from exhaustion or injury as illegal (*R. v. Orton et al.* [1878] 39 LT 293: *R. v. Coney* [1882] 8 QBD 534), to an acquittal of a manslaughter prosecution based on a fatality in the ring *not* caused by a boxing blow (*R. v. Roberts* (1901) *The Sporting Life*, 20 June, p. 8) and a bind over to keep the peace of the realm on the eve of a featherweight title fight (*R. v. Driscoll and Moran* (1911) *British Boxing Yearbook* 1985, p. 12).

In 1976, however, the Supreme Court of Victoria in Australia was required to formulate a criterion which ties in with the concurrent opinions expressed by Drs Adams, Wren and Whiteson (Chapter 18), and a well publicised precedent which occurred while these pages were being completed for the printers in November 1989. Adams and Wren at page 243 explain: 'Regulations are only as effective as those who implement them ... Improving the standards of the referees and other officials across the country is a slow and difficult process, but over the years a steady progress has been maintained. A fact which may surprise those outside the sport, and is a source of concern for the medical officers within it, is that it is not a requirement for these officials to maintain a valid first aid certificate. The fact that many other sports are in a similar position does not make that any more acceptable.' Dr Whiteson corroborates this impeccable medical approach with his advice and important qualification (p. 281): 'Providing the medical education of all referees is adequate and constantly being updated, as it is in this country, then the referee, in the opinion of the author, should continue to be in sole charge of the contest.' That important qualification 'as it is in this country' was particularly significant in relation to the World Championship Title Fight at London's Royal Albert

Hall during November 1989 between Azumah Nelson, the title holder, of Ghana, and Jim McDonnell, the challenger from Great Britain. The fight had been stopped in the twelfth round after McDonnell's right eye was badly injured and the events leading to this caused the respected and experienced columnist in the London *Observer*, Hugh McIlvanney, who is known for his sympathy to the boxing sport, to write in the issue for Sunday 12 November 1989; 'The fact that the challenger had fought with coolness, nerve, skill and energy through ten rounds (and seemed to me to be no more than a point or so behind ten at this stage) became heartbreakingly academic in the eleventh when his right eye closed suddenly into a ball of bruised flesh after what seemed to be a bang from the Ghanian's head. That injury represented a crippling handicap against a champion who, in spite of a largely torpid performance, had exhibited his famous capacity for havoc in the fifth round with a left hook that hurled a dazed McDonnell off his feet for the first count of his career ... Now began a series of misjudgments that could only provide encouragement for the abolitionist lobby. First, the referee, Joe Cortez, looked diligently into the sightless right eye and declined to intervene. Then, half-way through the eleventh, he did summon a Board of Control doctor, Ashwin Patel, to ringside to make an examination. From his home in New Jersey last week, Cortez said the doctor merely advised him to 'watch the eye' (ignoring it would have been some feat) and did not recommend that the fight should be stopped.

I find such a feeble response from the doctor incomprehensible; and the referee's contribution was underlined when he failed to endorse a stoppage after the first of two knockdowns in the twelfth.'

The potential significance medico-legally from Hugh McIlvanney's viewpoint was crystallised in the Supreme Court of Victoria. Mr Justice McInerney in *Pallante* v. *Stadiums Property Limited* (No. 1) [1976] VR 331 rejected a procedural application to strike out the statement of claim which formulated the documentary basis for a claim by a boxer who had received eyesight injuries when boxing under Australian Boxing Alliance Rules. He sued all persons other than his opponent, namely the promoter, his trainer, the matchmaker and the referee. The argument that the contest was a prize fight was the basis for the rejected application. The judgment as recorded in the summary of the report at p. 332 vindicated boxing as 'not an unlawful and criminal activity so long as, whether for reward or not, it was conducted by a contestant as a boxing sport or contest, not from the motive of personal animosity, or at all events not predominantly from that motive, but predominantly as an exercise of boxing skill and physical condition in accordance with rules and in conditions the object of which was to ensure that the infliction of boxing harm was kept within reasonable bounds, so as to preclude or reduce, so far as is practicable, the risk of either contestant incurring serious head injury, and to ensure that victory should be achieved in accordance with rules by the person demonstrating the greater skill as a boxer.'

The ultimate result of the claim was never disclosed, and in the absence of contrary information, should be treated as having been settled. Its existence as a live and modern precedent justifies and affirms the warnings and guidance built in to the contributions from Dr Adams, Wren and Whiteson in their respective contributions hereafter (Chapters 18 and 19).

A more clear-cut result occurred when the London High Court and Court of Appeal were required to consider an important schoolboy rugby injury case of significant consequence to all schools and their medical advisers as well as the victim.

The chronological sequence of dates (Table 1.2) is important for recognising and identifying the legal issues and consequences resulting from a policy decision by the Medical Officers' Schools Association (MOSA), and injuries suffered during an inter-house school match. This resulted in extensive litigation which, at the trial and on appeal, exonerated the school from coaching and insurance liabilities, but the medico-legal position is built in to the initiation and stimulus behind the underlying circumstances.

The action before Mr Justice Boreham lasted 26 days, and occupied 100 pages of a typescripted reserved judgment. Medical evidence relating to the injuries from a defective tackle blended with coaching evidence on rugby playing skills. Most significantly, the judgment relating to the insurance claim was based upon the principle that, because parents are under no obligation to insure, a corresponding duty cannot be placed upon schools. Since then, the Rugby Union has introduced a comprehensive scheme for rugby-playing schools under the terms of its Wavell Wakefield Charitable Trust, and the Central Council of Physical Recreation has pioneered a scheme on a wider basis.

The Van Oppen case raised many consequential legal issues not directly relevant to the medico-legal text, which I have discussed in the *New Law Journal* and also *Rugby World and Post* (*New Law Journal* **138**, 352, 29 July 1988 and *Rugby World and Post*, September 1988, p. 13 and [1989] 1 All ER 273: *Van Oppen v. Clerk*

Date	Action
1979 July	MOSA recommended insurance for all rugby-playing schools
1980 November	Simon Van Oppen injured in the tackle
1981 July	Bedford School implements MOSA report
1988 July	Mr Justice Boreham in London's High Court rejects claim for damages compensation. The claim being based on two grounds: **1** alleged negligent coaching of rugby techniques **2** alleged non-insurance as recommended by MOSA report
1989 April	Court of Appeal dismisses appeal and confirms judgment

Table 1.2 Events surrounding the Van Oppen school-boy rugby injury case.

to the Bedford Charity Trustees). In this perspective, however, it is significant that MOSA identified issues which in turn had their own consequential effects of alerting the sporting world to the necessity for adequate insurance cover at every active level.

Accordingly, those behind the scenes who do not discourage violent sporting misconduct cannot say that this does not put them on notice; and, if the medical profession and its associated disciplines recognise the issues and alert their patients sufficiently, collectively, individually and at administrative and governing body levels, they can contribute as much to the elimination of cheating by sporting violence as they have tried to contribute to at least the control, if not the elimination, of drugs in sport. A report from the Council of Europe dated 20 July 1989 cited the International Olympic Committee as having stated through its own medical commission in Seoul that doping can be considered as one of the factors causing violence. The Council of Europe's report* stated, without identifying the range or area of sources, 'Six out of 10 football players asked in March 1989 thought that a direct relationship exists between doping and violence on the pitch', and then concluded: 'If doping generates violence, one way to combat violence is to eradicate doping, through joint actions, both preventive and repressive, between governments and sports bodies at national and international level.'

*Dr John O'Hara, the experienced Chairman of the Football Association's Medical Committee, has emphasised to me that ten years of random drug testing within the FA's jurisdiction have found *no* player guilty of *deliberately* taking drugs (see also pp. 27–28).

Drugs

No need exists here to explain the highest possible profile which the drugs scenario commands on the public sporting medical stage. The Canadian Government inquiry into Ben Johnson's position and the much criticised attitudes of ambivalence of international athletics administrators at the Olympic Games and International Amateur Athletics Association, towards reinstatement of offenders against drug offences, are continuing issues at the time of writing. Another Canadian example and one from Scotland illustrate the problem which this particular area can create for doctors, administrators, participants and lawyers if the interaction between sporting regulations and lawfully prescribed drugs is not clearly recognised and defined.

An example of the necessity to understand clearly the true nature of the substances involved and their impact on sport and health was illuminated graphically during 1987 by a controversial public discussion about the use of beta-blockers. It was highlighted by a letter in the *Times* sports letters column from Dr I. M. James, Reader in Clinical Pharmacology at the Royal Free Hospital, Pond Street, NW3: 'A great deal of ill-informed comment has recently been voiced on the use of beta-blockers to obtain unfair advantage in certain competitive sports. The sports involved are those where the possession of a steady, non-tremulous hand is an advantage.

No one has pointed out that, whilst all beta-blockers have an effect on heart-rate, only certain members of this family of drugs have an effect on tremor. Basically beta-blockers can be divided into cardio-selective, where the effect on a tremor is minimal, and non-selective, where the effect on tremor is marked. Certainly in the case of Neal Foulds a cardio-selective beta-blocker was chosen. This seems to me to be a very clear evidence of a desire in his case at least not to obtain unfair advantage.'

These two cases from Canada and Scotland demonstrate the need for harmonious communications between so many different but interlocking areas concerned with this very sensitive but crucially important medico-legal penalty area.

Ron Angus and the British Judo Association

In 1984 the *Sunday Telegraph* announced, according to information from the British Judo Association, that a dope test on Ron Angus, winner of the under 78-kilo category in the All England Championship in December 1983, had proved positive. A sample contained traces of the banned substance pseudoephedrine.

Angus, who had dual Canadian–British nationality, claimed that the substance must have been contained in a sinus decongestant which he had taken under a lawful medical prescription by his Canadian doctor. Yet, because he had breached the Association's requirements, he was banned for life from competing in British championships.

Five months later, after he had taken legal advice, the *Daily Telegraph* reported that the High Court in London had lifted the ban with the Association's consent. It admitted that the absence of a hearing for Angus to explain his position breaches the rules of natural justice, and the life ban was duly rescinded. The Association's rules have now been tightened to place the onus on competitors and by implication, therefore, on their personal doctors, to ensure that lawful medication does not contain banned substances (*Daily Telegraph*, 15 June 1984).

Willie Johnston and FIFA (Fédération Internationale de Football Association)

In a different set of circumstances, the communication issue in the case of Ron Angus is in principle not dissimilar from that of Willie Johnston, the former Scottish international soccer player who was sent home in alleged disgrace from the 1978 FIFA World Cup competition in Mexico. In his book *On the Wing* he explained how his own English Football League doctor lawfully prescribed Reactivan pills for his nasal condition. His national team manager has explained in *The Ally Macleod Story: an Autobiography* how the Scottish FA doctor clearly warned Johnston about drugs; but the footballer patient had not realised that the pills contained a stimulant.

After the result was known Macleod has explained that the Scottish FA doctor asked the player sternly, 'Did you take Reactivan tablets before the game against Peru?' 'Yes,' came the immediate reply. 'But you told me you didn't take drugs,' said the doctor, puzzled as well as angry. 'They aren't drugs,' was the astonishing answer, and Johnston went on freely to admit that he had taken them 90 minutes before the game, as he had previously done at club level with West Bromwich Albion.

'Incredible as it may seem, it appeared that Johnston, a man of 31, who had been looking after himself for a long time in the tough world of professional football, had missed the whole point of the doctor's repeated warnings. I have thought about the matter a great deal over the months, and it is my view that he really believed that his Reactivan tablets were little more than smarties,' writes Macleod.

Both the Angus and the Johnston cases demonstrate the need for clear comprehension and understanding by athletes of the nature of any lawfully prescribed stimulant, and of any potential impact upon a sporting governing body's own regulations. They also prove the necessity for medical advisers to try to establish that comprehension and understanding by the patient; and if justice is to be achieved by administrators they should heed the provisions of the British Parliamentary statutory defence under Section 23(3)(b)(i) of the Misuse of Drugs Act 1971, that any accused person shall be acquitted of a drug offence 'If he proves that he neither believed nor suspected nor had reason to suspect that the substance or product in question was a controlled drug', i.e. one of which the use is controlled by the Act, and thereby unlawful generally.

That sub-section, like others comparable to it in principle, is laid down by Parliament, and illustrates the problems which face sports participants who require drugs lawfully for medicinal purposes.

I have attempted to resolve these problems by posing the following questions in Butterworth's *Sport and the Law* and Sports Council publications:

1 How are athletes and their personal doctors to know when a breach or potential breach of a sporting governing body's rules against drug abuse occurs?

2 How are sporting governing bodies to know that a failure to meet their own stringent rules for the protection of a particular sport does or does not arise from a lawful medicinal prescription?

3 How are lawyers to balance the interests of the sport in which they advise administrators with the need to respect the rights of individual competitors?

4 What is the patient to do when faced with what may become a conflict of personal health interests against the undoubted right in a free society to participate in healthy competition?

These questions cannot be shirked and have to be thought through within the framework of what lawyers recognise, usually in the international legal field, as a conflict of laws situation. Furthermore, with the explosion of international sport, and the concern of the World Health Organisation as well as international governing bodies about the problem, there is the added issue of international harmony for approaching solutions.

Suffice, therefore, that we should begin at home in the UK, by ensuring the following:

1 Doctors who treat patients competing athletically must familiarise themselves with the requirements of the particular sport in question, both at domestic and international level and pass on this information to their patients, the interested athletes.

2 Lawyers who advise administrators must see that any regulations to prevent cheating do not either transgress the rules of natural justice and the opportunity to be heard, or contravene the spirit of the British parliamentary defence that ignorance of the facts can be a defence in a drugs case.

3 Administrators should try, together with doctors, pharmacists, pharmacologists, lawyers and drug manufacturers, to attain a balance between the sport's rules and the individual's medicinal requirements, in the interests of fair play, health and the avoidance of cheating.

4 Competitors must familiarise themselves with their own medical requirements within the rules laid down by their particular sport.

As a last resort, because drug abuse is a national and international health hazard, the Government surely cannot opt out of taking an interest here, just as it is no longer ignoring its need to become involved with the problems of sporting crowd violence. As a start, consideration could be given to whether the lethal and recognised use of any known sporting drug substances, in addition to those which are already prohibited, should be outlawed alongside LSD, heroin, cocaine and other illegal substances. The proposal announced by the Home Office (in September 1987) that anabolic steroids were under consideration for being added to the lists of prohibited drugs is clearly a step in the right direction.

One long-term solution is offered by the Sports Nutrition Foundation which at present is housed in the London Institute of Sports Medicine under Dr Dan Tunstall Pedoe's jurisdiction at St Bartholomew's Hospital in London. It was created with the support initially of the Central Council of Physical Recreation, and its self-evident title points to a beneficial bodily health progression with long-term consequential effects. It does not and cannot claim to

no "lethal" drug can be legal

compete, however, with the short-term cheating advantages aimed for by drug takers.

Finally and by no means least in the never-ending struggle to reconcile bona fide drug medication with competitive sport, is the controversial impact of the contraceptive pill on the woman's athletic arena. Dr Ellen Grant in her challenging study, *The Bitter Pill: How Safe is the Perfect Contraceptive?*, published first in 1985, has explained how 'artificial derivatives of the male hormone testosterone are present in nearly all of today's pills' (p. 18, 1986 edition). The triple Olympic Games hurdler and Cambridge University blue, Peter Hildreth, commented in one of his *Sunday Telegraph* athletics correspondent's columns on 4 February 1986:

> 'There is evidence that women athletes who use it while not in breach of the rules are nonetheless reaping the benefits of illegal doping. The pill, a hormone, part of whose action is to reinforce the body's reserves at times of high physical demand, not only prevents loss of performance during menstruation, but also triggers a variety of advantageous side-effects. According to Dr John Guillebaud, author of the definitive textbook on the subject of the contraceptive pill, it stimulates an increase in the level of steroid hormone secretion from the adrenal and thyroid glands ...
>
> 'In sport the pill has served its users not merely in its intended role of protection against conception, but also by suppressing menstruation, in tiding them over those difficult times when training or competition would otherwise be curtailed. There was a time when the unlucky coincidence of the cycle with championship dates was known to have a decisive bearing on medals. The arrival of the pill meant that one of the variables accounting for loss of form was effectively mitigated, if not banished.'

No doubt there will be arguments against such contentions for which no definitive answer and solution can be assessed. What cannot be doubted is that the creation of the pill and its side-effects on athleticism in women should at least be considered, if only to be reflected alongside all other elements which demand the closest and most balanced approach by everyone identified here. We should be concerned with the manner in which the correct harmony between sport, medicine and the law can enhance the health of the individual alongside performance in sport.

3. Medical intervention for women in sport and the law

Separate and apart from the possible impact of the contraceptive pill as a performance-enhancing drug, two current developments have given the medical profession a wider relevance to the position of women in sport since the days when Mrs Martha Grace at Downend, near Bristol, bowled her three sons, E. M., G. F. and W. G. Grace, to cricketing immortality in the mid-1850s, and the daughters of John Willes, the Kent professional of that period, are attributed with inventing round-arm bowling because their skirts impeded their underarm deliveries. One is medical — the sex change operation; the other is social — the equal opportunities legislation. Both categories have been covered in depth in Butterworths' *Sport and the Law* in the chapter entitled 'Women in sport and the law', from where much of what follows is drawn.

London's High Court in 1970 witnessed a then unique claim to annul a marriage because of the sex change operation, when medical evidence proved that the "female" party to the marriage had been born a man. In *Corbett* v. *Corbett* (*ors. Ashley*) [1970] 2 All ER 33 Mr (later Lord Justice) Ormrod, himself trained as a doctor before being called to the Bar, was asked to adjudicate on this then unprecedented condition. In acceding to it he held that the party who had undergone a sex change operation 'is not a woman for the purpose of marriage but is a biological male and has been since birth.'

Around that period, unknown to many outside family circles a distinguished writer, then James Morris, underwent similar surgery to become Jan Morris; and five years later sport caught up with this new medical phenomenon in the year Parliament passed the Sex Discrimination Act. Dr Richard Rasskind, a New York ophthalmic surgeon, and a skilled tennis player, received similar surgical treatment to become after the operation Dr Renee Richards. Inevitably, the question emerged: what were the tennis authorities going to do about it? For the next two years Dr Renee Richards shunted between various US tennis tournaments which were sufficiently enlightened to accept "her" entries with the knowledge of her transsexuality. Those which were not, either rejected her outright, or conditionally upon chromosome tests being factually or conveniently satisfied. The world-wide International Tennis Federation invoked Olympic Games tests which the doctor was unable to satisfy. When the locally based tennis authorities also required such stringent limitations upon entry the New York's jurisdiction was invoked. In an action against the United States Tennis Association, the US Open Tennis Championship Committee and the Women's Tennis Association Inc., during 1977, Dr Richards claimed relief as a professional tennis player who had undergone sex reassignment surgery which had allegedly changed her sex from male to female. She sued for a preliminary injunction against the organisations

1 to prevent reliance on a sex-chromatin test for determination of whether she was female and thus

2 to permit her participation in the Women's Division of the US Open tournament.

The legal foundation of the action was that the condition breached the anti-discriminatory code built in to the New York State equal opportunities legislation. After hearing a battery of conflicting medical and tennis evidence, Judge Alfred M. Ascione held: 'when an individual such as plaintiff (*sic*), a successful physician, a husband and father, finds it necessary for his own mental sanity to undergo a sex reassignment, the unfounded fears and misconceptions of defendants (*sic*) must surely give way to the overwhelming medical evidence that the person before him is now female'. Accordingly, a requirement that the plaintiff pass the sex-chromatin test in order to be eligible to participate in the tournament was grossly unfair, discriminatory and inequitable, and violated plaintiff's rights under the New York Human Rights Law, and granted the injunctions (*Richards* v. *US Tennis ASSN & ORS 1977*: 400 NYS (2nd) 267).

Similar reliefs would have been available to Dr Richards at that time under British law if she had been subjected to similar conditions for a UK tournament. Not only could the Sex Discrimination Act 1975 have been invoked, as a result of the Court of Appeal's decision that acknowledged matrimonial sterilisation in *Bravery* v. *Bravery* [1954] 3 All ER 59 (where a wife failed to obtain a cruelty decree because the majority of the court held that she had consented to her husband's vasectomy), Dr Richards could have argued that the condition to undergo a sex-chromatin test would comprise an incitement to commit or to attempt to commit a battery.

By the time Dr Richards arrived in Britain, however, "she" came with an entirely different professional tennis status; as coach and adviser to the future Wimbledon champion, Martina Navratilova in 1977. This lasted for five years until Dr Richards retired from professional tennis and returned to her other profession, ophthalmic surgery. By then, 1982, English courts had begun to consider 'the average woman'.

In a different age group and in a different social setting a 12-year-old schoolgirl's wish to play soccer football with boys projected medical attitudes to women in sport via the Nottingham County Court to Lord Denning and Lord Justice Eveleigh and Sir David Cairns in London's Court of Appeal during 1978.

Section 44 of the Sex Discrimination Act as mentioned above contains the sole section identifying sport in a very limited manner. It comes within Part V of the Act under a general heading alongside other categories including charities, insurance and other circumstances nominated as 'General Exceptions from Parts II to IV', i.e. those covering employment, education and other unlawful discriminatory areas. It was enacted thus: 'Nothing in Parts II to IV shall, in relation to any sport, game or other activity of a competitive nature where the physical strength, stamina or physique of the average woman puts her at a disadvantage to the average man, render unlawful any act related to the participation of a person as a competitor in events involving that activity which are confined to competitors of one sex.' The key concepts here, of course, are the antithesis between 'the average woman' and 'the average man', and also 'competitors'. Both have been considered in the reported decisions of the tribunals and the courts. Both will doubtless have to be considered again. In a survey of the first decade's operation of the legislation from its inception on 31 December 1975, Lady Howe, the Equal Opportunity Commission's first deputy Chairman wrote in *The Financial Times*, 3 January 1986, 'The legislation was neither perfect nor comprehensive.' No reference was made to section 44. If it had been, the comment would have been justified that the first decade reflects an exploratory experience with a stop–go pattern. The reported cases illustrate a gradual move towards its beneficial application to sports women with the inevitable hiccups en route. Furthermore, a valuable survey by Dr Alice M. Leonard for the Equal Opportunities Commission of *The First Eight Years* (1976–83) (summarised in the *New Law Journal*, 31 January 1986) of the tribunal referrals identifies in its fuller text *sport* alongside 'Literary, artistic' in the applicants' occupations for claims under both the 1970 and the 1975 Acts; and for men as well as women only 1% of those who utilised the legislation are logged under these three comprehensive categories.

With such scant material no definable pattern can yet be traced; but the recorded cases in the various reported sources manifest a tentative approach bedevilled by the unrealistic delineation between 'the average woman' and 'the average man'. Women no less than men in sport demonstrate talents and qualities well above average which the slightest reflection can easily recognise. Indeed, this Parliamentary injection into sex legislation of the commercial shipping language of averaging suggests that the draftsman of the section and Parliament not only did not understand women in sport but could not have understood the above average skills which are the hallmark of true athleticism.

What is the 'average woman' and what is the 'average man' in *this* context has yet to be *fully* investigated by the courts. A tentative approach to it was made in the unreported decision of the Court of Appeal when it was concerned with whether or not a 12-year-old schoolgirl was discriminated against playing football with boys of her own age (see *Bennett* v. *The Football Association Ltd and The Nottinghamshire FA* [1978] CA 591). Tentative, because the issue and evidence called before the county court and accepted in the Court of Appeal was directed medically towards comparing and differentiating between boys and girls of 12 years of age, below and above the age of puberty; and a conclusion that the circumstances of the case proved existence of a disadvantage (the Act being silent on age levels). The playing merits do not appear to have been argued of the 12-year-old plaintiff-contender for a place in the boys' team for which she had been selected. Yet Lord Denning (at p. 2 of the transcript: no. 591 of 1978) said 'She ran rings around the boys'; and a witness as recorded in *The Daily Telegraph* report of the county court hearing said she was 'a vicious tackler and once tackled a 15-year-old so hard he had to be supported and taken from the field'. This pointed, of course, to this particular plaintiff *not* being put 'at a disadvantage to the average' boy! Concentrating on what appeared to be a diversion in evidence from doctors about puberty, and without apparent arguments on above average skills, the Court of Appeal overruled the Deputy County Court Judge who had adjudicated and awarded £250 in favour of the 12-year-old 'vicious tackler' of 'a 15-year-old'. Two years later in *Greater London Council* v. *Farrar* ([1980] ICR 266), the Employment Appeal tribunal at p. 272 C–D per Slynn J said, 'we read the decision of the Court of Appeal as applying to the particular facts before it'.

Certainly the imbalance between the medical evidence concerned with puberty and the apparent absence of argument on the evidence tending to prove the existence of above average athletic talents which did not disadvantage the female plaintiff leave this decision without any general guidance for future disputes in the manner stated above; and any schoolgirl footballers not caught through average talents by the exclusion clause in section 44 can at least consider their chances on different evidence and arguments of a replay.

4. Medical standards and medical negligence

The ordinary principles applicable generally to medical liabilities operate within the sporting context, subject to two crucial general considerations. One is the absence of any traceable pattern of liability arising out of medical services in the UK which contain a sporting flavour. The other is a corollary to it: the general public's and even judicial misapprehensions about claims for sporting injuries which have been expressed during the last three decades.

The limited researches of practitioners would have been responsible for the following observations of Lord Diplock as Diplock LJ in a claim concerning a photographer injured by a competitor's horse in the White City Horse of the Year Show and by Lord Donaldson as Sir John Donaldson, Master of the Rolls, in the negligent tackling soccer case. In *Wooldridge* v. *Sumner* [1963] 2 QB 43 at 65, Diplock LJ noted: 'It is a remarkable thing that in a nation where during the present century so many have spent so much of their leisure in watching other people take part in sports and pastimes there is an almost complete dearth of judicial authority as to the duty of care owed by the actual participants to the spectators', albeit in the context of that particular case where a professional photographer was the injured plaintiff; and, in *Condon* v. *Basi* [1985] 2 All ER 452, Sir John Donaldson said (p. 453): 'It is sad that there is no authority as to what is the standard of care which governs the conduct of players in competitive sports generally and above all, in a competitive sport whose rules and general background contemplate that there will be physical contact between the players, but that appears to be the position.'

Both statements are rebuttable by precedents which emerged during the years between the two World Wars from the realms of golf and motor racing: *Castle* v. *St Augustine's Links* [1922] 38 TLR 615 and *Cleghorn* v. *Oldham* [1927] 43 TLR 465 (golf); *Hall* v. *Brooklands Auto-Racing Club* [1933] 1 KB 205 (motor-racing); and *Brewer* v. *Delo* [1967] 1 Ll. Rep. 488 (golf). Nevertheless, this limited pattern emphasises the reluctance, in the UK at least, to invoke legal remedies for sporting injuries, during a period, of course, when the aggression inherent in modern competitive sport was less intense than it has become today, with the greater prize money and prestige that are associated in the manner identified in the chapter by Donald A. D. MacLeod.

KB: King's Bench (Law
Reports)
Ll. Rep.: Lloyd's List
Reports

Thus, the duty of care which a doctor and paramedical services owe to their charges, a breach of which alongside a reasonable foreseeable risk of injury or damage creates liability in negligence, should be recognised whenever a sporting injury requires treatment. The specialised medical sports injuries clinics and centres which are developing demonstrate a growing awareness of the need for such care. In these locations doctors are undoubtedly alerted to the obligation at all times to observe the risks within such a specialised sphere. Yet the risks may not necessarily be recognised or realised sufficiently or at all by the doctor or his associates, who may regard treatment of a sporting or sports-related injury by a casual or part-time participant, such as a sprained wrist suffered by a weekend golfer or tennis player, less seriously than that of an injured motorist or factory worker incapacitated from employment. 'You must give up golf, or tennis', is not unknown advice to such victims as the simplest treatment, without any recognition of the value of such activities to the patient and the long-term potentially dangerous consequences of such untreated situations. The weekend golfer or part-time cricketer with muscular ailments is no less entitled to the same level of medicine as any other patient; and the author's own legal and sporting professional experiences, information and observation confirm this trend among non-sporting medical practitioners who do not share their patients' sporting enthusiasms and interests.

Furthermore, the judicially recorded 'almost complete dearth of judicial authority' in the UK is not reflected in the more litigious climate across the Atlantic, as can be seen below; and this is compounded by the problems inherent in the evaluation of medical evidence, albeit for more complex general categories than those sporting medical science has produced in the courts so far. Recently, in *Wilshire* v. *Essex Health Authority* [1988] 1 All ER 871, the House of Lords directed a retrial with guidelines for the burden of proof because of judicial 'misunderstanding at the original hearing of evidence', and an 'irreconcilable conflict of medical opinion as to the cause of what was a complication in a premature birth, with substantial injurious consequences'.

A similar conflict of medical opinion associated with premature birth resulted in an earlier reversal by the House of Lords and the Court of Appeal of a £102 000 damages award, solely because the trial judge had drawn the wrong inferences of fact from the conflicting medical evidence. He had failed in the eyes of the appellate courts to distinguish between negligence and an error of judgement, for which no legal liability exists — the result in that case (*Whitehouse* v. *Jordan* [1981] 1 All ER 267). Together, these important House of Lords verdicts emphasise what Lord Scarman recorded in yet a third ruling from that ultimate judicial tribunal, as summarised in a contribution in the *All England Law Reports Annual Review*, 1987 (p. 179): 'What is remarkable about professional malpractice in the case of a doctor is that the courts have uniquely conceded to the medical profession the right to determine when there has been breach of that duty of care (*Sidaway* v. *Board of Governors of the Bethlem Royal Hospital and the Maudsley Hospital* [1985] 1 All ER 643 at 649).'

The areas within the sporting sphere where medical negligence can arise were considered in the chapter 'Sports medicine and the law' in Butterworths' *Sport and the Law*, taken from Butterworths' *Law and Medical Ethics* by Professor J.K. Mason and Dr R.A. McCall Smith. In their 1981 edition, and repeated in 1987, they identified eight situations, all of which are applicable to the sporting medical scene, which cannot be ignored by any medical practitioner, both generally and particularly in the present climate of spiralling aggressiveness of competition and risks in the playing of games at every level, from school age to senior citizenship. Thus, in *Affuto-Nartoy* v. *Clark & ILEA* (1984) *The Times*, 9 February, the defendant local school authority and its schoolteacher employee were held liable in negligence because an excessively enthusiastic games master innocently, and non-violently, tackled a smaller and less physically equipped pupil in a rugby game, with injurious consequences, and this principle was reiterated during preparation of this chapter with a similar decision by Leonard J in *Townsend* v. *Croydon Education Authority* (1989) *Daily Telegraph*, 13 April, p. 12. At the age of 14 the plaintiff had suffered a broken skull from an inadequately supervised playground 'kicking game' based on martial arts films. At the other end of the age scale, litigation is still pending between a retired golf-playing headmaster and a golf-playing opponent for an eye injury arising out of alleged negligence by playing a ball out of a bunker without sufficient warning. Such examples are sample illustrations of the extent to which sporting medical treatment can be required, extending beyond what was traditionally experienced by the average general medical practitioner before the sports explosion in a recreationally orientated society.

The following categories of negligence have been adapted from Mason and McCall Smith. Their application to the sporting scene can be summarised under each heading; but it should always be realised, adapting a judicial aphorism from the property world, that 'the categories of negligence are never closed':

1 Vicarious liability.
2 The reasonably skilful doctor; the usual practice; the custom test.
3 Misdiagnosis.
4 Negligence in treatment.
5 The problem of the novice.
6 Protecting the patient from himself/herself.
7 *Res ipsa loquitur.*
8 Injuries caused by drugs (*per se*, as distinct from the complex competition disciplinary issues already considered above).

Vicarious liability

Within this narrowly based chapter it is not necessary to consider the wider details of a superior's liability for another's wrongdoing within the scope of employment. This has long been established for hospitals, with the current administrative arrangements for apportionment of any damages awards between the various medical protection organisations and appropriate Government departments.*

For present purposes, an ideal example of the principles applicable to non-hospital and sporting medical malpractice emerges from the facts and awards by the British Columbia Court of Appeal. It upheld the trial judge's decision in favour of a claim by a 28-year-old professional ice-hockey player, Mike Robitaille, against his former employing hockey club, known as 'The Canucks' (*Robitaille* v. *Vancouver Ice Hockey Club Ltd* [1981] 3 DLR 288).

The Canucks club doctors and officials rejected continually sustained complaints of developing injuries suffered during play for the club. Negligence was proved because of what the court found to have been high-handed and arrogant forms of conduct, resulting in considerable loss and suffering. The doctors' legal nexus with the club to establish vicarious liability by the club comprised a relatively modest bonus of $2500: season tickets, free parking and access to the club lounge. The appeal court upheld the trial judge's evidential findings of fact that: 'The measure of control asserted by the defendant over the doctors in carrying out their work was substantial. The degree of control need not be complete in order to establish vicarious liability. In the case of a professional person, the absence of control and detection over the manner of doing the

* Since 1st January 1990 this has been superseded by National Health Service acceptance of damages liability within the service, but medical protection organisations and private insurance arrangements continue as before for liability outside the responsibility of the Health Authorities in England and Wales and Health Boards in Scotland and Northern Ireland.

work is of little significance.' In support of this proposition the court cited an English court's decision in *Morren* v. *Swinton and Pendelbury Borough Council* [1965] 2 All ER 349.

Of equal importance for sports men and women was a concurrent approval by the appeal court of the trial judge's conclusion that the plaintiff was contributorily negligent. He was held to be 20% at fault because of his failure to take any action, i.e. to complain to protect his own interest, was less than reasonable. There was evidence upon which Esson J could find that Robitaille was negligent, '... the trial judge correctly distinguished cases ... which dealt with factory workers ... dealing here with a highly paid experienced modern day professional athlete and not a factory worker responding to the mores of olden times' 124 DLR (3rd) at p. 204.

In the context of a 'highly paid experienced modern day professional athlete', this judicial approach was reflected four years later by the English Court of Appeal in *Condon* v. *Basi* (see p. 34) when it ruled that in respect of the duty of care element in a claim for negligence based upon a foul tackle 'there will be a higher degree of care required of a player in a First Division football match than of a player in a local league football match.'

In Robitaille's case it is arguable that the plaintiff's contributory negligence assessment by the court for not pursuing his medical complaints to agencies outside the negligent club's control earlier than he did was possibly harsh. Nevertheless, the judge heard extensive oral evidence, and his final awards, which included aggravated and exemplary damages, demonstrated his ultimate awareness of the plaintiff's overriding and justifiable grievances of medical neglect which created a clear-cut liability. The awards at 1981 levels comprised:

1 $175 000 for loss of professional hockey income.
2 $85 000 for loss of future income other than from professional hockey.
3 $50 000 for the traditional pain, suffering and loss of enjoyment of life."

The principles applied here would certainly be operated in the UK courts. The reciprocity with which Commonwealth countries apply and extend the traditional Anglo-Saxon Common Law was ideally exemplified in *Condon* v. *Basi*. In that landmark decision, extending and applying the concept of negligence to a violent foul soccer tackle, the Court of Appeal in London adapted and applied the judgments of two Australian judicial sources, Barwick CJ and Kitton from *Rootes* v. *Shelton* [1986] ALR 33, a negligence claim for injuries suffered from a water-skiing accident.

ALR: Australian Argus Law Reports

Sports doctors should therefore recognise that, even without a formal contract, elements of access to a club lounge, free parking, season tickets and a modest $2500 bonus can create cumulatively a sufficient degree of control to place them and their associated club jointly at risk if negligence can be established.

Nearer home, two examples from the professional football world pin-point potential vicarious liabilities if the facts merit such a conclusion. One concerned the Swansea City and Tottenham Hotspur Company clubs. The other related to litigation between Queen's Park Rangers and Sheffield Wednesday.

The commencement of the 1956–7 soccer season coincided with the arrival at the Welsh club of a player, Derek King, who was signed for £2000 without having undergone a medical examination. The Swansea club's history, 1912–1982, explains how 'He played only five games at the Vetch Field before being forced to give up the game as a result of a knee defect . . . the Swans claimed that King was unfit when he arrived, while the vendors held the opposite view. Unhappily for the Vetch men the contract was valid.'

The contractual terms were not identified, but the absence of any medical examination by a purchasing club would be unheard of today. Furthermore, if a club doctor were to misdiagnose an ascertainable medical flaw within the well-recognised medical legal criteria of Bolam's case (see p. 40) on an inspection before a transfer, and if within a reasonable time afterwards playing experiences should disclose such a medical flaw, the doctor personally could be at a substantial risk for any authentic loss suffered by the purchasing club, through loss of services or devaluation of the purchased player. Indeed, as these pages were being completed at the end of August 1989, a proposed £2 million pound transfer of Paul Ince from West Ham United to Manchester United was frustrated by ~~an~~ *the* apparent discovery of a pelvic injury upon a medical inspection.

In 1977, Queen's Park Rangers failed to satisfy Judge Laughton Scott in the High Court that Sheffield Wednesday had misled the London club into paying £55 000 for a player who had represented England's under-23 eleven, Vic Mobley, on the basis that his osteoarthritic knee condition had not been disclosed at the time of the transfer transaction. After a 20-day trial, and a reserved judgment, which covered extensive medical evidence, the Judge concluded that Mobley disclosed no osteoarthritic symptoms at the time of the transfer. No appeal against the decision was lodged.

While these pages were being prepared, a graphic illustration of how vicarious liability can arise for sporting organisations emerged in dramatic form when under-21 representative England midfield player, Paul Lake, playing for Manchester City, 'swallowed his tongue' after a collision with an opponent in a Football League match. The club physiotherapist successfully remedied the condition and the Manchester City Club doctor, Norman Luft, highlighted the fact that immediate availability of medical attention was essential. He advocated the desirability of doctors being located near the touch-line in the conventional dug-out, rather than being remotely sited in the grandstand.

The Football League rules insist that a doctor should be present at the grounds during every game. The absence of a doctor could create an ultimate civil liability, coexistent with the absence of facilities, an area which the Sheffield Wednesday Hillsborough inquiry will investigate. Less renowned clubs will not be able to afford such professional assistance. Nevertheless, the absence of first-aid facilities at even the most humble of occasions could, in appropriate circumstances, create a liability on the club for compensation.*

A further example in this area emerged during the last few days before these pages were sent to the printers. During the course of playing on Saturday 11 November 1989 for Arsenal against Millwall the England international player David Rocastle endured a similar experience to Manchester City's Paul Lake, and again relief was achieved by the club physiotherapist. On this occasion the referee in accordance with usual practice had allowed play to continue without immediately having any reason to be aware of the extent of the injury. He was criticised unfairly by reason of this unawareness in not stopping play for medical attention, although in comparable circumstances such delay could be fatal. The Arsenal team doctor in attendance to the patient–player was Dr John Crane who has contributed Chapter 26. At p. 336 under the sub-heading of 'Prevention of injury' he explains: 'Managers, coaches and referees have an important part to play in the prevention of injuries.' This complements the opinions of Drs Adams, Wren and Whiteson (Chapter 18) for amateur and professional boxing referees and Mr F. T. Horan in Chapter 28 at p. 344 under the sub-heading of 'The management of injuries' for cricket umpires. To adapt a well-known legal maxim to this particular area of accident prevention and vicarious liability, it may well be said that the categories of potential liability for player care and damage limitation are never closed.

The need for vigilance and caution in diagnosis and treatment for varying circumstances, ranging from *ad hoc* and emergency situations at one end of the scale to normal consultantcy circumstances at the other, cannot be stressed too strongly, and leads on to the next category identified by Mason and McCall Smith.

The reasonably skilful doctor; the usual practice; the custom test

Lord Scarman and the House of Lords restated time-honoured general principles in two oft-cited pages. In *Sidaway* v. *Bethlem* (see p. 36) he referred to a jury direction by McNair J in the leading case

---

*The doctor's liability can only arise if he is put on notice of lack of facilities and equipment and then fails to explain to the club the necessity of their existence. With varying degrees of equipment and facilities a doctor appointed by any club should be under a continuing duty to alert that club of the need for elementary medical resources consistent with the club's finance, membership and crowd capacity.

of *Bolam* v. *Friern Hospital Management Committee* [1957] 2 All ER 118: 'As a rule a doctor is not negligent if he acts in accordance with a practice accepted at the time as proper by a responsible body of medical opinion, even though other doctors adopt a different practice. In short, the law imposes a duty of care but the standard of care is a matter of medical judgment.'

In *Maynard* v. *West Midlands Regional Health Authority* [1985] All ER 635, he extended this: 'I do not think that the words of the Lord President [Clyde] in *Hunter* v. *Hanly* [1955] SLT 213 at 217 can be bettered: "In the realm of diagnosis there is ample scope for genuine difference of opinion and one man clearly is not negligent merely because his conclusion differs from that of other professional men ... The tried test for establishing negligence in diagnosis or treatment on the part of the doctor is whether he has been proved to be guilty of failing to act as a doctor of ordinary skill would act with ordinary care."'

SLT: Scots Law Times

A valuable illustration of failure to meet the criteria of this section comes from Dr John Betts's contribution on 'Scuba-diving and its medical problems: the role of the doctor' when he refers (pp. 295–6) to 'the problems which may befall the unprepared casualty officer' when confronted with an insulin-dependent diabetic business executive whose 'apparent response to sugar was misinterpreted'. On a claim by the widow of the deceased victim, who had committed suicide, 'Very substantial damages were awarded against the Area Health Authority and casualty officer while the BSAC and its members (who had accepted a dependent patient) were exonerated.'

A less satisfactory position for practical purposes is still on record from a first-instance judgment of nearly 40 years' antiquity in *Clarke* v. *Adams* (1950) CLYB 2707, 94 SJ 599. A physiotherapist's patient was warned when undergoing short-wave diathermy, 'When I turn on the machine I want you to experience a comfortable warmth and not anything more; if you do, I want you to tell me.' Expert evidence called from the Chartered Society of Physiotherapists confirmed that this was consistent with the normally prescribed practice. The patient did not report to the physiotherapist as requested that all was not well, and suffered burns. Slade J held that, having regard to the danger of burning to which the patient was being exposed, the warning given was inadequate and negligent. No appeal was lodged, but it is arguable whether a similar judgment would have resulted today.

CLYB: Current Law
Year Book
SJ: Solicitors Journal

Misdiagnosis

This category of potential liability is another where emergency pressures can extend the risk area. Mason and McCall Smith stake out the boundaries with the general comment: 'A mistake in diagnosis will not be considered negligent if the usual degree of dealings with patient's standards of care is observed but will be treated as one of the non-culpable and inevitable hazards of practice.' They also cited in a footnote a judicial observation: 'Unfortunate as it was that there was a wrong diagnosis, it was one of those misadventures, one of those chances, that life holds for people' (*Crinon* v. *Barnet Group Hospital Management Committee* (1959) *The Times*, 19 November).

Canada, however, again provides a direct example of liability which was established by the Ontario Court of Appeal. A 41-year-old tool and dye worker broke his right ankle when playing soccer with his son. A negligently erroneous X-ray prescription requiring attention to the right foot was compounded by a cascade of consequential errors involving several medical practitioners, including a radiologist, all of whom consolidated the earlier misdiagnosis. This resulted in the appellate court's confirmation of the trial judge's ruling that 'One negligent doctor could be liable for the additional loss caused by the other.' The appeal court also upheld the damages award of $50 000 for general damages, which included $34 465 for loss of income up to the date of trial (*Price* v. *Milawski* [1978] 82 DLR (3d) 130).

Dr John Betts's scuba-diving contribution also emphasises that 'the potential for mistaken diagnoses by both diver and doctor is large'; and this identifies a problem of communication which is as common to the lawyer seeking full factual foundation for a claim from a client, as to the doctor from his patient for treatment. It is also illustrated by Mr Richard Kendrick's contribution on 'Dental damage in contact sport: risk management for general dental practitioners' when he writes: 'Fractures of the cheek bone and mandible, however, show a much higher incidence in contact sports ... their diagnosis is important as further trauma before healing is complete can lead to marked displacement and complications ... important following a blow to the face or teeth that the appropriate X-rays should be taken to exclude such fractures. This may even apply after a blow to a tooth with no apparent loss of tooth substance. This emphasises the point that it is important to make a thorough examination of the patient who has been injured.'

Negligence in treatment

For this issue the formulae in the Sidaway case (see pp. 40–1) did not affect *Whitehouse* v. *Jordan* [1981] 1 All ER 267 when Lord Fraser explained at p. 281: 'The true position ... depends on the nature of the error. If it is one that would not have been made by a reasonably competent professional man professing to have the standard and type of skill that the defendant holds himself out as having, and acting with ordinary care, then it is negligence. If, on the other hand, it is an error that such a man, acting with ordinary care, might have made, then it is not negligence.'

With sports medicine evolving as a developing science and discipline with varying levels of experience for different sports and different parts of the anatomy and different ages and sexes, the possibilities of genuine conflicting and specialist opinions can easily exist. Speculation without real example cannot provide prophecy here. The legal formula has been laid down by the House of Lords in *Whitehouse* v. *Jordan* and is unaffected by the later opinions on Sidaway. Sports medicine must live with it until tested in the fire of evidentiary battles.

The problem of the novice

This issue is equally of concern to the club or organiser who does not provide for adequate facilities in accordance with conventional circumstance. The amateur club which permits an unqualified member to act as an *ad hoc* first-aid assistant without any professional experience, resulting in ultimate serious injury, is as much at risk as the hospital committee which is so unwise as to allow an inexperienced practitioner to carry out complex operations, usually reserved for mature and experienced staff. Thus a football club committee which employed an inadequate contractor to repair a grandstand, resulting in injury to spectators, was held personally responsible and liable in *Brown* v. *Lewis* [1986] 12 TLR 455.

where in this country could this happen?

Protecting the patient from himself/herself

The problem here is self-evident within the sporting scene; for instance excessively enthusiastic athletes striving to return to action when not fully fit or over-zealous coaches and team management committees, which are part of the recognisable pattern of command in every sporting discipline. Without firm medical guidance emphasising the harmful consequences of the zest for play overriding such medical advice, then a liability for negligence could well arise. The demands and stresses of competitive professional sport are particularly vulnerable in this category. Towards the end of 1988, a representative of Windsor Insurance Brokers Ltd, who act for the Football League and the FA explained, as recorded in the *Daily Mail*, 8 November 1988, that: 'Figures proved a third more players were forced out of the game than 10 years ago . . . The risk of serious injury problems began to get greater after the 1966 World Cup. Films of some of those Bobby Charlton goals show how much space players had then. Nowadays, teams squeeze the game into so limited an area of the pitch that there is bound to be more physical contact. It's the pace the players are running that increases the risk of serious injury.' Correspondingly, Dr John Crane in his chapter

'Association Football: the team doctor' emphasises: 'It is inexcusable practice in the care of footballers to inject any sprained ligament with local anaesthetic and let him carry on playing. Such a practice will merely convert a minor injury into a potentially serious injury.'

Res ipsa loquitur

This penultimate stage in Mason and McCall Smith's classification of medical negligence is identifiable by vivid critical and literal judicial commentaries on it. In the House of Lords, Lord Shaw of Dunfermline commented in *Ballard* v. *North British Railway Co.* [1923] SC (HL) 43 qt 46: 'If that phrase had not been in Latin, nobody would have called it a principle ... The day for canonizing Latin phrases has gone past.'

In a hospital negligence case Lord Denning as Denning LJ illuminated it with a judgment that the plaintiff before him on appeal was entitled to say: 'I went into hospital to be cured of two stiff fingers. I have come out with four stiff fingers and my hand is useless. That should not have happened if due care had been used. Explain it if you can' (*Cassidy* v. *Ministry of Health* [1951] 1 All ER 574 at 588).

Once again a Canadian precedent emphasises the point. The plaintiff entered hospital for treatment of a fractured ankle. He left with an amputated leg. No explanation existed. That evidence justified application of this principle with an inevitable judgment of negligence (*MacDonald* v. *York County Hospital Corporation* [1972] 28 DLR (3rd) 521).

Injuries caused by drugs

Laboratory developments, with their controversial conclusions evidenced by such publicised products as thalidomide and Opren, understandably led Mason and McCall Smith to comment:

> 'There is, first and foremost, a philosophical question as to the morality of providing an elaborate system of compensation for those who happen to be injured by drugs when others, who may have identical injuries caused by different factors, go uncompensated ...
>
> 'From the point of view of the doctor or the pharmacist, the major concern over strict liability laws along EEC lines lies in the need to ensure that the manufacturer can be adequately identified in order to avoid claims being made against himself. This might entail elaborate bureaucratic procedures and the fear has been expressed that it could lead to further development of the practice of defensive medicine. An interesting American twist is shown in *Oskehbolt* v. *Lederle Laboratories* (1983) Or. 656 P.2d 293.'

In the above-mentioned case, a doctor, having been successfully sued for prescribing a faulty drug, himself claimed against the manufac-

SC (HL): Sessions Cases (House of Lords) (Scotland)

Or. 656 P.2d: Pacific Reporter (Oregon, USA)

turers for negligently and fraudulently failing to warn physicians of possible harmful effects of prescription medicines.

From the point of view of the sports doctor, pharmacist and administrators, however, it is essential to emphasise once more: drug abuse and drug control within the world of sport demand special care from medical advisers. Any breach of that duty of care with risk of foreseeable damage or injury would create a prima-facie liability in negligence. They cannot now say that they have not been warned.

5. Sport's future for medicine and the law

The range of subjects covered in this volume demonstrates beyond doubt the interaction which exists between sports medicine and the law, for the benefit of sport and above all for the patients who are considered in respect of three areas: good health, education and self- or externally controlled discipline. The evidence from the medical profession and its associated activities ideally should form the guidelines for personal conduct and regulatory control. The control of cheating by drugs and violence is provided, not only by chemical testing in the former and referee control in the latter, but also by medical evidence which establishes the harmful and injurious consequences.

Public performance by athletes provides examples for future generations. This was confirmed by Alan Burns, the *Sunday Mirror*'s medical correspondent, in the issue of 16 April 1989. He cited the findings of the Institute for the Study of Children in Sport, where, according to its director, Martin Lee, a study carried out at Bedford College of Higher Education on 160 children disclosed that 'More than 33 per cent of ten year olds are prepared to commit a foul to gain an advantage', a percentage figure comparable to that disclosed by Davies and Gibson for injuries likely to be attributable to violent foul play resulting from their Guy's Hospital Athletics Injuries Clinic survey in 1978.

As the sporting scene and 'health and sport for all' campaigns expand yearly, sports medicine is well placed to monitor and steer developments for the benefit of society at large. Parliament gave a lead as long ago as 1970 when the Chronically Sick and Disabled Persons Act 1970 required public undertakings to provide access, parking and toilet facilities (including those relating to sport and recreation) which are practical and reasonable for a disabled person's needs. Section 5 of the Disabled Persons Act 1981 imposes duties on those who grant planning permission under Section 29 of the Town and Country Planning Act 1970 to draw attention to Section 4 and other provisions of that 1981 Act for the benefits required for the disabled.

At the time of writing in 1989 final conclusions are still awaited

from the Home Office and Parliament on the 1987 proposals referred to on p. 29 for anabolic steroids to be added to the lists of
proscribed drugs under the Misuse of Drugs Act 1971. Sporting
bodies' regulatory powers are limited to their own discretion.
Medical evidence for these particular substances' harmful consequences would impose more clearly identifiable sanctions on
cheating athletes than the present sporting regulations can create.

The Hillsborough Sheffield Wednesday judicial inquiry will contain recommendations for promotional and organisational requirements. It is likely that they will reiterate and re-emphasise what
has been on file and on record since earlier comparable inquiries
— into Wembley Stadium crowd problems in 1923 (Cmnd. 2088
(1924)), Bolton Wanderers disaster in 1946 (Cmnd. 6846 (1947)), the
Ibrox stand disaster (in 1971) and the Poppelwell Bradford City Fire
Disaster Reports — which led to incomplete and limited legislation.
Thus Parliament will fill the gaps on an *ad hoc* basis in the manner
it has previously manifested when responding to sporting disaster.

Conclusions and summary

Every chapter in this volume demonstrates the need for special care
in each sporting discipline. The requirements for boxers and jockeys
are different in detail from the needs to protect cricketers, footballers and athletes. Nevertheless, the level of care by doctors,
paramedical services, administrators and promoters and organisers
must inevitably interact upon each other. Parliament's entry into
these fields has been in the fragmentary manner identified here; and
this echoes the prognosis recognised by the creator of the role of
a Government minister with responsibility for sport, the former
Lord Chancellor, Lord Hailsham of St Marylebone, when he was
Minister for Science and Technology in Macmillan's Cabinet in the
early 1960s. He foresaw a need: 'Not for a Ministry but for a focal
point under a Minister for a coherent body of doctrine, perhaps even
a philosophy of government encouragement. My eloquence had its
effect on the Prime Minister and, before I knew where I was, I was
left to organise the first government of this kind.'

In the intervening quarter of a century no holder of that post
since then has held Cabinet office, and many different departments
in Whitehall, Health and Social Security, Environment, the Home
Office and Education, have fragmentarily been associated with the
sporting health of the community. While need remains to protect
communal health through the sporting scene, the one element
which binds all sports will always be the role of medicine harnessed
to the law at all its levels, playing, administrative and national.
Therein lies the future well-being of sport and its role in the international community.

Appendix 1.1. *Extract from recommendations in the interim report on the inquiry by RT Hon Lord Justice Taylor into the Hillsborough Stadium disaster [presented to Parliament August 1989]*

Co-ordination of emergency services

35 The police, fire and ambulance services should maintain through senior nominated officers regular liaison concerning crowd safety at each stadium.*

36 Before each match at a designated stadium, the police should ensure that the fire service and ambulance service are given full details about the event, including its venue, its timing, the number of spectators expected, their likely routes of entry and exit, and any anticipated or potential difficulties concerning the control or movement of the crowd. Such details should be readily available in the control rooms of each of the emergency services.*

37 Contingency plans for the arrival at each designated stadium of emergency vehicles from all three services should be reviewed. They should include routes of access, rendezvous points, and accessibility within the ground itself.*

38 Police officers posted at the entrances to the ground should be briefed as to the contingency plans for the arrival of emergency services and should be informed when such services are called as to where and why they are required.*

*These points were recommended to be carried out *before* the start of the 1989/90 soccer season. The rest of the recommendations in the report were recommended to be started forthwith and completed as soon as possible.

First aid, medical facilities and ambulances

39 There should be at each stadium at each match at least one trained first aider per 1000 spectators. The club should have the responsibility for securing such attendance.*

40 There should be at each stadium one or more first aid rooms. The number of such rooms and the equipment to be maintained within them should be specified by the local authority after taking professional medical advice and should be made a requirement of any Safety Certificate.

41 The club should employ a medical practitioner to be present at each match and available to deal with any medical exigency at the ground. He should be trained and competent in advanced first aid. He should be present at the ground at least an hour before kick-off and should remain until half an hour after the end of the match. His whereabouts should be known to those in the police control room and he should be immediately contactable.*

42 At least one fully equipped ambulance from the appropriate ambulance authority should be in attendance at all matches with an expected crowd of 5000 or more.*

43 The number of ambulances to be in attendance for matches where larger crowds are expected should be specified by the local authority after consultation with the ambulance service and should be made a requirement of the Safety Certificate.

Epilogue

The number of contemporaneous occasions illuminating the subject throughout this text, added between submitting the manuscript to the publisher and the final cut-off date for additions (12 November 1989), is indicative of the subject's developing potential. Three clear examples of this appear on pages 18, 24 and 47. During the time-lag between that cut-off date and the final date for proof corrections in mid-January 1990, the evolving pattern has not diminished. Football's world governing body, FIFA, banned Chile from the 1994 World Cup Competition and imposed severe sanctions on many of its medical advisers for falsifying medical reports about the condition of the national team goalkeeper and captain Roberto Rojas, who had feigned injury from a flare which had landed near him but did not strike him when the national team was losing 0-1 in a World Cup qualifying match against Brazil in Rio during September 1989. The English Football League announced its intention to appoint a supervising medical officer during 1990, and Lord Justice Taylor's anticipated *Final* Report will be required by protocol and precedent to be delivered to its commissioning Government Minister, the Home Secretary, who will decide upon its ultimate date for production after these pages have been finally corrected for publication. Furthermore, the Home Office is also the Government source dealing with prohibited drugs (and *not* the Department of the Environment which housed the Under-Secretary of State responsible for sport), which announced during early January 1990 that the Government intends to extend the Misuse of Drugs Act 1971 to make possession of muscle-enhancing anabolic steroids a criminal offence, two years after the Home Office announced in September 1987 its consideration for such an intention (pp. 29 and 46). As *The Times* recorded in a leading article on 29 December 1989, 'It has needed pressure from many quarters, particularly Mr Colin Moynihan, the Minister for Sport, and Mr Menzies Campbell, the Liberal Democrats' spokesman on sport, to put firmly en route to the statute book. They have done an important service'. Almost symbolically, a few weeks later in *The Times* Sports Letters pages for 11 January 1990 during a correspondence on the wider issue of British sport during the 1990s, the distinguished former international rugby referee and sports administrator, Air Vice-Marshal G.C. (Larry) Lamb, CB, CBE, AFC, explained the aim from his standpoint as General Secretary of the London Sports Medicine Institute in 'the closest consultation with the Sports Council, the BOA [British Olympic Association], BASM [British Association of Sports Medicine], and all other interested parties, including major governing bodies of sport, to translate this London orientated body into a national sports medicine institute serving the entire country.'

This target is consistent with what I have been increasingly aware of as the non-medical legal editor from my other editorial colleagues and sports doctors generally, namely the fragmented pattern of sports medicine throughout the UK. I had suspected this while I wrote the Introduction to my chapter 'Sports Medicine and the Law' in Butterworths' *Sport and the Law* (1988), without realising at the time that the concept had been first floated by Dr John O'Hara, Chairman of the Football Association Medical Committee. His initiative caused me to write then, 'The Football Association National Rehabilitation and Sports Injuries Centre has been opened at the National Sports Centre in Lilleshall, Shropshire; HRH The Princess Royal, as President of the British Olympic Medical Centre officiated at the opening of Northwick Park Hospital and Clinical Research Cantre in Harrow on the outskirts of North London; and London Sports Medicine Institute has been opened on the campus of St Bartholomew's Medical College. Yet Dr Dan Tunstall Pedoe, medical director of the Institute and medical adviser to the London Marathon explained to the *Daily Telegraph* (23 December 1986) "Sports Medicine has had virtually no official recognition or support from the health service. The average struggling athlete, let alone the serious amateur, is less well served here than in other countries, where there is government money for injuries and where there may well be well-established sports clinics."'

Throughout 1990, and beyond, successive Commonwealth Games and World Cup competitions in addition to countless other events will re-emphasize this justifiable complaint. Significantly, Larry Lamb's letter followed a three-part series in *The Times* assessing the world sports scene for the 1990s by Sebastian Coe and Daley Thompson in which they explained (5 January 1990) 'In many sports we still lose too many competitors too early through injury ... Ask any competitor what he or she most wants to see improved, and the answer will always be medical help.' I would extend that to anyone at *every* age and participatory level. Coe and Thompson claimed further, however, with words that could have been written intuitively with the following pages in mind.

> 'Doctors everywhere have to understand that they do not have all the answers. Sporting injuries require a multi-disciplinary approach. Often sports men and women need specialist insight and advice; for example, their reliance on a shoulder or knee is not that of most citizens. Few doctors have the knowledge and experience to treat every pull, strain, break or tear.
>
> 'Daley and I would like to see a national system in which specialists and interested doctors could co-operate effectively — aware of and able to call upon each other's help and guidance ... At any time, a wrong diagnosis, or treatment can ruin a career. Mistakes can never be wholly avoided. But what we need is an effective network, based perhaps on a central register, into which the best of our sporting talent (and their coaches and doctors) can plug themselves and get the best and the appropriate help when it is needed.'

If 'there is a tide in the affairs of men, Which, taken at the flood, leads on to fortune', then the pages which follow hereafter should provide a catalyst to cause the British Government to apply Lord Hailsham's general thoughts of the early 1960s (p. 46) of a need 'not for a Ministry, but for a focal point under a Minister for a coherent body of doctrine, perhaps even a philosophy of government encouragement', not only to the sporting scene in general, but to sports medicine in particular, for the general health and mental and spiritual health of the whole nation.

2 The nature and incidence of injury in sport

J. G. P. WILLIAMS

'I have nothing to offer but blood, toil, tears and sweat'
Winston Churchill

Understanding injury

The major problems confronted in dealing with injuries due to accidents in sport lie in a common lack of understanding of the nature of such injuries. There are generally speaking no such things as football injuries or rugby injuries or athletics injuries — only injuries! Respective sports, however, will have their own well-recognized patterns of damage and special requirements of the participants, usually involving an early return to activity.

Injury is damage to the body caused by a mechanical stress to which it cannot adapt in time or space. When confronted by such a stress the body essays to adapt by avoidance, transmission or absorption. When none of these is possible, either because the intensity of the stress is too great or because the duration is too prolonged, damage occurs. The nature of the primary damage is dependent on the type of stress applied. The body is able to 'distinguish' between different mechanisms of stress (for example, a direct blow, as opposed to a sudden stretch) and this is reflected in the consequent tissue damage (Fig. 2.1), but it cannot differentiate between the different situations in which such a stress may be imposed (for example, in a road traffic accident, in a domestic accident or on the sports field).

The type of activity in which the victim is engaged at the time of the injury will, however, largely influence secondary features of the pathological response. For example, in the case of a fracture of the tibia and fibula haemorrhage will be far greater in a footballer who sustains his injury in the middle of an active game than in the case of a sedentary passenger similarly injured in a motor-car accident.

Physical fitness developed for participation in sport not only influences the secondary effects of injury but also significantly affects the recovery process therefrom. A haematoma may be very much bigger in an athlete with high blood flow through exercising limbs, but the very process of training prepares the limb for the rapid reabsorption of extravasated fluid, and therefore haematomas are more rapidly absorbed in fit, athletic individuals than in sedentary people. The essential similarity, in terms of tissue damage, of

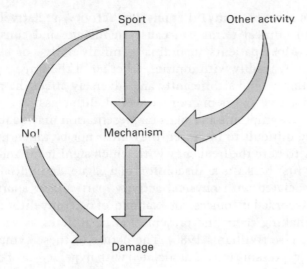

Sport   Other activity

No!   Mechanism

Damage

Fig. 2.1 Causal chain in injury.

the effects of similar stresses is particularly true in cases of instantaneous injury where relatively great external forces are applied, causing well-recognised damage patterns.

Problems, however, may arise in respect of overuse injuries (Corrigan 1968). These are due to internal stresses generated chronically during training and are relatively uncommon outside the sporting context, although they may be observed in the enthusiastic 'do-it-yourselfer' who suddenly engages in unaccustomed activity. They also occur in some areas of industry involving people who take up new jobs requiring unaccustomed repetitive activity, and they may also be met in 'high-performance' occupations, for example the armed forces, where the development of high levels of physical fitness are required. Until recently the aetiology, pathology and incidence of overuse injury were relatively uncertain, but there has been wide documentation of such injuries and a considerable literature in the English language is readily available (Williams & Sperryn 1976; O'Donoghue 1984; Helal *et al.* 1986).

In addition to specific injuries patients may present with clinical problems due less to specific stress overload than to secondary conditions, usually constitutional, which lead to biomechanical inadequacies for the activity performed, thus enhancing and multiplying the effect of what, for a normal person, would be acceptable stress levels. Examples include long-distance runners and joggers who have torsion of the tibia and excessively pronating feet, which on a day-to-day basis may cause no problems. Under the stresses of running or jogging, however, the faulty biomechanics makes the absorption of otherwise reasonable stress levels impossible, and breakdown occurs.

An important factor in injury in sport is that frequently symptoms and signs may be vague because presentation occurs in earlier states of the condition. In the trained, high-performance individual,

51

52

Chapter 2
The nature and
incidence of
injury in sport

whether in sport or in any other physical activity, a relatively minor problem in clinical terms can cause significant and considerable disability. Most patients in ordinary, mildly active or sedentary lives can cope readily with injuries, whether of the impact or over-use type, that would significantly and adversely affect the perform-ance of an active sports man or woman of élite class.

Although symptoms and signs on presentation may be relatively diffuse and difficult to interpret, they must not be taken lightly. It is salutary to note the frequency with which significant and serious pathology first presents as discomfort of a vague, and initially mild, nature associated with physical activity, particularly sport. There are many recorded instances, for example, of osteomyelitis and bone tumours making their first presentation in athletes as vague pain during exercise (Williams 1980). The nature of these symptoms is explained by pressure effects associated with hyperaemia of exercise. It is important for the attending clinician to make every effort to reach an accurate diagnosis and to be aware of the usual natural history of the condition diagnosed. Any variation from the familiar pattern of disease diagnosed should arouse suspicion and indicate the need for careful investigation.

Further complications arise when real injury occurs in patho-logical tissue. The case is recorded of an athlete who experienced sudden pain in the quadriceps muscle during training. On the face of it, this was a straightforward rectus femoris tear. There was no previous history. Clinically the patient had considerable swelling and bruising of the quadriceps with a tender mass in the front of the thigh. He was treated as a muscle tear and showed initially a good response. Subsequently, however, the swelling recurred without pain and the lesion proved to be a rhabdomyosarcoma. It was later demonstrated that there had been haemorrhage into the tumour mass and the muscle rupture had been of the sarcomatous rather than the normal muscle tissue. For such a lesion, however, it would be virtually impossible and probably undesirable to submit all patients with apparent muscle tears to ultrasound or computerised tomography (CT) scanning in order to detect rare malignancy. Cases of this sort nevertheless emphasise that things may not always be as they seem. The attending clinician must always maintain a degree of suspicion and at least be aware of the extent to which serious pathology may present as relatively innocuous injury.*

The vast majority of injuries in sport do not require any form of specialised knowledge or treatment. Even in a selected series at-tending specialist sports injuries clinics it has been shown that

*In the case described failure to detect the sarcoma at first presentation would be unlikely to be construed as negligence, on account of the rarity of the condition and the presence of another reasonable explanation for the presenting symptoms. The importance of careful follow-up for apparently innocuous conditions is, however, well demonstrated.

53
Chapter 2
The nature and
incidence of
injury in sport

more than 60% of cases could have been dealt with perfectly well by the patient's family doctor or by a recognised specialist in locomotor disorders (Sperryn & Williams 1975). Across the population of sportmen and women as a whole, the percentage of patients requiring highly specialist sports medical experience is substantially lower.

However, it must be remembered that a knowledge and understanding of the mechanics of injury in sport and its specialist management can only be acquired by formal study. Specific instruction in the peculiar problems of injured sports men and women should be obtained by doctors who seek to pursue a career in sports medicine.

One major difficulty facing the interested clinician is the plethora of anecdotal and otherwise unreliable material disseminated in both printed and verbal form. This has led inevitably to the encouragement and practice of ideas and treatment measures which do not always stand up to close inspection. Amongst these may be included the use of steroids by injection, the use of therapeutic ultrasound and even the use of cold for treatment. All these modalities of treatment are popular in the management of sports injuries, and all carry a significant element of risk. One of the depressing features of sports medical practice is the frequency with which patients present with iatrogenic problems related to the use of these and other forms of treatment.

Classification of injury in sport

Injuries in sport can be classified in a number of ways (Williams 1971). Classification by aetiology or causation is useful in that it assists in reaching the diagnosis through an appreciation of the mechanism of injury.

Essentially athletes and sports men and women present either with injuries sustained during sport which usually prevent further participation or alternatively with injuries sustained incidentally to the sports activity but which also interfere with subsequent participation. In the latter case injuries exist in a similar spectrum to those encountered in the population at large.

Injuries occurring in sport may be primary, that is to say the direct result of a specific stress or overload, or secondary, where the pathological condition has been itself provoked by some previous injury. For example, the anterior knee pain syndrome (chondromalacia patellae) may be secondary to some previous relatively minor knee injury which has caused quadriceps inhibition, which, through muscle imbalance, has in turn provoked the development of chondromalacia. Many causes of spinal pain, particularly in the low back, derive as secondary lesions from some previous relatively minor insult.

54
Chapter 2
The nature and
incidence of
injury in sport

King (1983) has also described a 'second injury' phenomenon. It occurs when an athlete or sports man or woman sustains a minor injury and continues to play instead of resting, thereby making himself/herself vulnerable to a second unrelated, but possibly more severe, injury.

Primary injury may derive either from forces generated outside the patient's body, in which case they are referred to as extrinsic, or from forces generated within, when they are described as intrinsic. Extrinsic injuries are usually instantaneous and cause more severe damage than intrinsic injury, because the mechanical forces involved are greater. Many of these injuries are similar to impact injuries in other activities, for example, dislocation of the shoulder occurs with monotonous regularity in rugby football as it does in domestic accidents. Various factors have been recognised in contributing to extrinsic injury, these being human, implemental, vehicular and environmental.

Intrinsic injuries derive specifically from the patient's own activities and may occur in a single incident or, more commonly, as a result of repeated stress overload. Single-incident injuries include sudden, complete rupture of the Achilles tendon, or a hamstring tear, whereas overuse injuries involve compartment syndromes, tendinitis and stress fractures.

As in all cases of injury, a carefully taken history should indicate the nature of the problem, particularly where there is adequate background knowledge of the natural history of the injury and of the mechanics of the sport. A common error of diagnosis — due specifically to lack of knowledge of its natural history — is misdiagnosis of sciatica as 'chronic hamstring strain', which occurs all too frequently. Pain, initially of gradual onset, experienced in the back of the thigh is not due to a 'pulled' muscle. A muscle tear occurs instantaneously and the onset of pain is therefore sudden. Gradual onset of pain in the back of the thigh during exercise is almost invariably sciatica, due to lumbar nerve root irritation. Too often practitioners, unaware of this simple fact, misdiagnose sciatica and patients are then subjected to more or less protracted periods of completely ineffective treatment directed to the hamstrings instead of to the primary cause in the lumbar spine.

Patterns of injury in sport

While it is true that there are no 'sport-specific' injuries as such, it is nevertheless possible to discern regular patterns of injury in different types of sport which are related to the mechanisms of stress within those sports (Weightman & Browne 1974). Indeed there may be changes in the patterns of injury within a given sport as a result of changes in the way that the sport is practised, often due to changes in the laws and regulations which govern it. In Rugby

55
Chapter 2
The nature and
incidence of
injury in sport

Union football, for example, there has been a reduction, both real and relative, in the incidence of cervical injuries as a result of changes in the laws relating to the scrummage (Burry & Calcinai 1988; see also Chapter 3). A further redefinition of the laws of this phase of the game would probably diminish further the risks of such injuries. At the same time there appears to be an increase in other types of contact injuries in rugby, in part caused by the practice of 'hyping up' teams before playing, so raising unnecessarily the level of aggression. The margin between what is fair and what is unfair and improper thus becomes progressively blurred. It is interesting to note that in rugby football 30% of injuries occur in a 'foul' situation (Davies & Gibson 1978).*

Patterns that may be clearly discerned across the whole spectrum of sports show that in Rugby Union and the other codes of football, in addition to judo, wrestling and boxing and indeed all 'body-contact sports', direct impact injuries are more common than in tennis or track and field athletics. Players in racket sports tend to have an increased frequency of injuries affecting the upper limbs, while track athletes show different patterns of injury according to the type of event in which they are competing. Sprinters, for example, tend to have upper leg-injuries, whereas in middle- and long-distance runners injuries tend to affect the lower leg.

It is tempting to classify injuries according to the sport, but this may be counter-productive in the sense that this tends to encourage fixed ideas as to what may or may not occur in a given sport. This often leads to conditions being missed because they were not regarded as being characteristic of the sport in question. What is needed in order to understand injury is a clear conception of its mechanism. Frequently the diagnosis becomes immediately apparent from the description of the way in which the injury occurred. Thus, for example, the football player who complains of pain and instability in the knee following an incident in which this foot was held in the ground by the studs of his boot while his body turned away from the knee, which was flexed, weight-bearing, abducted and externally rotated, would almost certainly have developed anteromedial rotary instability with damage to the medial meniscus and collateral ligament, capsule and possibly the anterior cruciate ligament. Given an accurate description from the patient himself or herself or from reliable witnesses as to how the accident occurred, the diagnosis usually becomes clear. To some extent this is also the case in an overuse injury; a clear description of the

---

*This to an extent may be something of a self-fulfilling prophecy, for the referee as the sole judge of fact on the field of play decides what is and is not 'foul play'. There remains scope, however, to further reduce the incidence of injuries during play by further alteration of the rules to avoid potentially dangerous situations, e.g. the 'pile-up', and by attempting to influence referees to become more discerning in distinguishing between legitimate enthusiasm and aggression constituting foul play.

56
Chapter 2
The nature and
incidence of
injury in sport

patient's training programme will often give a strong clue as to what is going wrong.

In the same way that a sound grasp of fundamental anatomy and biomechanics is required for the proper interpretation of case histories of injured sports men and women, so too is an understanding of the nature of the sport in question valuable. This is not to say that it is a prerequisite that the practitioner should necessarily have any specific experience of the sport. It is advantageous, however, to be able to interpret accurately the player's description of that phase of the game in which he was injured, and to this end it is useful but not essential to have at least a working knowledge of the rules and method of play.

In many instances injuries occur as a result of faulty technique, particularly in highly technical events (such as hammer-throwing), and correction of technique becomes an essential component of patient management. This is particularly so in a situation where as a result of injury the patient has developed bad habits. It is not necessarily every practitioner of sports medicine who is in a position to advise and coach patients out of their technical faults — but it is open to all to make certain that the patient is referred to a suitable authority in the sport for expert guidance for fault correction to prevent recurrence.

An important practical problem for the practitioner relates to the return of the patient to training and competition, particularly the latter. It is often said that the athletic patient 'wants to be 110% fit and he wants it yesterday'. Many athletes and sports men and women, particularly in the professional ranks, are often under severe pressure to return to sporting activity too soon. A major disadvantage of the system (in Association Football for example) of allowing substitutes on to the field is the temptation, to which managers frequently yield, of putting in a player who is far from fully fit, because the player in question has a considerable drawing power in terms of the number of spectators (and the financial benefits to the club accruing therefrom).*

There is in the pressure of the sporting situation a considerable temptation to take risks and cut corners in treatment so as to allow an undesirably rapid resumption of sporting activity. It is possible that in certain circumstances (particularly where the administration of drugs of one kind or another may be concerned) the practitioner may be pressurised into so inappropriate an attempt to restore the sports man or woman to competition that this may later be regarded as malpractice for which the practitioner might

---

* For the medical practitioner asked to advise in this situation, a dilemma may arise. The relationship between the doctor and the club is usually that the doctor is an agent of the club, receiving financial or other material reward for his services. The discharge of his duties toward the club, therefore, may conflict with the best interests of the 'patients'.

57
*Chapter 2
The nature and
incidence of
injury in sport*

be held liable for negligence (Ford 1980). There are times when the sports doctor finds himself walking a moral tightrope. It is important, therefore, that these issues should have been considered by the doctor, that he keeps good notes and that he feels confident that he would be able to justify his actions if subsequently challenged.

Misdiagnosis of injury

Until quite recently, and still in some instances today, sport as a human activity has been viewed with disfavour by medical practitioners. Patients who become injured in such activities thus often receive scant attention or sympathy from family doctors or hospital practitioners. Such an uncaring attitude invariably prejudices correct history-taking and a proper and careful examination. The attitude 'go away and rest it and don't bother me' is still too prevalent and may lead to disaster. Examples are regularly met of infection and tumours which first presented as pain in sport and have been left undiagnosed for too long because of a negative attitude to active treatment by the practitioner concerned. (Such attitudes and simple lack of care can of course be met in a variety of situations and do not always apply to sports men and women.)

Two clinical traps which have medico-legal implications and which occur commonly in sports men and women and non-sports men and women alike are the undiagnosed fracture of the waist of the scaphoid and the undiagnosed slipped upper femoral epiphysis (Hawkins 1985). These conditions are regularly featured in the annual reports published by the Medical Protection Society, and cautionary tales too often go unheeded.

Ignorance is perhaps the main reason why crises arise in the management of sports injuries. Most practitioners are able to deal effectively with major trauma, but apparently minor, yet nevertheless disabling, conditions remain inadequately diagnosed and treated.

There is an extensive and often excellent literature available at a variety of academic levels covering the whole spectrum of injury in sport, particularly those injuries which are not part of common orthopaedic or trauma practice. It is therefore remarkable how often these texts are unheeded (or perhaps not understood!) and even quite obvious pathologies misdiagnosed and consequently mistreated. One such example is complete rupture of the Achilles tendon (Medical Defence Union 1977). There should never be any difficulty in accurate diagnosis of this condition, yet it is frequently missed, patients being referred to physiotherapists for muscle strain. The condition is relatively uncommon but nevertheless should be familiar to general practitioners and accident and emergency department doctors.

58

Chapter 2
The nature and
incidence of
injury in sport

Mismanagement of injury

Over past years a plethora of new types of physical treatment has been introduced, the biological effects of some of which are still uncertain. Such methods of treatment are sometimes used with a worrying lack of discernment by various practitioners, particularly physiotherapists.

Ultrasound therapy is commonly used for soft tissue injuries without scientific measurement of the dose delivered or its direction. The therapist may have some idea of the output from the sound-head but has no means of determining the dose at tissue level or its biological effects. Studies by Dyson and others (Dyson *et al.* 1974; Dyson 1985) have indicated the type and extent of damage that treatment of this type may cause, yet it is still used in a rather haphazard fashion by practitioners who have only the sketchiest idea of its effects. Its value in some cases has been well established (Binder *et al.* 1985), but the number of clinical trials of this and other forms of physiotherapy that can be regarded as sound is very small. Histological examination, particularly of the ultrastructure of tendon material removed at surgery for chronic Achilles tendon pain, has indicated a significant degree of damage to the tendon. This accords remarkably closely with the damage observed by Dyson in experimental studies of tissues which had received excessive insonation. It may be that many cases of persistent Achilles tendon pain are partially iatrogenic in that lesions are possibly made worse by excessive insonation.

Another form of treatment in common use for sports injuries is cold, in the form of cold water baths, the application of a bag of frozen peas, endothermic commercial compresses and simple ice-bags. The risk to the integrity of the peripheral nerves in areas of cooling has been clearly defined (Bickford 1939; Pamchenko 1944). Furthermore, many patients show evidence of prolonged impairment of function after treatment with cold. It is dubious, therefore, whether such treatment specifically and favourably influences many of the conditions for which it is used, for example, ankle sprains or muscle tears.

The use of these treatment modalities has been hallowed, perhaps incorrectly, by years of practice without critical reappraisal. The sporting public's heightened expectations in respect of proper medical management may in future prove to be just the required stimulus to proper critical appraisal of methods of treatment currently in vogue which are popular without being rational.

Another form of treatment frequently but sometimes injudiciously practised by doctors and others is injection of local anaesthetic and steroid. The full effects of this type of treatment are also uncertain. There are many instances recorded in the literature of damage caused by such injections both in experimental and in therapeutic models (Ismail *et al.* 1969; Unverferth & Olix 1973; Kennedy &

59
Chapter 2
The nature and
incidence of
injury in sport

Baxter Willis 1976). The classic, perhaps, is complete rupture of the Achilles tendon following steroid injection for tendinitis. Ruptures can also occur at other sites, in addition to areas of scar breakdown and other pathological changes in injected tissues. Steroid stigmata including loss of subcutaneous fat, discoloration and scar stretching are well recognised and frequently seen in sports patients.

'Prevention is better than cure'

It has ever been the lesson of the Medical Protection Society and its sister organisations that prevention is better than cure. Prevention of unnecessary injury and damage in sports men and women demands a proper knowledge of sports traumatology and its correct application. The practice of sports medicine requires the same elements of care, dedication and study as any other branch of medicine.

References

Bickford R. G. (1939) The fibre dissociation produced by cooling human nerves. *Clinical Science* **4**, 159–65.

Binder A., Hodge G., Greenwood A. M., Hazleman B. L. & Page-Thomas D. P. (1985) Is therapeutic ultrasound effective in treating soft tissue lesions? *British Medical Journal* **290**, 512.

Burry H. C. & Calcinai C. J. (1988) The need to make rugby safer. *British Medical Journal* **296**, 149–50.

Corrigan A. B. (1968) Sports injuries. *Hospital Medicine* **2**, 1328–34.

Davies J. E. & Gibson T. (1978) Injuries in Rugby Union football. *British Medical Journal* **2** (6154), 1759–61.

Dyson M. (1985) Therapeutic applications of ultrasound. In *Clinics in Diagnostic Ultrasound*, vol. 16, *Biological Effects of Ultrasound*, ed. W. L. Nyborg & M. C. Ziskin, pp. 121–33. New York: Churchill Livingstone.

Dyson M., Bond J. B., Woodward B. & Broadhurst J. (1974) The production of blood all stasis and endothelial damage in the blood vessels of chick embryos treated with ultrasound in a stationary wave field. *Ultrasound in Medicine and Biology* **1**, 133–48.

Ford P. G. T. (1980) Ethics in sports medicine — some medico-legal considerations. *British Journal of Sports Medicine* **14**, 90–1.

Hawkins C. (1985) *Mishap or Malpractice?* Oxford: Blackwell Scientific Publications.

Helal B., King J. B. & Grange W. J. (1986) *Sports Injuries and their Treatment*. London: Chapman & Hall.

Ismail A. M., Balakrishnan R. & Rajakumar M. K. (1969) Rupture of patellar ligament after steroid infiltration. *Journal of Bone Joint Surgery* **51B**, 503–5.

Kennedy J. C. & Baxter Willis R. (1976) The effects of local injection of steroids into tendons — a biomechanical and microscopic study. *American Journal of Sports Medicine* **4**, 11–21.

King J. B. (1983) Second injury syndrome (Letter). *British Journal of Sports Medicine* **17**, 59–60.

Medical Defence union (1977) *Annual Report 1977*. London: Medical Defence Union.

O'Donoghue D. H. (1984) *Treatment of Injuries to Athletes*, 4th edn. Philadelphia: W. B. Saunders.

Pamchenko D. I. (1944) Retrograde changes in the spinal cord in frost bite of the extremities. *American Review of Soviet Medicine* **1**, 440–3.

Sperryn P. N. & Williams J. G. P. (1975) Why sports injuries clinics? *British Medical Journal* **3**, 364–5.

Unverferth L. J. & Olix M. L. (1973) The effect of local steroid injection on tendons. *Journal of Sports Medicine and Physical Fitness* **1** (4), 31–7.

Weightman D. & Browne R. C. (1974) Injuries in Association and Rugby Football. *British Journal of Sports Medicine* **8**, 183–7.

60
Chapter 2
The nature and
incidence of
injury in sport

Williams J. G. P. (1971) Aetiological classification of injury in sportsmen. *British Journal of Sports Medicine* **5**, 228–30.
Williams J. G. P. (1980) *A Colour Atlas of Injury in Sport.* London: Wolfe Medical.
Williams J. G. P. & Sperryn P. N. (1976) *Sports Medicine,* 2nd Edn. London: Edward Arnold.

The doctor's contribution towards safety in sport — an exercise in preventive medicine 3

D. A. D. MACLEOD

'Beneath the rule of men entirely great the pen is mightier than the sword'
From *Richelieu II*, ii, by E. C. Lytton

Prologue

The identification of risk factors and their eradication both for healthy living and in sport are exercises in preventive medicine. So much has been written about whether sports medicine really is a speciality or specialism. If one considers, however, the two main components of sports medicine — the physiological assessment of fitness or exercise medicine, and the prevention and treatment of injuries — then sports medicine, albeit dealing with a particular healthcare population, is in itself an exercise in preventive medicine.

In Rugby Union football, besides the identification of risk factors through epidemiological and clinical injury surveys, the structure of injury care is itself a challenge in preventive medicine.

Most rugby games, apart from senior international and represention matches, are unattended by doctors or physiotherapists. The grass roots matches in many parts of the country and the world are watched by one man and his dog, if that!

Two rugby playing countries have tried to overcome the problem of first-aid cover at matches, but both in different ways and for some different reasons. In Wales, with a playing population of over 30 000 each weekend, many games are attended by members of the Welsh Association of Sports Trainers. This is an association of members of the lay-public in general, who are given courses and lectures on sports first-aid, are given accreditation and who play an invaluable role in the primary care of the injured played. If necessary, the paramedical and medical professions are the second part of contact, and hospitalization and surgery are the third. This tripartite structure serves the rugby playing community well.

In Japan, where there are over 120 000 players each weekend, rugby players have the same problem as the Japanese golfers, an inadequate number of playing pitches. To counteract this logistical problem, there are some playing grounds throughout Japan where several matches are played on the same pitch on the same day, starting at 6.00 a.m. in the morning and continuing until the evening! As rugby is also played nearly all the year round, most of the playing surfaces are devoid of any grass. The Kento Medical Society in Japan is a society of over 300 rugby doctors who ensure that most of these pitches each have an ambulance, a doctor and

62

Chapter 3
The doctor's
contribution
towards safety in
sport

paramedical personnel in attendance throughout the day. The society consists mainly of primary care practitioners, orthopaedic surgeons and rehabilitationists, and holds annual conferences on rugby medicine.

One can always learn from other countries and other sports to introduce safety factors. In Sweden for instance, every sporting participant has to be licensed by the respective governing body to partake in that sport. The licence is linked to an accident and injury insurance scheme which is compulsory and is underwritten and insured by one company only, Folksam. This company, through their computerised programme, have statistics on all injuries in every sport and in turn provide information on risk areas to each governing body who may introduce legislation to make the sport safer.

The philosophy of the Scandinavian countries on the whole is similar to that in the UK with regard to the ethics of sport and fair play, and this also applies to the question of drugs in sport.

International rugby, through the World Cup and, at the time of writing, possible changes in the laws appertaining to amateurism, is facing its biggest challenge yet. Administrators and the rugby medical profession, by continual monitoring of risk factors in the game, epidemiological surveys and worldwide introduction of randomized dope testing, should ensure wherever possible that rugby keeps to the Olympic ideal of sportsmanship and fair play.

John E. Davies

All responsible governing bodies in sport should ensure that the common patterns of injury that are associated with their particular discipline are identified and minimised, wherever practical, by appropriate changes in the laws of the sport concerned. Any change in the laws under which a sport is conducted ought to be introduced with an appropriate educational programme involving participants, coaches and officials.

It is important not to lose sight of the fact that sport must at the same time retain its inherent challenge and character. These qualities lead inevitably to a degree of risk, which will be associated with a certain number of unavoidable injuries.

Exercise programmes designed to promote the physical well-being of individuals, irrespective of their age, should be structured in such a way that risk is minimal and the prospect of injury eliminated.

Individuals participate in sport for many different and complex reasons. The majority of sports men and women participate in sport to promote their physical fitness and for fun, enjoying the camaraderie of the event or the club to which they belong. This applies in both individual pursuits and team games. Inevitably there is an increased risk of injury in contact and collision sports, compared with individual activities and racket sports.

Many leisure activities which are undertaken on an individual and unsupervised basis such as hill-walking, horse-riding and swimming are associated with significant risks of both catastrophic and minor injuries. The real dangers associated with these activities are constantly underestimated and this is particularly true with regard to hill-walking in the Scottish mountains, where approximately 20% of 'call-outs' of the Scottish Mountain Rescue Teams are to recover the dead (McGregor 1988).

Although most sports men and women pursue their pastime 'for fun', by comparison, a proportion of amateur sports men and women constantly strive to achieve greater and greater peaks of performance. Irrespective of the nature of the sport in which they are involved, there is an inevitable sharp increase in the risk of injury associated with increasing demands of training and competition when the athlete is striving to reach the very limits of his or her potential. It is well recognised that the greater the number and intensity of training sessions and competitions undertaken by international athletes, the greater is the risk of injury in both amateur and professional sport. These injuries may be due to fatigue, physical stress, overuse, psychological burn-out or simply increased opportunities for damage. In professional sport, there is additional pressure on the athlete to 'perform', irrespective of any niggling minor injury or illness that may be present: 'No play — no pay'. The additional financial pressures placed on professional athletes to perform to entertain and to win are inevitably associated with very different attitudes towards their injuries and their sport.

Sport, whether it is undertaken for fitness, for fun, or as a profession, should not be associated with avoidable risks of injury or illness during either training or competition. Most athletes' active participation in sport, particularly if they are the élite striving for success or are professionals, tends to be relatively short-lived because of the physical and psychological demands placed upon them. Participation in sport at the top level in the twenties or early thirties age-groups should not inevitably mean permanent disability or premature ageing. The psychological stresses of retirement from sport are sufficiently distressing in themselves without having to face the additional burdens of disability that could have been avoided by appropriate training programmes and coaching techniques, as well as by education or sports legislation designed to minimise the risk of injury, and good medical care. Athletes striving for success should not be considered as experimental physiological preparations, and the pressures to which they are subjected by enthusiastic coaches and sports scientists should be monitored by appropriately trained and committed doctors.

Role and responsibilities of doctors

One of the significant problems that has deterred doctors from undertaking studies to identify the risks in association with sport is the difficulty in agreeing a definition of 'an injury'. There is no

63
Chapter 3
The doctor's
contribution
towards safety in
sport

64

Chapter 3
The doctor's
contribution
towards safety in
sport

difficulty with major injuries, but with minor and moderate injuries it can be extremely difficult to agree with both the athletes and the coaches involved in the sport under consideration. Many athletes would include impaired performance in the definition of an injury. Performance is linked to both psychological and physical factors. The same applies to a definition based on time lost from training; from this point of view the definition of an injury might relate to whether or not the athlete sought medical advice. Such a definition is not reliable, however, as it would also have to take into account the availability of a doctor for consultation at the time of perceived need. Many athletes prefer to take their injuries to a physiotherapist or other practitioners of alternative medicine.

It has been agreed in rugby football that studies undertaken to identify the causative factors resulting in injury should only include those injuries which prevent the player participating in the sport one week after the injury occurred, or if the player has been admitted to hospital. This definition eliminates many of the minor grazes, lacerations and bumps and bruises that are concomitant with collision sport and are assumed to be part of the ordinary risk of participating in rugby football.

In the future, it seems likely that increasing pressure will be placed on the governing bodies of sport as the number of participants in both leisure and sporting activities increases. With each succeeding generation, the population as a whole tends to get bigger and stronger. Training programmes and modern coaching techniques improve the overall fitness of athletes participating in sport at all levels, as well as changing the attitudes of athletes involved in an activity. In these circumstances, any governing body which fails to review the changing pattern of risk associated with their sport will lose the confidence of their participants. Equally, any law change produced by the governing body must be monitored closely from the point of view of safety to ensure that the hoped-for change which was sought by the alteration in laws is not associated with an increased risk of injury.

Increasing consumer sophistication among athletes and coaches will place increasing pressure on the medical profession to ensure that their knowledge of exercise physiology and sports medicine is of the highest standard. It is inevitable that doctors involved in sport will be subjected to continued monitoring of their standards of clinical practice. This will have to be associated with improved formal teaching programmes at both undergraduate and postgraduate level, examinations to monitor performance and the eventual development of a recognised speciality in exercise and sports medicine. This speciality would be equivalent in status to occupational health or accident and emergency medicine and surgery.

In 1987 the Scottish Sports Council published a short guide for governing bodies of sport on the provision of medical advisory services. In this guide, the Scottish Sports Council recommended that an effective medical service would identify, document and analyse risk factors associated with injury or illness in their sport, and then recommend appropriate measures that could be taken to minimise the risks. The medical team would have to possess a substantial knowledge of the sport in question and establish a close liaison with the participants, coaches, officials and administrators responsible for the designing of safe laws for that activity. The medical team will be expected to give advice about first-aid requirements for players. The medical team might also be involved in the development of safe and effective protective equipment for participants in the sport which could not in any way harm an opponent. The medical team would ensure that the environment in which the sport was undertaken was safe and practical, with, for example padded posts and, where appropriate, flexible non-shattering poles at goal-lines, for corner flags, etc. The playing surface and the immediate surrounds should not be cluttered with dangerous 'street furniture' such as advertising boardings and spectator barriers into which an athlete might accidentally crash. The medical team would have to clarify whether they were to undertake responsibility for the safety of spectators as well as players. Spectator safety presents vastly different problems and requires liaison with different agencies and emergency services (see Chapter 1).

Athletes participating in sport accept the obvious and foreseeable risks that might reasonably be associated with the activity in question, assuming that the event is undertaken within the rules, and that the rules have been designed to ensure fair and safe competition. Sporting behaviour by athletes would ensure that they honour these rules and respect both their opponent and the decisions of the officials. Unfortunately, in the present day and age, sporting behaviour has a tendency to be replaced by 'gamesmanship' and many athletes and coaches devote considerable time and energy to devising techniques which will overcome their opponents by playing to the limit of the rules and sometimes beyond. The presence of the doctor at training sessions as well as matches can help emphasise the importance of adopting safe techniques.

Doctors involved in sport have an ethical and legal duty to provide competent professional services and to ensure that they practise medicine to a high standard with appropriate facilities. The doctor has an additional ethical responsibility with regard to the prevention of injury by advising that appropriate protective equipment is worn by the players, the environment is safe, and vulnerable individuals do not participate in an event when there is a risk of aggravating a primary injury or sustaining a second, invariably more serious, injury. If a doctor recognises a pattern of events leading to injury, he has an ethical duty to draw this to the attention of the players, coaches and legislators, in the hope that this pattern can

65

*Chapter 3
The doctor's
contribution
towards safety in
sport*

66
Chapter 3
The doctor's
contribution
towards safety in
sport

be broken and the injuries minimised. On occasion, the doctor may be faced with a situation where an injury has resulted from violence outside the rules of the game. This may occur as a result of careless of thoughtless play, but may be the result of deliberate cheating, recklessness or violence and, in these circumstances, the doctor has a duty both to treat the injured player and to protect other players from similar violence by informed liaison with the relevant official in the event, club or sport and the individuals concerned.*

Minimising the dangers of sport

The player who elects to participate in a sport accepts the ordinary risks of this activity. In many sports, significant dangers do exist and all players must accept the responsibility of minimising serious injury. A resurgence of the old-fashioned concept of sporting behaviour, in which an athlete respected the opponent, played within the spirit and laws of the game, and honoured the officials, would go a long way towards making the life of sports legislators and the doctors involved in sport a lot easier.

American football

Many sports have made major achievements adopting the principles outlined above. In 1964, the American Association of Neurological Surgery initiated a series of studies into catastrophic injuries in American football. Over the subsequent years, detailed analysis of these catastrophic injuries, which included death and permanent paralysis, was undertaken. In 1968, 36 fatalities occurred in 1.25 million American football players. As a result of detailed co-operation and scientific research initiated by the medical profession in conjunction with American football coaches, a series of modifications to the laws, equipment and coaching techniques has achieved a dramatic improvement in the situation and only four catastrophes occurred in 1983. The achievements of the medical profession working with the governing bodies of American football make inspiring reading and are reviewed in detail in Schneider *et al* (1985).

Rugby

In 1978, the International Rugby Football Board established a Medical Advisory Committee to advise the board on the incidence of injuries occurring in Rugby Union with a view to identifying

---

* A conflict of interests between the doctor and his patient and the doctor and the controlling body arises here. This may be overcome by anonymous reporting of incidents or probably more practically by analysis and reporting of trends of injury coupled with suggested changes in the laws where appropriate.

67

Chapter 3
The doctor's
contribution
towards safety in
sport

relevant risk factors and modifying the laws of the game. Since that date, a number of major law changes in Rugby Union, in conjunction with a series of resolutions and recommendations, have been made on the basis of improving player safety. Among these changes are the following:

1 Elimination of the 'high tackle'.
2 Changes in the laws relating to scrummaging to improve the stability of the scrum, reduce the impact or collision forces as the scrum is formed, and penalise attempts to pull down or collapse the scrum. The range through which the scrum may rotate, has also been controlled by legislation.
3 Changes in the laws relating to the tackle, the ruck and the maul, encouraging quick release of the ball and ensuring that players stay on their feet.
4 International rugby has accepted the need for doping control to eliminate cheating by the taking of drugs. Rugby has, in addition, included in its recommendations a statement that players should not participate in rugby if they require drugs or injections for relief of acute illness or injury. Doping control in rugby includes testing for the presence of injectable local anaesthetic agents.
5 Detailed recommendations have been made with regard to the appropriate matching of players participating in rugby at school, during youth and at under-18 and under-21 levels, stressing the importance of assessing an individual player's maturity rather than solely judging his abilities on age.
6 The International Rugby Football Board has repeatedly advised players to purchase and use individually fitted dental mouth-guards to protect their teeth and reduce the risk of both orofacial and concussional head injuries.
7 The International Rugby Football Board has stressed the recommendation that any player who has been concussed should not participate in a rugby match for a minimum of three weeks after his head injury, and only when an appropriate medical examination has been undertaken.

Boxing

Boxing as a sport has been subject to considerable criticism by certain medical groups. Much work has been undertaken by the medical profession in assessing the damaging effects of both amateur and professional boxing and the consequences or cumulative brain injury. The design of the boxing glove has been significantly altered to reduce impact. In both amateur and professional boxing, the referee, trainer and doctor will stop a fight earlier than used to occur. In amateur boxing outside the UK, many competitions now insist on the participants wearing protective headgear, but these have not been subjected to the same detailed scrutiny to check their efficacy

68
Chapter 3
The doctor's
contribution
towards safety in
sport

as has been applied to the skull-cap worn by jockeys and the helmets worn in American football or ice-hockey (see Chapter 18).

Ice-hockey

Ice-hockey is a fast, exciting sport, inevitably involving contact through collision. Violence has all too readily been accepted, if not actively encouraged, to draw in the crowds. This violence has been associated with well-documented cases of catastrophic injury, particularly in North America, and this has led to increasing medical concern as to the standard of supervision of the sport and the enforcement of the rules under which it should be played. Ongoing studies continue into the incidence of serious injury in ice-hockey and there is great concern associated with the number of players suffering quadriplegia following a crash into the boards at the side of the rink, after they have been pushed or 'checked' from behind.

International sport

International travel in sport and the consequent problems of alteration in the participant's biorhythm due to jet lag, acclimatisation and changes in altitude are other areas in which the interested doctor can be involved in the prevention of injuries or illness. Detailed studies in this field have been undertaken, particularly with regard to athletics and cycling. These studies have shown that even the fittest athletes must allow one day's recovery for every three- to four-hour adjustment in their 'time clock', whether they are travelling east or west from their normal time-zone environment. Additional stresses will be placed on athletes if they ascend to an altitude of over 1000 m, or if there is a significant change in either the temperature or the humidity. A doctor helping prepare athletes for a significant competition on the other side of the world or in another environment will be involved in detailed planning with the athlete and his or her coach, with regard to modification of the athlete's training programme, diet, salt and water intake during the crucial acclimatisation period, as well as ensuring that the athlete rapidly returns to a normal pattern of sleeping and waking. Failure to undertake this planning inevitably results in overuse injuries, principally to muscles and tendons, an increased vulnerability to direct injury as a result of fatigue, and the danger of 'metabolic collapse'.

Hill-walking

The report prepared by the Medical Adviser to the Scottish Mountain Rescue Committee on the nature of causes of injuries sustained in 190 Scottish mountain accidents is a prime example of what can be achieved as a result of informed analysis of appropriate injuries. This report highlights a series of risk factors among which it states that the commonest cause of injury while hill-walking in Scotland is a simple slip or stumble and that there is a need for increased awareness among the public of the risks that they take. Avalanches are a major cause of winter mountain accidents in Scotland and widespread education initiatives have been taken to draw attention to the frequency, causes and risks of avalanches in Scotland throughout the winter. An avalanche, in conjunction with the failure to carry and to be competent in the use of crampons or ice-axes, invariably leads to a fatal accident.

69
Chapter 3
The doctor's
contribution
towards safety in
sport

Conclusion

Many governing bodies in sport have yet to develop appropriate medical advisory services. Such a service will have various administrative and organisational responsibilities but one of the most worthwhile contributions that the medical profession can make to sport is to undertake relevant research into the incidence of injury and illness associated with that sport, with a view to identifying risk factors that result in injury that can readily be eliminated from the sport in question without altering the character of that sport. Sport for all need not necessarily mean minor injuries for many, moderate injuries for some, permanent disability for a few and the occasional death, if the sports legislators have the relevant risk factors drawn to their attention by informed and committed doctors working with them.

References

McGregor A. R. (1988) The nature and cause of injuries sustained in 190 Scottish mountain accidents. *Scottish Sports Council Research Digest*, No. 1.
Schneider *et al.* (1985) *Sports Injuries: Mechanisms, Prevention and Treatment*, eds Schneider *et al.* Bultimore: Williams & Watkins.

4 Fatalities associated with sport

BERNARD KNIGHT

'Death is the great leveller'
J. Kelly, Scottish proverb

In the other chapters of this volume, authors with an expert knowledge of a variety of sports discuss the morbidity associated with their particular sport. Thankfully only a small proportion suffers the ultimate morbidity — death — and it is solely this aspect which will be considered here.

Incidence of fatalities

No reliable overall mortality statistics are available for sporting activities. Apart from the inherent errors in all mortality figures, due to inaccurate certification, many sport-associated deaths are not identifiable as such in official statistics. For example, 'natural' deaths precipitated by exertion are usually registered solely under the disease process. Deaths of spectators may not be categorised under a sport index — and many deaths directly attributable to sporting activity may not be identifiable from the raw statistical material.

Where legal inquiries are made, primarily coroner's inquests in England, Wales and Ireland, a study of the annual returns provides reliable information — but, where the cause of death is recorded as 'natural causes', no such inquest is held.*

Though overall statistics are unsatisfactory, some idea of the relative risks to life of the various sports may be gained from figures attributed to certain categories, and these will be mentioned later under the appropriate headings. In general, the greatest single cause of mortality associated with sporting activities is undoubtedly pre-existing natural disease exacerbated by exertion. This far exceeds trauma and other causes directly attributable to the performance of sport.

*Certification of death should be made by the 'ordinary medical attendant' of the patients, in cases where the death is not reported to the coroner. For further details, see p. 70.

The legal aspects of sporting fatalities

Before discussing the actual causes of death in various sports, the legal consequences must be surveyed. There are a number of aspects which may affect the doctor, whether he or she is a team medical officer, the medical attendant of an individual competitor or merely a doctor who only becomes involved when some tragedy occurs.

or a spectator

70

Death certification

If the death undoubtedly appears due to natural disease, then certification will depend upon the particular circumstances. If the deceased's own medical attendant is called, he or she may — and indeed may be obliged to — provide a medical certification of the cause of death if it is known that the patient suffered from some potentially fatal disease and he or she had attended the deceased at some time in the two weeks before death. If the doctor considers that the circumstances are quite consistent with death from the pre-existing disease, then certification must proceed as in any other natural death, irrespective of the sporting connection. It is debatable whether or not a team doctor can be considered to be 'the medical attendant', if the victim has another regular doctor such as a home general practitioner. Before any doctor can sign a death certificate, acceptable to the registrar of births and deaths, he or she must have seen the deceased in a professional capacity during the 14 days immediately preceding the death, which also means that he or she must be fully aware of the medical history, if any.

Probably, if a person dies whilst taking part in an event taking place near home, his/her own GP should sign the certificate if he or she saw the deceased during the past fortnight, provided that the death is not to be reported to the coroner. If death occurs at some sporting event away from home, then it will depend on the attitude of the local coroner as to whether he or she would consider the team medical officer to be 'the medical attendant'. In many (probably most) cases, the coroner would require the death to be formally reported to him or her, so that an autopsy could be conducted. If death occurs abroad, then the local regulations will apply, and these will vary from country to country.

Reporting to the coroner

Even where death seems due to natural causes, if it is sudden and unexpected, most will need to be reported to the coroner, in England, Wales, Ulster and the Irish Republic. In Scotland, the Procurator-fiscal is the corresponding law officer.

Only if the deceased had a well-diagnosed disease which was recognised as lethal — and the doctor had attended him/her professionally during the past 14 days and the circumstances of the death seem consistent with the diagnosis — can a coroner's inquiry be avoided. In most cases associated with sport, this would hardly apply, as someone with such recently diagnosed and treated serious disease is unlikely to be indulging in strenuous activity — although of course it does happen (see Chapter 8).

Reporting a death to the coroner is usually carried out by the police where trauma or other accident has occurred. If natural disease is suspected, but the doctor cannot provide a valid certificate, either because of the 14-day rule or because it is felt that the sporting activity has had a contributory effect, he or she may well telephone the coroner, usually via the coroner's officer or other policemen.*

*In cases of doubt it is always wiser for the doctor concerned to discuss the case with the coroner via the coroner's officer. The doctor may wish to seek advice initially from his protection organisation.

In jurisdictions other than Britain, the local regulations will apply. In the USA, some states have a coroner system, but many have a Medical Examiner Office, where the forensic pathologist is also the equivalent of the coroner, combining the medical and circumstantial investigation.

In many parts of the Commonwealth, the British coroner system remains a legacy of empire, but in most of Europe, the police and a judge assume the central role in the investigation of sudden, unexpected or traumatic deaths.

Whatever the system, witnesses will be required to give statements of their knowledge of the events surrounding the death and one of the prime witnesses will be the doctor. He or she will have to relate the medical knowledge of the deceased, including the clinical history and the mode of death, etc.

Medical confidentiality is not usually a consideration in a coroner's inquiry, as all witnesses can be obliged by subpoena to attend an inquest and be compelled to divulge any information to which they are privy, on pain of penalties for contempt of court.

In all cases of traumatic or unnatural death, an inquest will be held, almost inevitably after an autopsy. Unless a doctor has been able to issue a death certificate in the cases of natural death, these will also be reported to the coroner and an autopsy performed. If the latter reveals that death was due to natural disease, the coroner will dispose of the case and issue a certificate, in most cases without an inquest. However, some natural deaths associated with sport will still go to a public inquest, either because the law statutorily requires this or because the coroner's discretionary powers persuade him or her to hold an inquest.

For example, a man who suddenly drops dead playing squash and whose autopsy reveals a recent myocardial infarct is unlikely to be the subject of an inquest. However, the death of the same man whose infarct causes him to crash his competition glider must go to an inquest — and an inquest with jury — as this is statutorily classed as an aviation fatality. Yet again, if the same man died during the same squash game, with the same infarct, but his wife complained that the doctor was negligent in not diagnosing his coronary disease the previous month, then the coroner may well exercise his or her discretion in holding an inquest to clarify the situation.*

* At such an inquest the family of the deceased may well be represented by solicitors and/or barristers. Such 'high-profile' proceedings may well indicate the subsequent intention of civil proceedings directed against the medical attendant(s) of the deceased. If the doctor finds himself unexpectedly under attack at an inquest, it is advisable to request an adjournment to permit the doctor to seek legal advice and/or representation.

When a death is reported to the coroner, whether or not an inquest is held, the doctor has no further part to play other than providing a statement and probably appearing as a witness. The doctor does not sign a death certificate or a cremation certificate, as these are provided by the coroner.

Civil liability

Where one person brings a legal action for damages against another, the suit is a civil matter as opposed to criminal proceedings, in which one party is the State, acting in the name of the sovereign.

In sport it has been accepted for centuries that someone who voluntarily participates does so under the mutual understanding that he or she accepts any risk arising from that sport, including the actions of other players who are participating in the game. A rock-climber who falls from a cliff-face cannot sue the owner of the mountain; nor can a boxer who suffers a subdural haematoma sue his opponent. This concept is embodied in the maxim *volenti non fit injuria*.

= If you stick your neck out, do not complain if the axe descends.

Of course, injuries or death sustained during a sporting activity only come under this dictum if they were suffered during the normal course of the sport. If a rugby player has some ribs broken in a legitimate tackle, he cannot sue the other player — but, if the other player breaks his jaw with a deliberate punch, this would be grounds for an action in tort — and perhaps also for a criminal prosecution (see pp. 14–26).

This long-standing 'gentlemen's agreement' has gained the force of law over the years, it being accepted that every sports man or woman carries his or her own risks. However, this has been challenged in recent years by an increasing number of cases in which injury or death has been blamed on the actions of others. The injured party or the personal representatives of a dead player may sue another player for negligence or assault, relying mainly on a departure from the accepted rules and conduct of the game, to avoid the *volenti non fit injuria* concept, for the basis of their case.

Of course, civil actions may also be brought against the manufacturers of allegedly faulty equipment which has led to mishaps — the snapping of a weak wire on a hang-glider or a badly designed face-mask on an American footballer may lead to an action in contract or tort against the manufacturer, or an action under any relevant product liability legislation.

In all these matters, the doctor may become involved in giving an opinion on the mode of causation of the injury or death or in describing his or her part in attempted resuscitation and treatment. The doctor may alternatively be the party sued, if it is alleged, for example, that he or she:

1 allowed an unfit player to go on the field or participate in some hazardous activity such as diving or climbing, etc. (see Chapter 20);

2 was negligent in diagnosis, treatment or resuscitatory measures after the mishap occurred.

The fact that a team or club doctor is usually an unpaid volunteer makes no difference to his duty of professional care to a patient. The three essentials of negligence — medical or otherwise — are that:

1 the defendant (doctor) has a duty of care to the plaintiff (patient), and

2 there is a breach of that duty, by an act either of commission or of omission, and

3 the patient suffered damage as a result — in this context, death. Though the deceased patient is obviously unable to take legal action him or herself, the personal representative of the deceased may sue, the bulk of the potential damages being recompense for lost earning capacity for benefit of dependent relatives.[*]

Criminal proceedings

Until very recently, it was virtually unheard of for criminal proceedings to arise from injuries in sport, as the spirit of the *volenti non fit injuria* principle made it even less likely that the State would interest itself in such a matter. Though not involving deaths, several recent events of a somewhat shameful nature on the rugby field have ended in criminal prosecutions and convictions (see pp. 14–26). This unhappy development is perhaps symptomatic of the erosion of the sporting ethos consequent upon the increasing pressure to win, rather than the rather more old-fashioned acceptance of 'taking part' as the important feature of sport.

Violently frayed tempers may lead to personal combat on the field and the cases referred to criminal proceedings have included the partial biting off of an ear and other injuries sustained in a common assault. The only relevance to the doctor involved in these types of cases would be the probability of his being called either as a witness as to fact from seeing what happened or, more likely, as a professional witness to describe the original nature of the injuries.

Natural disease and sporting deaths

The great majority of sport-associated fatalities are due to pre-existing natural disease, rather than trauma and other unnatural processes. The deaths are usually sudden and unexpected, as people

---

[*] This is because sport as a leisure activity is predominantly a pastime of young, fit, employed individuals. Loss of earnings — usually calculated as the annual sum lost (the multiplicand) multiplied by the remaining life expectancy in years (the multiplier) — is often a large sum of money, for which the doctor may be liable if negligence and causation are proven.

with overtly dangerous symptoms are unlikely to indulge in strenuous sporting pastimes.

As with most sudden unexpected deaths, the prime cause lies in the cardiovascular system, even if the blood vessels responsible lie not necessarily in the thorax, but in the cranium or abdomen.

Coronary atherosclerosis

This is not exactly synonymous with 'ischaemic heart disease' because other cardiac diseases, such as hypertension, aortic valve disease and some congenital abnomalies, also cause myocardial ischaemia. Nor is it equivalent to 'coronary thrombosis' or 'myocardial infarction', both of which, where no autopsy has been performed, are over-diagnosed as causes of sudden death. In fact, the mode of coronary death likely to be associated with strenuous sporting activity is not that of a myocardial infarct, which is usually a sequel to thrombus formation or an atheromatous stenosis.

The coroner's pathologist sees a different population of coronary victims than does the hospital physician, and is forced to assume that sudden, unexpected death is more often due to an arrythmia, such as ventricular fibrillation, producing cardiac arrest. People who die from established coronary thrombi and infarcts are more likely to die in front of their television sets than on a jogging circuit, though of course it cannot be denied that some such deaths are precipitated by exercise when morphological myocardial damage already exists.

The effect of catecholamines, noradrenaline, etc., is probably relevant to sudden death in sport, because adrenal activity from emotion, excitement and competitive exertion is more likely to induce ventricular arrythmias in susceptible individuals. Recent observations on the use of injected catecholamines in attempted resuscitation have shown that myocardial fibres can be rapidly damaged, with the formation of fragmented myofibrils with contraction bands. The cardiac arrythmias seen in solvent abuse have been shown to be due to these substances sensitising the myocardium to noradrenaline.

It is beyond the scope of this text to describe the symptomatology and pathology of coronary artery disease, but suffice to say, that numerically, it forms the greater part of sport-associated sudden deaths.

Within this group, the doctor must be alert for the victim of familial hypercholesterolaemia because of the need for subsequent diagnosis and prophylactic measures amongst the surviving family. This diagnosis will rest on autopsy findings, and all young persons dying of coronary atheroma below the age of 35 should have post-mortem cholesterol levels measured. It is one of the few biochemical analyses which give reliable results *post mortem* and is an example of the community health benefits that can flow from coroner's pathology.

Other cardiac conditions

In older age-groups, hypertensive heart disease and calcific aortic stenosis are relatively common causes of sudden unexpected death. In younger persons, the whole range of cardiomyopathies may be encountered, including asymmetric septal hypertrophy or hypertrophic obstructive cardiomyopathy (HOCM). These are usually unsuspected and therefore undiagnosed in people who are characteristically asymptomatic and thus well enough to participate in active sports.

Some years ago, 'isolated, Fiedler's or Saphir's myocarditis' was a favourite diagnosis for sudden deaths in young subjects, being based on the histological detection of foci of chronic inflammatory cells in the myocardium. Many of the diagnoses were based on insufficient evidence and some published surveys of traffic fatalities have shown that similar patchy cellular infiltrates are present in control populations.

Congenital cardiac lesions are occasionally found in sport-associated deaths, especially atrial septal defects, patent ductus arteriosus, coarctation of the aorta and various valve defects. Death may occur even when these conditions are already diagnosed: the risk of acute cardiac failure can be underestimated. Other cases are found for the first time at autopsy.

Obscure cardiac deaths

Every coroner's pathologist sees a few deaths each year in which the most exhaustive investigation fails to reveal the cause of death. Even excluding the most common group of this type, namely the so-called 'cot deaths' in infants, most of the obscure cases are in young people, both teenagers and young adults. This section of the population will obviously contain some sport-related deaths simply because the age range coincides. One cannot, however, deduce any causal relationship with sport in these fatalities.

It is probable that these obscure deaths occur also in older subjects, but there is often an overlay of chronic degenerative cardiovascular disease, notably coronary atheroma, which provides an acceptable and convenient, if not always wholly convincing, reason for the death.

These deaths of occult cause may occur on or off the sports arena. In some instances, a footballer or runner may literally drop dead on the field, obviously the victim of a cardiac arrest. Due to the lack of any premonitory symptoms, there is no opportunity to determine whether some arrythmia preceded the collapse. In other cases, the death may occur some time after the actual sporting exertion and here it is extremely questionable as to whether the fatality can be linked in any way with the activity. For example, the author dealt with the death of a previously fit young man of 21, who played a Saturday afternoon game of club rugby. He celebrated in moderation that evening, then awoke during the night with non-specific complaints of feeling unwell — then promptly died. A full autopsy with histology, virology, toxicology and microbiology failed to reveal the slightest abnormality and the death had to be recorded as 'unascertained'.

Lesions of large arteries

Rupture of an aortic aneurysm is a common cause of sudden, un-expected death in the general population but again is relatively unlikely to be seen very often in active participants of the more strenuous types of sports, because these lesions are more common in advancing age. However, many men in their fifties and sixties may be at risk whilst jogging, playing squash or taking part in strenuous exercise, especially if it is unaccustomed.

The most common type of aortic aneurysm occurs as a result of an atheromatous degeneration. This is most commonly found in the abdominal segment of the vessel, though it can occur in its thoracic course.

Less often, a dissection of an aorta suffering from medionecrosis may occur, although the event is precipitated by a tear through an atheromatous plaque on the inner surface. Dissecting aneurysms are usually in the thoracic aorta, though they may rapidly spread upwards and downwards, often leading to aortic incompetence and cardiac tamponade if the upper extension enters the pericardial sac.

Rarely, a young person may be struck with a dissecting aneurysm as part of a Marfan-type syndrome.

Cerebral aneurysms — subarachnoid haemorrhage

One of the major causes of sudden disability and death in young and middle-aged adults is subarachnoid bleeding, almost always from a ruptured berry aneurysm on the circle of Willis.

This affects both sexes and, because of the relative immunity of younger women from fatal coronary disease, it is one of the first causes to consider in the sudden unexpected death of a woman under the age of 45 — the other causes being pulmonary embolism and complications of pregnancy.

The pathology is well known and needs no further elaboration here. The aneurysms are sometimes called 'congenital', but this description is not accurate, as they develop as age progresses. The weakness in the arterial wall, however, is congenital, probably due to fenestration in the elastic laminae at the site of atrophied foetal vessels.

In a small proportion of 'spontaneous' subarachnoid haemorrhage (i.e. known to be unassociated with trauma), no aneurysm is detected at autopsy, but this is in part due to the difficulties of identifying a small lesion after rupture. About 15% of non-traumatic subarachnoid haemorrhages are not associated with a discoverable aneurysm.

The precipitating factors in the rupture of a cerebral aneurysm are only partly understood. A rise in blood-pressure is undoubtedly a potent factor and, in view of the number of dramatic collapses and some deaths that have occurred on the sports field, it seems likely that strenuous physical exertion must be related. Whether it is a rise in systolic and diastolic blood-pressure or a marked increase in heart rate and cardiac output is not known.

~~Obviously~~ excitement and emotion, with their adrenal response, *may be* ~~are~~ as potent as muscular exertion. Of course, as with coronary and other cardiovascular disease, a berry aneurysm can rupture at rest, but proof that intense and perhaps unaccustomed exercise is a factor is shown by the not uncommon history of collapse and sometimes death during sexual intercourse.

There is a controversy in the forensic world about the role of alcohol in the rupture of a berry aneurysm. It is claimed, unconvincingly, that alcohol both increases the blood-pressure and dilates the cerebral vessels: in fact, alcohol widens the pulse pressure somewhat, but may actually lower the diastolic pressure. As for dilating cerebral vessels, the completely fibrotic sac of a cerebral aneurysm is quite incapable of muscular vasodilatation.

More pertinent than alcohol in relation to sports fatalities is the role of trauma in ruptured cerebral aneurysms. It is hard to deny that an expanded, thin-walled aneurysmal sac is vulnerable to the physical trauma that accompanies many sports, especially boxing and rugby football. Only a few years ago, a rugby player of international renown was struck down during a match with a ruptured 'berry' aneurysm, thankfully surviving long enough to undergo successful neurosurgery. It may be noteworthy, however, that the haemorrhage which occurred was unassociated with head trauma immediately prior to the player's collapse on the field of play.

In the criminal sphere, which might have future relevance to sporting injuries, it has been a matter of considerable controversy as to whether the perpetrator of an assault which was followed by a fatal rupture of a cerebral aneurysm could be charged with homicide. In England (as opposed to Scotland or the Continent), it was formerly held that there was reasonable doubt about the causative connection between a ruptured berry aneurysm and head trauma, but several cases in recent years have tended to strengthen the association between the two.

The issue of causation, in berry aneurysm, is of relevance in the sporting context, when it has to be decided, either by a coroner, a court or some internal sporting inquiry, whether the fatality was indeed a consequence of a head injury. Because of the undoubted association with exertion and emotion, which may be impossible to separate in time from the actual injury, it may be difficult indeed to decide on causation.

Another important association with subarachnoid haemorrhage is trauma to the side of the neck. Unrecognised until a few years ago, this probably accounted for some of the cases of 'spontaneous' subarachnoid bleeding where no aneurysm was found. The pathologist in a proportion of these occult cases probably missed deep bruising in the neck muscles behind and below the ear, as this is an area which is not usually dissected by the pathologist unless there are specific indications. The lesion in these catastrophes is a tear in a vertebral artery, which allows blood to track into the cranial cavity at the level of the foramen magnum. Most of the early published cases had a fracture of the transverse process of the atlas vertebra, but later it was shown that such a fracture is not necessary for the damage to the vertebral artery either in the osseous tunnel or where it perforates the dura. The injury to the neck need not be severe — it seems to be the specificity of the target area that is important, causing acute lateral flexion and rotation of the head on the upper cervical vertebrae, with possibly stretching of the atlanto-occipital membrane. The lesion is seen quite often in criminal assaults and, although no case has been reported in the forensic literature as having occurred in a sporting context, it is likely that some past subarachnoid haemorrhages have been misdiagnosed, where the relatively mild injury to the neck has been unrecorded.

he means its lateral mass

Other natural causes

Though persons with chronic diseases in general have to either avoid or reduce their participation in sporting activities, there has been a marked trend recently for people with all kinds and degrees of disability to involve themselves in many types of sport (see Chapters 8–10). Here the doctor has a vital role in tailoring their activities to their capabilities and in detecting early signs of their exceeding their threshold of safety.

However, even with the most vigilant monitoring, sudden deterioration, even to the point of death, may occur in a variety of natural diseases. For example, sudden death may supervene, in a sporting context as well as elsewhere, in patients with bronchial asthma or epilepsy. An asthmatic may die quite unexpectedly, even if he or she is not in status asthmaticus or perhaps not even suffering an attack. Once again, the sensitisation of the myocardium by adrenergic bronchodilators must always be suspect as a cause of sudden arrythmia and arrest — a syndrome which caused many deaths some 20 years ago, until intense medical publicity reduced the usage of adrenergic drugs in the treatment of asthma. Even where such toxic effects can be excluded, asthma can still lead to unexpected death, and the same applies to epilepsy, where a sudden fatality may be unassociated with status epilepticus or even a solitary fit.

In summary, many types of natural disease may cause death, either in the infinite variety of situations of daily life or in the sporting context. It may be impossible to distinguish these, as it may be sheer chance that a probably inevitable death happened to occur whilst the victim was indulging in some sporting activity.

The many spectators who die of cardiovascular disease and those who die whilst performing some non-strenuous pastime would perhaps have died elsewhere at the same time. However, the wrestler who dies of acute cardiac insufficiency during a bout or the weight-lifter who ruptures an aneurysm whilst in competition almost certainly has had his fatal event precipitated by exertion.

Intermediate between these is the situation where, though the physical stress is minimal, there is an element of excitement and emotion which may mediate itself through the adrenal response to trigger the fatal episode. In determining the cause and effect, which may well have legal repercussions of greater or lesser degree, the facts of each tragedy must be assessed in an individual way.

Further reading

Cameron J. M. & Mant A. K. (1972) Fatal subarachnoid haemorrhage associated with cervical trauma. *Medicine, Science and Law* **12**, 66–70.
Coast G. C. & Gee D. J. (1984) Traumatic subarachnoid haemorrhage — an alternative source. *Journal of Clinical Pathology* **37**, 1245.
Karch S. B. (1987) Resuscitation induced myocardial necrosis, catecholamines and defibrillation. *American Journal of Forensic Medicine and Pathology* **8**, 3–8.
Simonsen J. (1988) Massive subarachnoid haemorrhage: report of six cases and a review of the literature. *American Journal of Forensic Medicine and Pathology* **9**, 23–31.

HIV disease and sport 5

C. LOVEDAY

'*Venienci occurite Morobo*' (meet the disease as it approaches)
Aulus Persius Flaccus

Human immunodeficiency virus (HIV) disease is a chronic retroviral infection of human T-helper lymphocytes resulting in the gradual but remorseless destruction of the immune system. Acute infection

Continent	Country with more than 250 cases	Number of AIDS cases[a,c]
Africa[b]		10995
	Burundi	960
	Central African Republic	254
	Congo	1250
	Kenya	964
	Malawi	583
	Rwanda	901
	Tanzania	2369
	Uganda	1608
	Zaïre	335
	Zambia	536
	Zimbabwe	380
Americas		62536
	Brazil	2325
	Canada	1517
	Dominican Republic	352
	Haiti	912
	Mexico	713
	USA	55167
Asia		231
Europe		10677
	Belgium	297
	Denmark	251
	France	3073
	Holland	420
	Italy	1619
	Spain	789
	Switzerland	355
	UK	1344
	West Germany	1848
Oceania		834
	Australia	758

Table 5.1 Cases of acquired immunodeficiency syndrome (AIDS) reported world-wide up to 31 March 1988

[a] HIV antibody-positive individuals are 30–50 times this number.
[b] Actual cases very much higher as early cases are unrecognised, and case reporting is probably still not accurate.
[c] At time of going to press in September 1989 all numbers have doubled.

81

with HIV is followed by many years of chronic infection with no symptoms and few signs. As the disease progresses there is evidence of moderate immunodeficiency with recurrent common infections having an altered natural history and associated with constitutional symptoms and signs. End-stage disease, acquired immunodeficiency syndrome (AIDS), presents with opportunistic infection, unusual tumours and evidence of severe immunodeficiency.

Most acute HIV infections occur without symptoms. Development of anti-HIV antibodies occurs 4–12 weeks after infection and persists for life. Virus may be found in most body fluids but concentrations are highest in blood, semen and cervical secretions. Evidence suggests viral antigenaemia may fluctuate, being high early and late in the course of the disease with additional episodes of antigenaemia during the long asymptomatic phase of infection. Thus it is probable that in individual's infectivity is variable and difficult to predict.

One hundred and thirty-three countries in the world have now reported cases of AIDS (85273 March 1988) and it is certain there must exist an even larger unidentified population (30–50 times the AIDS cases) of asymptomatic HIV antibody-positive individuals (5–10 million world-wide) capable of transmitting the virus (Table 5.1).

Epidemiological data indicate that infection is spread by sexual contact and percutaneous and transplacental routes. Early in the epidemic high-risk groups (homosexual/bisexual men, intravenous drug users, haemophiliacs, transfusion recipients, prostitutes and sexual partners of all these) were identified, but infection has now spread outside these groups into the heterosexual population and it is no longer possible to predict reliably those who may be at risk.

At present there is no cure or vaccine available to treat the disease. Education is the only measure available to control the spread of infection.

Risk to sports competitors

Sports people, like any other individuals, are subject to general risks of infection by HIV, the greatest risk being that of sexual transmission. Thus, it is important that the number of sexual partners should be restricted and condoms used, especially when visiting countries where there is a high prevalence of HIV disease in the male and female populations (Table 5.1). The sharing of facilities (changing-rooms, showers, toilets, etc.), normal social contact and swimming pools constitute no danger of infection. Sharing of towels, razors, toothbrushes and 'bucket and sponge'* is a source of potential risk of all infections and should be discouraged.

---

*The 'bucket and sponge' communally used to 'treat' injuries in a wide variety of team sports must now be viewed as a mode of transmission of the virus, especially where bleeding has occurred. Sensible medical advice must therefore discourage the use of this traditional item of equipment and ban its use completely in areas of high risk (see table).

Medical facilities in developing countries may not be presumed to be equivalent to those in the UK, and where HIV disease is prevalent must pose a further potential risk of infection. For sports people travelling and competing in such countries, 'immediate care packs', including sterile needles, syringes and intravenous fluids (blood substitutes), are available to take from the UK.

There is no documented evidence that contact sports (rugby, judo, etc.) have resulted in the transmission of HIV infection, but this area merits special consideration. HIV does not survive long in the open but there are a few documented cases of seroconversion following infected blood coming into contact with open skin lesions. With relatively low numbers of infected cases so far in existence, lesser modes of transmission may not be in evidence from epidemiological studies, but theoretically it must be conceded that a bleeding skin wound on an HIV-infected person must pose a risk to an opponent, in the event that infected blood comes into contact with or rubs against an open lesion on the skin of the uninfected opponent. If this (theoretical) risk becomes a reality considerable difficulties will exist for 'contact' sports in the future unless the HIV status of competitors is known. Such an undertaking is not without its own problems, e.g. who organises testing? is it mandatory? are individuals counselled? how often should individuals be tested?*

Clearly these will relate to activities in which there is significant potential for blood loss in one or more of the participants, and will be especially concerned with whether a bleeding participant may continue to play and therefore run the risk of making direct physical contact with another player or players. Where blood from an infected player is spilt on to an open wound of another player there exists the risk of transmission of the virus. The necessity for precautions to eliminate this risk of cross-infection will naturally depend on the prevalence of the disease amongst participants. In parts of the world where significant numbers of the population are affected it would be prudent to advise sports men and women of the individual risks that they run. Players known to be positive should perhaps be excluded from selection and players who suffer significant wounds during play should either have these covered or be excluded from further participation. Preactivity testing for HIV status is fraught with legal and ethical problems and is probably not a practical proposition, but However, if thought to be desirable, it should be coupled with full medical counselling of the implications of having the test.

*This is an entirely new problem for the world of sporting activity and, in due course, must be addressed by individual governing bodies of respective sports which are at greatest risk.

Risk to first-aid workers, sports marshals and stewards

Many sporting activities involve the possibility of trauma and the resulting injuries pose risks to those who deliver immediate care to the competitors. The risks of HIV transmission in this setting may be put into perspective by considering the cases of occupationally acquired HIV disease so far documented. World-wide, a small number of cases of health-care workers infected during their work have been reported. These include: a female nurse in the UK who sustained a needlestick injury inoculation of approximately 1 ml of patient's blood, a female nurse in the USA receiving a deep intramuscular needlestick injury, a female nurse from Martinique who sustained a needlestick injury without injection, a female nurse from France who sustained a superficial needlestick injury during thoracocentesis, a female nurse working ungloved with chapped skin whose hand was in contact with a patient's blood for 20 minutes during a cardiac arrest, a female phlebotomist with severe acne having blood splashed in her face, a female technologist who spilled contaminated blood on to her ungloved hands while carrying out plasmapheresis, and a male surgeon following work in Africa. Weighed against these cases are the results of follow-up studies of thousands of health-care workers who have had accidental contact with infected blood (Table 5.2), and only two seroconversions are documented here after at least one year's follow-up.

Thus the risks to those with unbroken skin coming in contact with infected blood are very small but do exist. These risks may be reduced further by the following recommended precautions:

1 Assume all casualties are HIV antibody-positive (never try to predict who may be positive).
2 Wear gloves for all procedures that involve contact with blood or other body secretions.
3 Cover all cuts or abrasions on hands with dressings before going on duty.
4 Wear glasses for procedures when blood may be splashed into the face.
5 Wash skin immediately after contamination with patient's blood or secretions.

Table 5.2 Outcome of some studies of health-care workers exposed to HIV-infected blood

	Number of staff	Type of exposure	Seroconversions at one year
Center for Disease Control, Atlanta, USA	1097	Needlestick, sharps, splash	1
National Institute of Health, USA	332	Needlestick	0
University of California, USA	63	Needlestick	0
Thames Health Regions, UK	150	Needlestick, sharps, splash	1

6 Dispose of potentially infectious sharps safely; never attempt to resheathe needles.

7 Dispose of waste materials by burning.

8 Clothing soiled with blood or secretions should be washed in a hot-cycle washing-machine, with a presoak for 30 minutes in hot soapy water at 70°C. If clothes cannot withstand these temperatures they can be soaked for 30 minutes in household bleach (1 in 10) or Milton solution diluted according to instructions.

9 Any other equipment or surfaces contaminated with blood may be treated with household bleach (as above).

10 Generally maintain sensible standards of hygiene.

11 Communal items such as a bucket and sponge have no further place in the care of injured sports people.

No cases of HIV infection resulting from mouth-to-mouth resuscitation have been described, but nevertheless it is recommended that one of the simple devices that are available for carrying out mouth-to-mouth ventilation (Table 5.3) with no direct contact between operator and patient is provided for use (i.e. carried by every first-aid worker or available at every marshal/first-aid post at sporting events).

It is essential that training programmes for all personnel are available to educate about risks of HIV infection and how to avoid them, and these should be repeated at intervals to ensure knowledge is up to date and to reduce complacency.

Summary

1 Sports people generally have the same risks of infection as the general population.

2 Certain contact sports pose a theoretically higher risk of virus transmission from one competitor to another. These risks are proportional to the prevalence to HIV-infected individuals in a given

Laerdal pocket mask	Laerdal Medical, Stavanger, Norway	**Table 5.3** Devices to assist in mouth-to-mouth ventilation
Sussex valve airway	Tandisdale Medical, Forest Row, Sussex, UK	
Brook airway	G. H. Wood, Toronto, Canada	
Resusciade	Portex Ltd, Hythe, Kent, UK	
Sealeasy/Venteasy mask–airway	Respironus, Monroville, PA 15146N, USA	
Dual aid	Vitalograph Ltd, Buckingham, UK	

population, which varies markedly from country to country (see Table 5.1).

3 Potential risk of infection of first-aid workers, sports marshals and stewards is small but does exist. However, these risks can be reduced further by carrying out routine recommended precautions when caring for the injured.

Uses and abuses of drugs in sport: the athlete's view 6

T. J. ANSTISS

'Better to hunt in the fields for health unbought than fee the Doctor
for a nauseous draught'
John Dryden

Introduction

A knowledge of the relationships that exist between athletes and
pharmacologically active compounds is of vital importance to the
medical practitioner involved with athletes. Efficient prescribing
can reduce both time off training and ameliorate the impact of illness on performance. The practitioner must also be aware of the
fact that many athletes self-administer non-prescribed drugs in an
attempt to improve their performance on the playing field or in the
arena.

Prescribing for illness in athletes

Athletes are prone to suffer from the same cross-section of illnesses
that may affect any other group or patients. In this respect they
should be provided with the same treatment as anyone else attending their doctor. Care should be taken, however, with preparations likely to affect adversely the athlete's training (including their
sleep and dietary habits), and also with drugs in any of the five
classes banned by Olympic sports (see Appendix 6.1). The Sports
Council will gladly advise where uncertainty exists.

It should be remembered that self-medication with certain over-
the-counter preparations (most notably cough and cold remedies)
can result in a failed urine test. It is the athlete's responsibility to
know the rules and avoid such preparations,* as well as preparations about which he or she is uncertain. Ignorance of the rules is
no defence. To prevent inadvertant ingestion of banned substances
the Sports Council has produced a card the size of a credit card with
information for athletes, and a more comprehensive list of permiss-
able drugs (with their foreign names) for doctors (Appendix 6.2).
However, if an athlete has an illness for which only a drug from the

---

* Professional advice sought by athletes on the subject of the admissibility of the use
of non-proprietary preparations in sports does not fall under the provisions of the
NHS. Such advice should therefore be sought on a 'private' basis and is subject to the
common law standards for accuracy and competence.

88

*Chapter 6
Uses and abuses
of drugs in sport:
the athlete's view*

banned list will do, then a letter should be sent to the governing body of the athlete's sport informing them of the date of commencement and likely date of cessation of treatment. This is preferable to a letter sent after a positive urine test, which may be viewed with some suspicion by the powers that be.

Inflammatory problems

Most athletes in training are no strangers to musculo-skeletal inflammation, and a short course of aspirin (600 mg q.d.s.) is often of use in helping symptoms settle and expediting return to full training. Piroxicam may be the drug of choice, however (Heere 1988). The medical practitioner must take care to establish the athlete's current analgesic consumption, since many athletes will have self-medicated with over-the-counter non-steroidal anti-inflammatory drugs (NSAIDs), e.g. ibuprofen.

For musculo-skeletal inflammatory conditions which have not responded to an adequate trial of conservative therapy (i.e. rest, ice ultrasound, etc.) a local corticosteroid injection may prove effective. 1–2 cm³ of hydrocortisone acetate in 5% lignocaine is infiltrated into or around the affected region as appropriate using aseptic technique, and the area rested for 48 hours before commencement of a suitable rehabilitation programme (Roy & Irvine 1983).* Since local anaesthetics are one of the 'classes of drugs subject to certain restrictions', if an athlete is to have a local anaesthetic before or during a competition some sports require written submission of the diagnosis, dose and route of administration. The practice of prescribing parenteral corticosteroids to promote recovery from overtraining is not recommended.

Performance-enhancing substances

'We consider this [doping] to be the most shameful abuse of the Olympic ideal: we call for the life ban of offending athletes: we call for the life ban of coaches and the so-called doctors who administer this evil' (Sebastian Coe, Olympic Congress at Baden–Baden) (Donohue & Johnson 1986).

Brief history

The use of drugs for non-therapeutic purposes is both widespread and ancient. Man has cultivated vines, hemp, poppies, coca and tobacco plants to produce substances which alter perception and

---

*The risks associated with the procedure should be carefully explained to the athlete, and a record of this placed in the athletes notes. There is an increased risk of tendon rupture following repeated steroid injections.

89

*Chapter 6
Uses and abuses
of drugs in sport:
the athlete's view*

mood for thousands of years, and has been seeking naturally occurring substances to improve psychomotor performance for centuries.

South American Indians have used cocaine to decrease hunger and improve stamina on long marches and it is believed that West African peoples have used cola accuminata for similar purposes (Prokop 1970). It is thought that both third-century Greek athletes and the fierce Nordic Beserkers ingested psychotropic mushrooms prior to competition/combat (Prokop 1970, Todd 1987). So ingrained is the belief in the existence of such substances that modern mythology finds Popeye ingesting cans of spinach, and Asterisk impotent *– not so.* against the Romans without a draft from Getafix, the druid's brew.

More recently, in 1865, several swimmers in a canal race in Amsterdam were charged with taking performance-enhancing substances, and in 1869 cyclists were known to be using 'speedballs' of heroin and cocaine. Burk's (Todd 1987) claims that use of caffeine, alcohol, nitroglycerine, ethyl ether, strychnine and opium were common among athletes in the late nineteenth century, whilst French cyclists of the period are alleged to have used Vin Mariani (Murray 1983), a mixture of coca leaf extract and wine called the wine of athletes. Amphetamines replaced other stimulants in the competitive arena in the 1940s and 50s (though as late as 1956 at the Melbourne Olympics, doctors reported spasms in one competitor characteristic of strychnine poisoning), and anabolic steroid use is believed to have begun in the early 1960s. Testosterone and its esters became popular in the late 1970s, whilst growth hormone and human chorionic gonadotrophin have become the magic potions of the 1980s.

Current prevalence

Official estimates of the prevalence of drug taking are based on the failed urine test rate at major championships — usually about 2% of all samples. This is generally recognised to be a considerable underestimate resulting from sample bias, i.e. it represents only those athletes unlucky or stupid enough to get caught. Over 20 years ago, US Hammer-thrower George Fenn stated 'I cannot name one guy, and I know just about all of them, who is not using steroids'. Further evidence for the prevalence of such behaviour comes from an unofficial survey conducted at the 1972 Munich Games by Olympic discus thrower Jay Silvester (Silvester 1973). He sampled fellow athletes from seven nations and reported that 61% admitted using anabolic steroids in the six months prior to the Games. More recently, in the 1983 Pan-American games in Caracas, Venezuela, 19 athletes from ten different countries failed the dope test (Neff 1983). Twelve members of the US track-and-field team flew home after the announcement of the first positive results from the weight-lifting competition, and a large number of other competitors withdrew

90
Chapter 6
Uses and abuses
of drugs in sport:
the athlete's view

with sudden injury or performed well below standard, possibly to avoid being tested.

Doping control

Following the amphetamine-related deaths of several cyclists in the late 1960s, the International Olympic Committee (IOC) set up a medical commission charged with eradicating drug abuse in Olympic sports. Testing was first introducèd in the Grenoble Games in the winter of 1968, and more comprehensively in the Mexico Games the following summer. The first Olympics in which testing for steroids took place was Montreal in 1976 after the development of a reliable radio-immunoassay technique by Professor Raymond Brooks, of St Thomas' Hospital, London. Six athletes were found to have traces of anabolic steroids in their urine at this festival. Testing at European track meets in 1979 caught several female athletes, including three of the world's top middle-distance runners. In 1982 the IOC Medical Commission added exogenous testosterone to its list of banned substances; testosterone abuse being deduced from an abnormal testosterone : epitestosterone ratio.

Various devices have been used by athletes and their aides to enable continued drug use without risk of disqualification. Traditionally the authorities have focussed their attention on attempts to detect traces of banned substances in the athletes urine at the time of competition. Athletes would switch to steroids with a more rapid excretion as the competition approaches, attempt to flush out the drug and/or use masking substances to effect excretion and make analysis more difficult. Athletes may also perform (or have performed for them) their own assay prior to departing for the competition, and then withdraw if found to be still excreting. Other techniques rumoured to have been used include the submission of clean samples from bottles left behind the cistern, from a bag in the axillae via fine tubing taped to the body all the way down to the meatus, or the allegedly stimulating but risky technique of 'urinary infusion' in which a close friend (if not before, then definitely afterwards) passes urine into the athlete's catheterised bladder.*†

* 'You've passed the dope test sir, but you are three months pregnant!'

Both the definition of doping and the list of banned substances have evolved over the years as athlete and chemist have tried to outwit each other.

Currently, doping may be defined as: '... the administration of, or the use by, a competing athlete of any substance foreign to the body, or of any physiological substance taken in abnormal

---

† Doctors have a moral obligation to decline to be hired by any such athlete in these circumstances, there is no guarantee, however, that the unscrupulous technically qualified entrepreneur would not benefit from such a situation. Perhaps the answer lies with the legislators of the sports governing bodies to institute random year-round testing with severe penalties for offenders.

quantity* or taken by an abnormal route of entry into the body, with the sole intention of increasing in an artificial manner his performance in competition' (Donahue & Johnson 1986).

The IOC bans five pharmacological classes of agents, three practices, and places restrictions on the use of three other classes of drugs.

91

Chapter 6
Uses and abuses
of drugs in sport:
the athlete's view

Class A. Stimulants

These drugs — which include sympathomimetic amines and CNS stimulants — have proved popular with competitors in both endurance-based sports (e.g. cycling) and sports requiring explosive power and aggression (e.g. field events, weight-lifting, contact sports) due to their capacity to act simultaneously on the central and autonomic nervous system, musculo-skeletal system (improving muscular contractility) and metabolic systems (e.g. increasing the release of free fatty acids, FFAs). Their misuse has probably declined from a peak in the 1960s.

In Belgium in 1965, tests revealed that over 57% of professional and 23% of amateur cyclists were taking amphetamines, and in 1966 the first five competitors in the World Professional Road Race refused to take a doping test. One of the five (Jacques Anquetil) (Donahue & Johnson 1986) later said, 'everyone in cycling takes dope himself, and those who claim they don't are liars'. On the other side of the Atlantic, in a very different sport, the extent of amphetamine abuse in American football (and the adverse behavioural and psycho-social consequences of such abuse) have been well documented by psychiatrist Arnold J. Mandell (1976) in his fascinating book of the same period *The Nightmare Season* and in a paper entitled 'The Sunday syndrome' (Mandell 1979).

The psychological effects sought by athletes from these substances include enhanced alertness and ability to concentrate, decreased sense of fatigue, elevation of mood, increased self-confidence and increased aggression. Undesirable effects include interference with timing in technical events (e.g. hammer-throwing, pole-vaulting), an increased risk of injury due to overconfidence and excessive aggression, unpredictable and potentially devastating psychological consequencies (e.g. schizophrenic-like psychosis) in vulnerable individuals, and death. It was the amphetamine-related death of 29-year-old British cyclist Tommy Simson during the televised climb in the 1967 Tour de France which contributed to the setting up of the IOC Medical Commission to eradicate drug abuse.

---

*This would include the use of 'blood doping or autologous transfusion, i.e. removal of a quantity of the athlete's blood in the 'training' phase for storage and replacement just prior to the event, producing temporary supranormal oxygen-carrying capacity of the blood.

92

Chapter 6
Uses and abuses
of drugs in sport:
the athlete's view

Class B. Narcotic analgesics*

The psychological effects of opium may have been known to the Sumerians, but the first accepted reference to poppy juice is in the writings of Theophrastus in the third century BC. In 1680 Thomas Sydenham wrote that 'amongst the remedies which it has pleased Almighty God to give to man to relieve his sufferings, none is so useful and efficacious as opium' (Goodman & Gilman 1985).

Nevertheless, these potent analgesics are banned by sports governing bodies to prevent athletes competing with the pain of injury masked: a situation which might lead to worse damage. They have little ergogenic potential, and are not heavily abused by the injury-free. The issue of pain relief to enable competition is dealt with in a later section.

Class C. Anabolic steroids

Biochemistry. 1771 saw John Hunter induce male characteristics in the hen by transplanting testes from the cock, and in 1849 Berthold demonstrated that the typical results of castration could be prevented by implanting gonads into castrated roosters. The belief that testicular failure was the cause of ageing in man led to attempts to isolate the active testicular principal, thought to be an elixir of life. Brown-Sequard claimed increased vigour and work capacity from a preparation in 1889, but it is unlikely that his aqueous extract had any significant quantity of hormone. Butenant obtained 15 mg of androstenedione from 15 000 l of male urine in 1930, and the active testicular prncipal itself was isolated shortly after. Elucidation of the chemical structure and synthesis of the hormone was achieved in 1935, to which the name testosterone was given (Goodman & Gilman 1985).

Originally developed for the treatment of patients with medical conditions, e.g. Fanconi's anaemia, hypogonadism or severe catabolic conditions, anabolic steroids are the result of structural manipulations of the testosterone molecule.† 17α-alkylation reduces first-pass metabolism and facilitates oral administration, whilst

---

*Not only are opiate drugs banned in the eyes of the IOC Medical Commission, they are also drugs which are illegal to possess in most parts of the world, unless prescribed or administered by a medical practitioner. In the UK controlled drug regulations apply. These drugs are of course invaluable therapeutic agents in conditions of severe pain, e.g. fractures. The practitioner should remember that if these drugs are administered to an athlete the clinical indication for treatment should be recorded as well as the type and amount of the drug given, in case the decision should later be challenged by the athlete, or the sport's governing body. A dose of opiate analgesic before or during an event effectively disqualfies the athlete from competition.

† Anabolic steroids are synthetically-produced compounds whose structure and function are similar to naturally produced male sex hormone by chemical manipulation. However, the molecule can be modified to make it have a longer-lasting effect and greater efficiency in stimulating protein (muscle) synthesis.

93

Chapter 6
Uses and abuses
of drugs in sport:
the athlete's view

esterification of the 17-hydroxyl group increases lipid solubility and permits depot administration. Both testosterone itself and its anabolic steroid derivatives may be esterified, with testosterone being available in proprionate, cyprionate and enanthate forms. Enzymic de-esterification leads to the slow release of the testo-sterone or steroid molecule, with the length of the ester chain determining the duration of action.

Androgens increase protein synthesis by both increasing the amount of mRNA produced by the cell nucleus, and by counteract-ing the inhibitory effect of cortisol on ribosomal protein synthesis-ing activity. Athletes would like this effect to be limited to muscles, tendons and ligaments, but unfortunately (especially for female athletes) protein synthesis is also stimulated in other tissues — notably those associated with secondary sexual characteristics.

Nevertheless, anabolic steroids do differ in the relative balance of androgenic to anabolic effects they induce — this being measured by bioassay in 21-day-old castrated male rats. The effects of a seven-day period of steroid administration is assessed on the mass of both the levator ani muscle and the seminal vesicles, and this result expressed as a ratio; the 'therapeutic index'.

Regrettably, one still hears health professionals (and the British National Formulary) claiming that anabolic steroids do not provide advantages for athletes. Expressing such an opinion to individuals who know otherwise not only fails to change their behaviour, but also serves to reduce the credibility of medical opinion in their eyes. After sufficiently heavy training, athletes will often go into negative nitrogen balance. This is the result of stress-induced ACTH/cortisol release from the hypothalamic–pituitary axis. Since a major com-ponent of the action of anabolic steroids is to counteract the de-crease in muscle ribosomal activity brought about by corticosteroids (Bullock *et al.* 1968) it is not surprising that these compounds will only benefit athletes training hard enough to go into negative nitro-gen balance. The studies which failed to demonstrate improved training gains for subjects taking steroids generally failed to use sufficiently intense training and used non-specific methods for eval-uation of strength (see Haupt & Rovere 1984 for an excellent review).

History of use. It has been suggested that members of the SS were given testosterone to increase their aggression (Silverman 1984). The earliest evidence of hormone abuse in a more sporting context comes from Dr John B. Zeigler (Todd 1983), the US team physician at the 1954 world weight-lifting championships in Vienna, who claimed that the Russian team doctor disclosed that some his team were on testosterone. A few lifters in the US then commenced this practice for themselves, switching to the anabolic steroid Dianabol (methandrosterone) when this was put on the market by Ciba-Giegy

94

*Chapter 6
Uses and abuses
of drugs in sport:
the athlete's view*

in the late 1950s. In 1962, Bob Hoffman of the York Barbell Club contributed a piece to *Health and Strength* magazine entitled 'The most important article I ever wrote' claiming tremendous gains for athletes using isometric strength training principles. He neglected to mention that several of them were also taking anabolic steroids, but when this became more widely known, anabolic steroid abuse began to spiral and isometrics went the way of the 'hula-hoop'.

Athletes had opened a pharmacological Pandora's box, and in many sports it became difficult to make the national team if you

Table 6.1 Adverse effects associated with anabolic steroid use

Hepatic
  Peliosis hepatis
  Hepatoma
  Cholestatic jaundice
  Elevated liver function tests

Endocrine
  Decreased luteinising hormone
  Decreased follicle stimulating hormone
  Decreased testosterone
  Testicular atrophy
  Acne
  Gynaecomastia
  Altered glucose tolerance
  Hyperinsulinism
  Decreased spermatogenesis
    Decreased motility
    Amorphous sperm
  Masculinisation in women
    Hoarsening of voice
    Hirsuitism
    Menstrual irregularities
    Enlarged clitoris
    Decreased breast size
    Alopecia

Cardiovascular
  Elevated blood pressure
  Increased low-density lipoprotein cholesterol
  Changes in triglyceride concentrations
  Fluid and water retention

Skeletal
  Epiphyseal closure

Subjective
  Aggressiveness
  Changes in libido
  Irritability
  Muscle spasm
  Nervous tension
  Headache
  Changes in hair growth
  Dizziness
  Nausea
  Euphoria
  Rash
  Changes in appetite
  Urethritis
  Scrotal pain
  Increased urine output

Originally published in Kibble M. & Ross M. (1987) Reprinted with permission from the American Society of Hospital pharmacists.

95

Chapter 6
Uses and abuses
of drugs in sport:
the athlete's view

remained drug free, let alone compete successfully in major championships. Drug testing on the day of competition did nothing to decrease drug use in the off-season, when steroids are of more use anyway in enabling more work to be done. Rumours abounded that drug testing was not always as random as it might have been, since officials and organisers were reluctant to catch big names who drew in the crowds. The 1977 statement of the American College of Sports Medicine (basically stating that these compounds were of no use to athletes, who must be mad to use them in view of the horrendous side-effects), drastically reduced the credibility of the medical profession in the eyes of many athletes who knew otherwise.

The increase in the prevalence and sophistication of drug testing, the hepatotoxicity of the orals and long half-life of injectable steroids led to a resurgence of interest in testosterone and its undetectable esters about ten years ago. There is speculation that this change led to increases in the rupture of biceps and quadraceps tendons resulting from either increased aggression, disproportionate strength gains compared to connective tissue hypertrophy, or a combination of the two.

Side-effects of steroids. Common and less common side-effects associated with anabolic steroid use are listed in Table 6.1. Users of these compounds sometimes claim that the dangerous side-effects have only been documented in already ill patients being treated with large doses of 17α-alkylated steroids for prolonged periods. However, there is a growing awareness of an association between sports-related steroid use and fatal and potentially fatal complications — notably, ischaemic heart disease and severe liver disease including tumours. Minor side-effects are exceedingly common, however, including virilisation in women. Psychological changes may be profound, including uncharacteristic violent behaviour and mood swings which may lead to strain and even break-up of marriages and relationships. A recent paper (Pope & Katz 1988) reports a frighteningly high frequency of psychotic episodes in regular users of anabolic steroids. A large retrospective study (JAMA 1987) is underway to examine for long-term adverse health consequences (especially in the cardiovascular and hepatic systems) amongst individuals who used steroids in the 1970s.

Steroid usage patterns.[*] Sophisticated patterns of drug taking have evolved in order to maximise gains, keep side-effects to a minimum

---

[*]This section has been included to provide an insight into the practices which are indulged by some athletes aspiring to the top level in their sport. To the medical practitioner who may have to treat the aftermath of this form of unsupervised self-medication the details and extent of abuse that can occur may be of technical interest. The authors and editorial board wish to emphasise that medication to enhance performance with banned drugs such as anabolic steroids is a practice which

96
*Chapter 6
Uses and abuses
of drugs in sport:
the athlete's view*

and beat the drug tests. Steroids are usually taken in *cycles* of between four and 12 weeks to enable endogenous testosterone levels and Liver Function Tests (LFTs) to return to normal between cycles. '*Stacking*' involves the taking of two drugs simultaneously — commonly an oral with an injectable (e.g. an Anavar/Deca-durabolin stack) whilst '*Shotgunning*' is the dubious practice of taking several preparations at once. '*Plateauing*' results from steroid receptor down-regulation, manifesting itself as failure to continue making gains at that dosage. '*Staggering*', or switching to a different steroid after plateauing on the first, attempts to combat this, but there is little evidence for its efficacy (unsurprisingly). *Human chorionic gonadotropin* (e.g. Profasi 5000) is used by some to expedite the return of endogenous serum testosterone levels to normal after stopping steroids (a kind of wake-up call for the testicles). Athletes on steroids will commonly switch to preparations with shorter half-lives (i.e. orals) as competition approaches, and may even be aware of their bodies clearance times (i.e. how long it takes for them to become 'clean'). The recent development of a test for exogenous testosterone administration (via testosterone : epitestosterone ratio estimation) may have led to some athletes administering testosterone/epitestosterone mixtures.

Supply. Athletes usually obtain their drugs from the black market, though steroids remain freely available over the counter in some countries (including, I understand, some EEC ones). Gymnasia form a major distribution point, where a word in the right ear and a few fivers can result in a selection of tablets, phials, syringes and bad advice. Mail order businesses exist, though not on the same scale as they do in North America (Taylor 1987), where a raid on a flat of a black marketeer uncovered over $2 million worth of steroids, including 3053 vials of Deca-durabolin, 84 vials of veterinary grade steroids and 2344 bottles of dianabol tablets. The athletic drug market is big business, as witnessed by the recent conviction of ex-British 400 m champion David Jenkins for running a drug smuggling enterprise in California.

Information sources. Athletes are commonly well aware of which preparations or combinations of steroids they do well on, and some keep meticulous records of dosages, training gains, mood changes

Continued from p. 95
is to be deplored on medical, ethical and philosophical grounds. The various regimes that are described are likely to increase the chances of serious side-effects. It is the view of the editorial board that doctors should take no part in providing any such drugs for these purposes. Furthermore, if pressurised or coerced into so doing they should report the matter to the relevant governing body of the sport concerned, whilst at the same time maintaining the anonymity of the individual 'patients' concerned.

97
Chapter 6
Uses and abuses
of drugs in sport:
the athlete's view

and side-effects, often going back several years. Other information comes via word of mouth from other users, coaches and health professionals* and from perusal of the medical and underground literature. One manual in the latter category provides a particularly useful insight into the attitudes of some of the hard-core steroid-taking fraternity. In it the authors review the latest drugs on the market, giving tablet data, availability, side-effects, black market price, etc. (a veritable *mims* for the gym). 'Straight facts' include: 'the more you take, the more you grow' 'the less toxic a steroid is for your liver, the less effective it is for growth', and 'there is no such thing as too much steroid'. There is no need to emphasise the dangers of such rubbish. Their advice on injecting is sound, however: 'if you insist on using anything larger than a 21 G for an injection, run your arm up the inside to make sure there aren't any mice living in it.'

Growth hormone. Growth hormone became popular in the late 1970s to early 1980s, due to the more rapid and more permanent gains it was alleged to produce in combination with its undetectability. Severe and permanent side-effects abound, however, including diabetes, acromegaly, arthritis and myopathy. Whilst the risk of Jakob–Creutzfeld disease has been eliminated with the development of biosynthetic forms of the hormone, early synthetic forms had an additional methionine group resulting in antibody formation in 30% of children treated (MacIntyre 1987). The long-term consequences of this are unknown.

Some athletes may attempt to increase the secretion of growth hormone from the pituitary gland by ingestion of certain drugs (including propranolol, vasopressin, clonidine and levodopa) or certain amino acids such as ornithine, arginine, lysine and tryptophan. The effectiveness of such methods is unknown, in marked distinction to the potential hazards.

Class D: Beta blockers[†]

The chronotropic action and peripheral reduction of physiological tremor produced by these drugs is thought to confer advantages

---

* The doctor's input into this situation must inevitably be negative, as there can be no justification for doctors to play any part in the provision of anabolic steroids for use in enhancing athletic performance. Any athlete seeking advice must be dissuaded and counselled regarding the risks attaching to this form of drug abuse (*vide infra*).

† There is little in the way of danger to health that can be attributed to the use of β_2-blockers, other than in overdosage. It may indeed be difficult to justify withholding these drugs where they are medically indicated, e.g. in a hypertensive patient, who takes part in a sport when the drug is banned, e.g. snooker. As always, a good medical history and examination well recorded, will distinguish the case where the drug is legitimately prescribed from that in which the competitor seeks to gain unfair advantage.

98
Chapter 6
Uses and abuses
of drugs in sport:
the athlete's view

in precision sports (Kruse 1986). Competitors in some of the more sedentary sports may require β-blockade for cardiovascular reasons, hence the governing bodies dilemma in separating those with *bona fide* therapeutic indications from the cheats.

Class E. Diuretics

Diuretics have long been abused by athletes in sports with weight restrictions (e.g. jockeys, wrestlers, weight-lifters) and also by body-builders to improve muscular definition ('cutting-up') before a competition. The potential for electrolyte disturbance is minimised by prudent rehydration and nutritional practices. Spironolactone may possibly have been used as an anti-androgen to decrease the virilising effects of androgens in women. Carbonic anhydrase inhibitors can supress or inhibit urinary excretion of sympathomimetics, and for this reason urine is pH tested in the initial screen.

Miscellaneous compounds

Probenicid (Benemid) is used to supress urinary excretion of certain drugs prior to competition (a 'masking' agent) and cyproheptadine hydrochloride (Periactin) may be used to increase appetite and facilitate weight-gaining. Thyroxine is sometimes used to assist weight loss, and ACTH may assist in recovery from overtraining and inflammatory problems. Dimethyl sulphoxide (DMSO), a carrying agent, was in vogue a few years ago as a panacea for all kinds of injury problems but seems to have fallen out of fashion. To increase further the risks associated with such drug-taking behaviour, they are commonly procured from the black market which is not renowned for its quality-control mechanisms.

Blood doping

The possibility of autologous transfusion (blood doping or blood packing) by athletes prior to competition came to the public attention during the 1972 Munich Olympics, when rumours circulated that the Finnish athlete Lasse Viren had used this technique to good effect. Mr Viren, however, attributed his 5000 m and 10 000 m victories to reindeer milk, and this author, for one, accepts this explanation. More recently, seven members of the US Olympic cycling team, including four gold medallists, admitted to having had pre-race transfusions (Gledhill 1982). There was a degree of coercion involved, with the coach hinting that those who would not agree might find their selection chances reduced. Further, instead of re-infusion of the athletes own previously venesected packed cells, in some cases this involved transfusion of whole blood from a relative,

99

*Chapter 6
Uses and abuses
of drugs in sport:
the athlete's view*

carried out in a hotel room close to the velodrome. So much for the Olympic Ideal.

The studies looking into the benefit to athletes of erythrocytaemia have, like the steroid studies, produced conflicting results (Buick *et al.* 1976, Gledhill 1982, Thomson *et al.* 1983). Again, this is likely to be the result of methodological shortcomings in the studies showing no effect. The theory behind the practice is that increasing the haemoglobin by transfusion will increase oxygen delivery to the working muscles and the capacity for aerobic work, providing that oxygen delivery is the limiting factor and cardiac output and blood distribution to the muscles is not adversely affected by the increased viscosity. Studies demonstrating no benefit (Gledhill 1982) have generally used inadequate re-infusion volumes and/or re-infused too early after withdrawal — before the body had replenished the loss. Also, the blood was more commonly refridgerated, which is known to result in greater erythrocyte loss than if it had been frozen. In summary, those studies which have shown improvements in aerobic capacity (Taylor 1987) appear much more likely to have induced an adequate erythrocytaemia.

Ethical issues

Is drug abuse by individuals engaged in sport so dangerous or immoral that those involved should be condemned? What grounds are there for so restricting an individual's liberty to do what he wants with his body?* John Stuart Mill strongly attacked any form of paternalistic restriction of individual liberty but only for fully autonomous adults. So one question to be asked is are drug taking athletes fully autonomous — or are they in some way coerced into drug taking? It is this author's experience that many athletes taking drugs would prefer not to, but since they suspect their rivals are drug-taking they feel that they must in order to compete without disadvantage. It is not considered cheating, just doing what everybody else does in order that the years of sacrifice and discipline are not all for nothing. Any reassurance to athletes that their rivals are not using drugs in the off-season would be a welcome development, and it is good to see that many sports are progressing down this road. Britain should be congratulated on implementing random off-season testing for its own athletes in advance of developments in other countries. The recent success of the British athletics team may partly be accounted for by a reduction in the chemically inflated per-

---

*The question of drug abuse in sport for the purpose of gaining unfair advantage presents a moral dilemma. The question facing the medical practitioner, society at large and sport in general, concerns the relative dangers that are presented by the use of powerful drugs in a non-therapeutic situation, when there exists because of them the possibility of damage to the individual through serious side-effects of the drugs, damage to the sport through the introduction of unfair competition, and damage to society at large through the erosion of its moral fabric.

100

Chapter 6
Uses and abuses
of drugs in sport:
the athlete's view

formances of other nations, as more effective drug-testing strategies begin to bite.

Pain relief

What should the doctor do when asked to provide pain relief to enable an athlete to continue competition? There can be no hard and fast rules here, each situation requiring individual appraisal (Anstiss 1989). Factors to be considered include:

1 Is the injury likely to get worse if the pain is masked? (Broken nose or severe ankle sprain).

2 Does the athlete really want to continue, or is he or she being psychologically pressured by family, team mates or coach?

3 How important is the competition to the individual — is it his/her last chance for a British title, or just the street championships?

4 What other measures can be taken, e.g. equipment modification, changes in technique, protective taping?

5 Is the athlete intelligent enough to understand the risks and give informed consent?

6 Does the sport forbid or place restrictions on the contemplated practice?

For instance, if a 30-year-old wrestler in his final competitive year sustained a mild ankle sprain in the warm up prior to a major competition, and the resulting pain was obviously inhibiting his mobility, I would consider a local infiltration of anaesthetic followed by supportive taping, whereas I would not consider providing a similar service for, e.g. a young rugby player in an unimportant game that his team was losing.

Steroid prescription

What should a general practitioner do if an individual enters his or her surgery requesting anabolic steroids by prescription, and/or regular monitoring of blood pressure and LFTs? Some physicians have argued that their wishes should be complied with, since the patient will otherwise take black market preparations of dubious quality. Arguments against this position abound, including the fact that athletes are unlikely to stick to the dosages prescribed, that such assistance might be interpreted as condoning·the practice of drug-taking for performance enhancement, and that medico-legal consequences may result if recipients of prescribed steroids develop serious side-effects, as has happened in the USA (Thomson *et al.* 1983).

Such a consultation, however, provides an opportunity to assess the individual's knowledge and experience in the area, and disabuse him or her of any factually incorrect and possibly dangerous beliefs.

101

Chapter 6
*Uses and abuses
of drugs in sport:
the athlete's view*

Appendix 6.1: International Olympic Committee list of doping classes and methods

I. Doping classes

A   Stimulants
B   Narcotics
C   Anabolic steroids
D   Beta-blockers
E   Diuretics
F   Peptide hormones and analogues

II. Doping methods

A   Blood doping
B   Pharmacological, chemical and physical manipulation

III. Classes of drugs subject to certain restrictions

A   Alcohol
B   Marijuana
C   Local anaesthetics
D   Corticosteroids

Note

The doping definition of the IOC Medical Commission is based on the banning of pharmacological classes of agents. The definition has the advantage that also new drugs, some of which may be especially designed for doping purposes, are banned.

The following list represents examples of the different dope classes to illustrate the doping definition. Unless indicated, all substances belonging to the banned classes may not be used for medical treatment, even if they are not listed as examples. If substances of the banned classes are detected in the laboratory, the IOC Medical Commission will act. It should be noted that the presence of any drug in the urine constitutes an offence, irrespective of the route of administration (25 May 1989).

Examples and explanations

I. Doping classes

A. Stimulants

Amphetaminil	Benzphetamine
Amiphenazole	Caffeine*
Amphetamine	Cathine

102

Chapter 6
Uses and abuses
of drugs in sport:
the athlete's view

Chlorphentermine
Clobenzorex
Clorprenaline
Cocaine
Cropropamide
Crotetamide
Diethylpropion
Dimethylamphetamine
Ephedrine
Etafedrine
Ethamivan
Ethylamphetamine
Fencamfamin
Fenethylline
Fenproporex
Furfenorex
Meclofenoxate
Mefenorex

Methoxyphenamine
Methylamphetamine
Mehtylphenidate
Morazone
Nikethamide
Pemoline
Pentetrazol
Phendimetrazine
Phenmetrazine
Phentermine
Phenylpropanolamine
Pipradol
Prolintane
Propylhexedrine
Pyrovalerone
Strychnine
And related compounds

*For caffeine the definition of a positive depends on whether the concentration in urine exceeds 12 mg/ml.

Stimulants comprise various types of drugs which increase alertness, reduce fatigue and may increase competitiveness and hostility. Their use can also produce loss of judgement, which may lead to accidents to others in some sports. Amphetamine and related compounds have the most notorious reputation in producing problems in sport. Some deaths of sports men and women have resulted even when normal doses have been used under conditions of maximum physical activity. There is no medical justification for the use of 'amphetamines' in sport.

One group of stimulants is the sympathomimetic amines of which ephedrine is an example. In high doses, this type of compound produces mental stimulation and increased blood flow. Adverse effects include elevated blood pressure and headache, increased and irregular heart beat, anxiety and tremor. In lower doses they, e.g. ephedrine, pseudoephedrine, phenylpropanolamine, norpseudo-ephedrine, are often present in cold and hay fever preparations which can be purchased in pharmacies and sometimes from other retail outlets without the need of a medical prescription. *Thus no product for use in colds, flu or hay fever purchased by a competitor or given to him should be used without first checking with a doctor or pharmacist that the product does not contain a drug of the banned stimulants class.*

Beta-2 agonists. The choice of medication in the treatment of asthma and respiratory ailments has posed many problems. Some years ago, ephedrine and related substances were administered quite frequently. However, these substances are prohibited because they are classed in the category of 'sympathomimetic amines' and therefore considered as stimulants.

103
Chapter 6
Uses and abuses
of drugs in sport:
the athlete's view

The use of only the following β_2-agonists is permitted in the aerosol form:
Bitolterol
Orciprenaline
Rimiterol
Salbutamol
Terbutaline

B. Narcotic analgesics

Anileridine	Dipipanone
Buprenorphine	Methadone
Codeine	Morphine
Dextromoramide	Pentazocine
Dextropropoxyphene	Pethidine
Diamorphine (heroin)	Phenazocine
Dihydrocodeine	Trimeperidine
	And related compounds

The drugs related to this class, which are represented by morphine and its chemical and pharmacological analogues, act fairly specifically as analgesics for the management of moderate to severe pain. This description, however, by no means implies that their clinical effect is limited to the relief of trivial disabilities. Most of these drugs have major side-effects, including dose-related respiratory depression, and carry a high risk of physical and psychological dependence. There exists evidence indicating that narcotic analgesics have been and are abused in sports, and therefore and IOC Medical Commission has issued and maintained a ban on their use during the Olympic Games. The ban is also justified by international restrictions affecting the movement of these compounds and is in line with the regulations and recommendations of the World Health Organisation regarding narcotics.

Furthermore, it is felt that the treatment of slight to moderate pain can be effective using drugs — other than the narcotics — which have analgesic, anti-inflammatory and antipyretic actions. Such alternatives, which have been successfully used for the treatment of sports injuries, including anthranilic acid derivatives (such as mefenamic acid, floctafenine, glafenine, etc.), phenylalkanoic acid derivatives (such as diclofenac, ibuprofen, ketoprofen, naproxen, etc.) and compounds such as indomethacin and sulindac. The Medical Commission also reminds athletes and team doctors that aspirin and its newer derivatives (such as diflunisal) are not

104

*Chapter 6
Uses and abuses
of drugs in sport:
the athlete's view*

banned but some pharmaceutical preparations where aspirin is often associated with a banned drug such as codeine should be used with caution. The same precautions hold for cough and cold preparations which often contain drugs of the banned classes.

Dextromethorphan is not banned and may be used as an antitussive. Diphenoxylate is also permitted.

C. Anabolic steroids

Bolasterone	Nandrolone
Boldenone	Norethandrolone
Chlordehydromethyltestosterone	Oxandrolone
Clostebol	Oxymesterone
Fluoxymesterone	Oxymetholone
Mesterolone	Stanozolol
Methandienone	Testosterone*
Methenolone	And related compounds
Methyltestosterone	

*For testosterone the definition of positive depends on the administration of testosterone or the use of any other manipulation having the result of increasing the ratio in urine of testosterone : epitestosterone to above 6.

This class of drugs includes chemicals which are related in structure and activity to the male hormone testosterone, which is also included in this banned class. They have been misused in sport, not only to attempt to increase the muscle bulk, strength and power when used with increased food intake, but also in lower doses and normal food intake to attempt to improve competitiveness.

Their use in teenagers who have not fully developed can result in stunting of growth by affecting growth at the ends of the long bones. Their use can produce psychological changes, liver damage and adversely affect the cardiovascular system. In males their use can reduce testicular size and sperm production; in females, their use can produce masculinisation, acne, development of male pattern hair growth and suppression of ovarian function and menstruction.

D. Beta-blockers

Acebutolol	Nadolol
Alprenolol	Oxprenolol
Atenolol	Propranolol
Labetalol	Sotalol
Metoprolol	And related compounds

The IOC Medical Commission has reviewed the therapeutic indications for the use of β-blocking drugs and noted that there is now a wide range of effective alternative preparations available in order to control hypertension, cardiac drug arrhythmias, angina pectoris and migraine. Due to the continued misuse of β-blockers in some sports where physical activity is of no or little importance, the IOC Medical Commission reserves the right to test those sports which it deems appropriate. These are unlikely to include endurance events which necessitate prolonged periods of high cardiac output and large stores of metabolic substrates in which β-blockers would severely decrease performance capacity.

105

Chapter 6
Uses and abuses
of drugs in sport:
the athlete's view

E. Diuretics

Acetazolamide	Diclorphenamide
Amiloride	Ethacrynic acid
Bendrofluazide	Frusemide
Benzthiazide	Hydrochlorothiazide
Bumetanide	Spironolactone
Canrenone	Triamterine
Chlorthalidone	And related compounds

Diuretics have important therapeutic indications for the elimination of fluids from the tissues in certain pathological conditions. However, strict medical control is required.

Diuretics are sometimes misused by competitors for two main reasons, namely: to reduce weight quickly in sports where weight categories are involved and to reduce the concentration of drugs in urine by producing a more rapid excretion of urine to attempt to minimise detection of drug misuse. Rapid reduction of weight in sport cannot be justified medically. Health risks are involved in such misuse because of serious side-effects which might occur.

Furthermore, deliberate attempts to reduce weight artificially in order to compete in lower weight classes or to dilute urine constitute clear manipulations which are unacceptable on ethical grounds. Therefore, the IOC Medical Commission has decided to include diuretics on its list of banned classes of drugs.
NB: For sports involving weight classes, the IOC Medical Commission reserves the right to obtain urine samples from the competitor at the time of the weigh-in.

F. Peptide hormones and analogues

Chorionic gonadotrophin (HCG — human chorionic gonadotrophin). It is well known that the administration to males of human chorionic gonadotrophin and other compounds with related activity leads to an increased rate of production of endogenous androgenic steroids and is considered equivalent to the exogenous administration of testosterone.

106
Chapter 6
Uses and abuses
of drugs in sport:
the athlete's view

Corticotrophin (ACTH). Corticotrophin has been misused to increase the blood levels of endogenous corticosteroids notably to obtain the euphoric effect of corticosteroids. The application of corticotrophin is considered to be equivalent to the oral, intramuscular or intravenous application of corticosteroids. (See section IIID).

Growth hormone (HGH, somatotrophin). The misuse of growth hormone in sport is deemed to be unethical and dangerous because of various adverse effects, for example, allergic reactions, and acromegaly when applied in high doses.

All the respective releasing factors of the above-mentioned substances are also banned.

II. Methods

A. *Blood doping*

Blood transfusion is the intravenous administration of red blood cells or related blood products that contain red blood cells. Such products can be obtained from blood drawn from the same (autologous) or from a different (non-autologous) individual. The most common indications for red blood transfusion in conventional medical practice are acute blood loss and severe anaemia.

Blood doping is the administration of blood or related red blood products to an athlete other than for legitimate medical treatment. This procedure may be preceded by withdrawal of blood from the athlete who continues to train in this blood depleted state.

These procedures contravene the ethics of medicine and of sport. There are also risks involved in the transfusion of blood and related blood products. These include the development of allergic reactions (rash, fever, etc.) and acute haemolytic reaction with kidney damage if incorrectly typed blood is used, as well as delayed transfusion reaction resulting in fever and jaundice, transmission of infectious diseases (viral hepatitis and AIDS), overload of the circulation and metabolic shock.

Therefore the practice of blood doping in sport is banned by the IOC Medical Commission.

B. *Pharmacological, chemical and physical manipulation*

The IOC Medical Commission bans the use of substances and of methods which alter the integrity and validity of urine samples used in doping controls. Examples of banned methods are catheterisation, urine substitution and/or tampering, inhibition of renal excretion, e.g. by probenecid and related compounds.

107

*Chapter 6
Uses and abuses
of drugs in sport:
the athlete's view*

III. Classes of drugs subject to certain restrictions

A. Alcohol

Alcohol is not prohibited. However breath or blood alcohol levels may be determined at the request of an International Federation.

B. Marijuana

Marijuana is not prohibited. However, tests may be carried out at the request of an International Federation.

C. Local Anaesthetics

Injectable local anaesthetics are permitted under the following conditions:
1 that procaine, xylocaine, carbocaine, etc. are used but not cocaine;
2 only local or intra-articular injections may be administered;
3 only when medically justified (i.e. the details including diagnosis, dose and route of administration must be submitted immediately in writing to the IOC Medical Commission).

D. Corticosteroids

The naturally occurring and synthetic corticosteroids are mainly used as anti-inflammatory drugs which also relieve pain. They influence circulating concentrations of natural corticosteroids in the body. They produce euphoria and side-effects such that their medical use, except when used topically, requires medical control.

Since 1975, the IOC Medical Commission has attempted to restrict their use during the Olympic Games by requiring a declaration by the team doctors, because it was known that corticosteroids were being used non-therapeutically by the oral, intramuscular and even the intravenous route in some sports. However, the problem was not solved by these restrictions and therefore stronger measures designed not to interfere with the appropriate medical use of these compounds became necessary.

The use of corticosteroids is banned except for topical use (aural, opthalmological and dermatological), inhalational therapy (asthma, allergic rhinitis) and local or intra-articular injections.

Any team doctor wishing to administer corticosteroids intra-articularly or locally to a competitor must give written notification to the IOC Medical Commission.

108
Chapter 6
Uses and abuses
of drugs in sport:
the athlete's view

Appendix 6.2: Information for athletes, coaches and medical practitioners on the permissible use of drugs in amateur sport
(From the IOC Medical Commission)

Introduction (please read this section carefully before using this guide)

The only legitimate use of drugs in sports is under the supervision of a physician for a clinically justified purpose. The International Olympic Committee (IOC) and international sports organizations initiated drug testing to protect amateur athletes from the potential unfair advantage that might be gained by those athletes who take drugs in an attempt to increase performance. Drug testing is also meant as deterrent to protect athletes from the potential harmful side-effects which some drugs can produce.

The list of banned drugs contains a very small percentage of the currently available pharmacological arsenal and does not hinder the proper treatment of athletes for justifiable therapeutic reasons.

The following list of *permitted classes of drugs* is offered to the international sports community as a guide only. It is not comprehensive. Part I is a partial compilation which gives examples of drugs and preparations widely used in some countries or on some continents. Part II lists the generic names of corresponding drugs.

The list covers a number of therapeutic and/or pharmacological classes which are considered to be the most useful and which are used in the treatment of some ailments fairly common in those individuals who practice sport. The IOC Medical Commission wishes to state that the inclusion of brand names does not constitute in anyway an endorsement of the product nor a recommendation of the efficacy of the various substances these products contain. Furthermore, the absence of a product from the list does not constitute an unfavourable judgment, on the part of the Medical Commission, nor a recommendation against its use. Again, the list is provided for information purposes only.

The list mainly comprises drugs available on prescription from a medical doctor. It should be realized that a number of preparations containing banned drugs are available, from pharmacies in many countries, without a prescription. Care should be exercised particularly when obtaining treatment for pain, colds, headaches and nasal and bronchial problems. Likewise, preparations containing only an antibiotic or an antihistamine are permissible. However, care should be taken not to use an antihistamine tablet or liquid preparation which contains ephedrine or another sympathomimetic amine.

Very often, the same brand name covers different preparations, one or many of which may contain a banned drug. Some vitamin

109

Chapter 6
Uses and abuses
of drugs in sport:
the athlete's view

preparations sold in some countries also contain banned drugs such as psychomotor stimulants or anabolic steroids. Also remember that the rules of some International Federations may not allow the use of certain substances (such as tranquillisers) which are permitted in some sports. The IOC Medical Commission encourages individual countries to use this guide for establishing their own list of permissible drugs.

The IOC Medical Commission invites all those involved in sports to be cautious with drugs. During the Olympic Games, more information may be obtained from the Medical Commission by leaving a message in a specially identified box in the Olympic Village.

Part I

1. Antacids and some other gastrointestinal agents like anti-diarrhoeals

Acinorm (DEN), Alcap (ITA), Aldrox, (ARG), Alka-2 (USA), Allulose (NOR), Altacit (GBR), Aludrox (GBR), Alumag (S.AFRI), Aluminox (HOL), Amphojel (ARG, CAN, S. AFRI), Andursil (GBR), Antepsin (GBR, ARG, ITA), Cantil (AUS, CAN, FRA, USA), Colofac (AUS, GBR), Diarsed (FRA), Diloran (GBR), Diovol (GBR), Donnagel (CAN), Duspatal (FRG, HOL, ITA), Equilet (USA), Gamma-gel (ITA), Gastridine (ARG), Gaviscon (AUS, GBR), Gelusil (CAN, GBR), Hi-Ti (JPN), Imodium (AUS, BEL, CAN, DEN, FRA, FRG, GBR, HOL, ITA, S.AFRI, SUI, USA), Kaomycin (GBR), Kaopectate (GBR), Lomotil (AUS, CAN, S. AFRI, USA), Maalox (GBR, CAN), Milid (FRG, ITA, S.AFRI, SUI), Nacid (JPN), Palmicol (FRG), Pepto-Bismol (GBR), Prodexin (GBR), Promid (JPN), Reasec (ITA, SUI), Rinveral (ESP), Riopan (CAN, ITA, FRG, USA), Riopone (S.AFRI), Robalate (CAN, USA), Sulcrate (CAN), Talcid (FRG), Titralac (GBR), Tralanta (JPN), Ulcerban (USA), Ulcermin (JPN), Ulsanic (S.AFRI), Unigest (GBR).

Beware

Do not take preparations containing codeine or opium e.g. Diban, Donnagel-PG capsules.

2. Anti-asthmatic agents and anti-allergenic agents

*Albuterol (USA), Aldecin (AUS, BEL, GBR, JAP, SUI, SWE), *Alotec (JPN), *Alupent (ARG, CAN, FRG, S.AFRI), Aminodur (USA), Asmafil (ITA), *Asmaten (ARG), *Asmatol (ARG), *Asmidon (JPN), *Astmopent (POL), *Astop (ISR), Atrovent (AUS, BEL, FRG, HOL,

110
Chapter 6
Uses and abuses
of drugs in sport:
the athlete's view

SUI, SWE), Beclovent (CAN, USA), *Beconase (AUS, BEL, CAN, FRG, GBR, HOL, SUI), *Becotide (AUS, BEL, CAN, ESP, GBR, JAP, NOR, S.AFRI, SUI, SWE), *Bitolterol mesylate (USA), *Bricalin (ISR), *Bricanyl (ARG, FRG, GBR, SWE, S.AFRI), *Bristurin (JPN), Bronkodyl (USA), Cardophyllin (AUS), Choledyl (AUS, CAN, DEN, S.AFRI, USA), Corophyllin (CAN), *Dosalupent (ITA), Euphyllin (FRG, S.AFRI), Euspirax (FRG), *Feevone (AUS), Intal (ARG, AUS, CAN, ESP, FRG, GBR, JAP, SUI, USA), Lomisdal (BEL, DEN, FRA, HOL, ITA, S.AFRI, SUI, SWE), *Metaprel (USA), *Pulmadil (AUS, BEL, DEN, S.AFRI), *Salbutan (ITA), *Salbutol (TUR), *Sultanol (FRG, JPN), *Terbasmin (ITA), Theocoline (JPN), Theo-Dur (CAN), Theolair (BEL, CAN, HOL, SWE), Theovent (USA), *Ventolin (ARG, CAN, ITA, S.AFRI, USA).

Beware

These β-agonists are permitted in aerosol (inhalation form) only. Refer to the IOC list of banned classes and methods for restrictions regarding these drugs and the use of corticosteroids for the treatment of asthma.

3. Anti-nauseants and anti-emetic agents

Anaus (ITA), Antivert (USA), Aviomarine (POL), Bonamine (CAN), Dramamine (AUS, BEL, CAN, ESP, FRA, FRG, HOL, S.AFRI, USA), Emetrol (CAN), Gravol (CAN, GBR), Ibikin (ITA), Maxolon (AUS, BEL, FRA, S.AFRI, SUI), Neptusan (DEN), Nibromin-A (JPN), Postafen (DEN, HOL, NOR), Primperan (AUS, BEL, FRA, S.AFRI, SUI), Reglan (CAN), Scop (transdermal) (AUS), Stemetil (CAN), Tigan (USA), Torecan (ARG, CAN, FRA, FRG, ITA, USA), Transderm (CAN), Vertigon (GBR), Vomex A (FRG), Yesdol (JPN), Yophadol (JPN).

4. Anti-ulcer drugs

Biogastrone (AUS, BEL, CAN, FRG, GBR, HOL, JAP, S.AFRI, SUI), Burimamide (GBR), Cimetum (ARG), Gastromet (ITA), Metiamide (GBR), Metoclol (JPN), Primperan (AUS, BEL, DEN, FRA, GBR, HOL, NOR, S.AFRI, SUI), Reglan (CAN, USA), Tagamet (ARG, BEL, CAN, ESP, FRA, FRG), Zantac (GBR).

5. Aspirin and similar analgesic (non-narcotic) and anti-inflammatory non-steroidal agents

Acetamol (ITA), Acetard (DEN, SWE), Acetylin (FRG), Adiro (ARG, BEL, HOL, ESP), Alcacyl (SUI), Allopydin (JPN), Aluprin (USA),

Anaprox (USA), Aquaprin (S.AFRI), Arlef (AUS, BEL, FRA, FRG, ITA, S.AFRI, SUI), Asatard (ITA), Aspasol (S.AFRI), Aspirin, Benortan (BEL, DEN, FRA, FRG, HOL, SUI), Benotabol (ARG), Ben-U-Ron (BEL, FRG, SUI), Bonabol (JPN), Brufen (AUS, BEL, DEN, FRG, JPN, S.AFRI), Bufemid (BRA), Calip (ARG), Capisten (JPN), Cinnamin (JPN), Cinopal (ITA, S.AFRI, SUI), Clinoril (ARG, AUS, BEL, CAN, DEN, GBR, ITA, HOL, S.AFRI, SUI, USA), Cresopirine (FRA), Desinflam (ARG), Dirox (ARG), Dispril (BEL, NOR, SWE, SUI), Dolisal (PER), Dolobid (AUS, GBR, ITA), Dorbid (BRA), Droxaryl (BEL, HOL), Ecotrin (AUS, CAN, USA), Ennagesic (S.AFRI), Enteretas (ARG), Entrophen (CAN), Enzamin (JPN), Feldene (GBR), Flanax (BRA, MEX), Flosint (ARG, ITA, S.AFRI), Glifanan (ARG, BEL, FRA, HOL, FRG, ESP, S.AFRI, SUI), Hyprin (JPN), Idarac (ARG, BEL, CAN, FRA, ITA, S.AFRI), Imotryl (FRA), Indacin (JPN), Indocid (ARG, AUS, BEL, CAN, DEN, FRA, ITA, S.AFRI, SUI, USA), Istopirine (HUN), Motrin (CAN, USA), Naixan (JPN), Nalfon (DEN, ESP, SUI, USA), Naprosyn (ARG, AUS, CAN, DEN, GBR, FRG, S.AFRI, USA), Norfemac (CAN), Orudis (CAN, DEN, ITA, JPN, ESP, S.AFRI), Paloxin (S.AFRI), Panadol (AUS, GBR, FIN), Paramidin (JPN), Pasalin (JPN), Pentosol (ESP), Ponstan (AUS, CAN, BEL, GBR, S.AFRI, SUI), Ponstel (USA), Pontal (JPN), Prinalgin (S.AFRI), Profenid (ARG, FRA, SUI), Progesic (GBR), Prolix (S.AFRI), Prolixan (BELG, DEN, FRA, FRG, HUN, ITA, HOL, SUI), Rheumox (GBR), Rhonal (ARG, BEL, CAN, JAP, HOL, S.AFRI), Salitison (JPN), Sedalgin (AUS), Sedapyren (S.AFRI), Sulindac (GBR), Superpyrin (TCH), Tamas (ARG), Tandearil (CAN, SUI), Tanderil (ARG, AUS, BEL, DEN, FRA, FRG, ITA, HOL, ESP, S.AFRI, SUI), Tantum (ARG, AUS, DEN, FRG, HOL, ITA, S.AFRI), Tolectin (BEL, CAN, DEN, FRG, S.AFRI), Tylenol (BEL, CAN, SUI, USA), Voltaren (ARG, BEL, DEN, FRG, ITA, JPN, ESP, SUI), Winolate (S.AFRI), Zubirol (ARG), Zumaril (ITA).

111
Chapter 6
Uses and abuses
of drugs in sport:
the athlete's view

Beware

Do not take preparations containing codeine, morphine, heroin, opium, ephedrine.

6. Contraceptives

Anacyclin (FRG, SUI), Brevinor (AUS, GBR, S.AFRI), Conova 30 (GBR), Demulen 50 (CAN, GBR, S.AFRI, SWE, USA), Eugynon (ARG, BEL, DEN, FRG, GBR, HOL, ITA, NOR, SUI), Exluton (ARG, BEL, FRA, HOL, S.AFRI), Femulen (GBR, S.AFRI), Micronovum (FRG, S.AFRI, SUI), Minilyn (GBR), Nordiol (ARG, AUS, S.AFRI), Ortho-novum (AUS, BEL, CAN, FRG, HOL, ITA, SUI, USA), Ovostat (BEL, HOL, SUI), Ovral (ARG, CAN, S.AFRI, USA), Ovulen (ARG, AUS, ESP, FRA, FRG, HOL, GBR, SUI, USA).

112

Chapter 6
Uses and abuses
of drugs in sport:
the athlete's view

7. Decongestants and nasal preparations

Afrazine (GBR), Beconase (AUS, BEL, CAN, FRG, GBR, HOL, S. AFRI, SUI), Iliadin (GBR, FRA, S.AFRI), Lidil (ARG), Nafrine (CAN), Naphazoline HCl (ARG, AUS, BEL, BRA, JPN, USA), Nasivin (FRG, ITA, HOL), Otrivin(e) (AUS, BEL, CAN, DEN, ITA, HOL, NOR, S.AFRI, SUI, USA), Rynacrom (AUS, BEL, HOL, S.AFRI), Soframycin (BEL, FRA, GBR), Tyzine (AUS, BEL, DEN, ESP, FRG, S.AFRI, SUI, USA).

Beware

Do not use preparations containing 'sympathomimetic amines' such as pseudoephedrine, phenylpropanolamine, etc.

8. Expectorants and cough suppressants

Syrups: Balminil DM (CAN), Bisolvon (AUS, BEL, DEN, FRG, GBR, HOL, ITA, JAP, LUX, NOR, S.AFRI, SWE, SUI), Cosylan (GBR), Dextphan (JPN), Muflin (GBR), Reorganin (FRG), Resyl (BEL, CAN, ESP, SWE, SUI), Robitussin plain (AUS, CAN, GBR, ITA), Sancos (GBR).

Tablets: Astomin (JPN), Bisolvon (AUS, BEL, DEN, FRG, GBR, HOL, ITA, JAP, LUX, NOR, S.AFRI, SWE, SUI), Bractos (ARG), Hustazol (JPN), Lysobex (ITA), Respirex (ESP), Sinecod (BEL, FRG, ESP, ITA, SUI), Tessalon (CAN, NOR, SWE, SUI, USA), Tessalin (NOR).

Lozenges: Balminil pastilles (CAN), Bradosol (CAN, DEN), Cepacol (AUS, CAN, USA), Coricidin throat lozenges (CAN), Merocets (GBR), Neo-Bradoral (SUI).

Suppositories: Demo-Cineol (CAN), Medicil (ITA), Plausitin (ARG, ITA).

Beware

Most cough syrups contain one or several banned drugs.

9. Griseofulvin and other antifungal agents

Ancotil (ARG, AUS, CAN, DEN, FRA, FRG, JPN, NOR, SWE, SUI), Batrafen (BRA, JPN), Canesten (AUS, CAN, DEN, FRG, GBR, HOL, ESP, ITA, NOR, S.AFRI, SUI, SWE), Empecid (ARG, JPN), Eparol

113

Chapter 6
Uses and abuses
of drugs in sport:
the athlete's view

(FRG), Fasign (ARG, AUS, GEL, DEN, HOL, NOR, S.AFRI, SUI, SWE), Fulcin (FRA), Fulvicin (CAN, USA), Fungilin (AUS, DEN, GBR, ITA), Fungo-Polycid (ESP), Grisovin(e) (AUS, GBR, AFR, SUI, SWE), Monistat (CAN, GBR, SUI, USA), Mycostatin (ARG, AUS, CAN, DEN, FRA, ITA, NOR, ESP, S.AFRI, SUI, USA), Pimafucin (AUS, BEL, FRG, GBR, ITA, NOR, S.AFRI, SUI), Tinactin (CAN, SUI, USA), Tinaderm (ARG, AUS, GBR, ESP, ITA, S.AFRI).

10. Haemorrhoidal preparations

Anucaine (GBR), Anusol (GBR), Cinkain (DEN, SWE), Nestosyl (GBR), Nupercainal (BEL, CAN, DEN, ITA, SUI, USA).

Beware

Some anti-haemorrhoidal preparations contain hydrocortisone. See the IOC list of banned classes and methods regarding the use of corticosteroids.

11. Hypnotics, sedatives and tranquillisers

Abasin (FRG), Adalin (FRG, HOL), Amytal (AUS, BEL, CAN, HOL, ITA, USA), Ativan, (AUS, CAN, GBR, S.AFRI, USA), Benzolani (URS), Brovarin (JPN), Chloralol (CAN), Dalmadorm (FRG, HOL, NOR, AFR, ITA, SUI), Dalmane (AUS, CAN, GBR, USA), Dalmate (JPN), Doriden(e) (BEL, CAN, DEN, ITA, USA, GBR), Dormogen (TCH), Equanil (AUS, CAN, DEN, FRA, GBR, S.AFRI, USA), Euhypnos (AUS, GBR), Evidorm (GBR), Evipan (FRG), Gardenal (BEL, CAN, FRA, ITA, ESP, S.AFRI), Halcion (BEL, CAN, DEN, GBR, S.AFRI, SUI), Haldol (BEL, CAN, FRA, FGR, GBR, SUI, SWE, USA), Largactil (AUS, BEL, CAN, DEN, ESP, FRA, GBR, HOL, ITA, NOR, S.AFRI, SUI), Levanxol (BEL, ESP, HOL, S.AFRI), Lexotan (AUS, BEL, DEN, ITA, JPN, S.AFRI), Librium (AUS, BEL, CAN, DEN, FRA, FRG, GBR, HOL, ITA, NOR, S.AFRI, SUI, USA), Mebaral (CAN, USA), Medomin (CAN, FRG, GBR, HOL, SUI), Mogadon (ARG, AUS, BEL, DEN, FRA, FRG, GBR, ITA, NOR, S.AFRI, SUI), Nembutal (AUS, BEL, DEN, FRA, FRG, GBR, HOL, ITA, SUI, USA), Noludar (BEL, CAN, DEN, FRG, GBR, S.AFRI, SUI, USA), Noctec (AUS, CAN, GBR, USA), Normison (AUS, GBR, S.AFRI), Prominal (AUS, BEL, GBR, ESP, ITA), Restoril (CAN, USA), Restwel (S.AFRI), Schlafen (JPN), Serenid (GBR), Serepax (AUS), Sobile (ESP), Soneryl (AUS, BEL, CAN, DEN, FRA, HOL, S.AFRI, SUI), Sopental (S.AFRI), Stelazine (AUS, CAN, GBR, S.AFRI, USA), Theobromine (—), Tranxene (AUS, BEL, CAN, FRA, GBR, HOL, NZL, S.AFRI, USA), Tuinal (GBR, CAN, USA), Valamin (FRG), Vallium (ARG, AUS, BEL, CAN, DEN, FRA, FRG, GBR, HOL, ITA, NOR, S.AFRI, SUI, USA).

114
Chapter 6
Uses and abuses
of drugs in sport:
the athlete's view

12. Insulin and other antidiabetic agents

Daonil (ALG, ARG, AUS, BEL, DEN, FRA, HOL, ITA, NOR, S.AFRI, TUN), Diaben (ARG), Diabinese (ARG, AUS, BEL, CAN, GBR, HOL, ITA, NOR, S.AFRI, USA), Diamicron (AUS, FRA, GBR, ITA, S.AFRI), Dibotin (GBR), Dimelor (ARG, AUS, BEL, CAN, GBR, ITA, S.AFRI), Dipar (ESP, S.AFRI), Gilemal (HUN), Glucophage (AUS, BEL, CAN, DEN, FRA, FRG, HOL, ITA, NOR, S.AFRI, SUI, SWE), Gludease (JPN), Glutril (DEN, FRA, FRG, GBR, S.AFRI, SWE, SUI), Insoral (AUS, S.AFRI), Insulin (—), Islotin (ARG), Nadisan (ARG, BEL, FRG, ESP, SWE, SUI), Nigloid (JPN), Nogluc (ARG), Ordimel (HOL, SWE), Orinase (CAN, USA), Promide (AUS), Rastinon (AUS, BEL, DEN, GBR, ITA, NOR, S.AFRI, SUI), Silubin Retard (BEL, ESP, S.AFRI, SUI), Tolinase (AUS, BEL, ESP, HOL, SUI, SWE, USA).

13. Muscle relaxants

Aneural (FRG), Carisoma (GBR), Dantamacrin (FRG), Dantrium (AUS, BEL, CAN, FRA, GBR, HOL, NZL, S.AFRI, USA), Distalene (ARG), Equanil (AUS, CAN, DEN, FRA, GBR, S.AFRI, USA), Flexeril (CAN, USA), Lyseen (ARG, BEL, FRG), Maolate (USA), Methocabal (JPN), Mydocalm (DEN, FRA, HOL, HUN, SUI), Norflex (AUS, BEL, CAN, DEN, FRG, GBR, S.AFRI, SUI, SWE, USA), Rinlaxer (JPN), Robaxin (ARG, AUS, CAN, DEN, GBR, HOL, NOR, S.AFRI, SWE, SUI, USA), Sinaxar (AUS, BEL, DEN, S.AFRI), Soma (CAN, ITA, USA).

14. Ointments/creams/lotions

Baciguent (CAN, USA), Bacitracin (—), Caladryl (GBR), Debrisan (AUS, DEN, GBR, HOL, NOR, NZL, S.AFRI, SWE, USA), Iduviran (FRA, SUI), Myciguent (AUS, CAN, S.AFRI, USA), Neosporin (GBR), Retin-A (AUX, GBR, ITA, NZL, S.AFRI, SUI, USA), Soframycin (AUS, CAN, DEN, GBR, HOL, S.AFRI, SUI), Stoxil (AUS, CAN, S.AFRI, USA), Vioform (AUS, CAN, FRG, GBR, S.AFRI, SUI, USA), Zostrum (EIRE, FRG).

15. Ophthalmic and otic preparations

Albucid (ARG, AUS, GBR, S.AFRI), Auralgen (—), Auraltone (GBR), Collyrium (GBR), Disine (AUS, GBR, ITA, SUI, USA), Iduviran (FRA, SUI), Maxitrol (GBR), Myciquent (AUS, CAN, S.AFRI, USA), Opticrom (AUS, CAN, FRG, GBR, NZL, SUI), Ototrips (GBR), Otrivine-Antistin (GBR), Phenazone (ARG, AUS, BEL, BRA, HUN, JAP, MEX, POL, RUS, TCH, USA), Polyfax (GBR), Prontamid (ITA),

Sodium Sulamyd (CAN, USA), Vasosulf (S.AFRI), Xerumenex (GBR).

115
Chapter 6
Uses and abuses
of drugs in sport:
the athlete's view

16. Penicillins and other antibiotics

Achromycin (AUS, CAN, DEN, FRG, GBR, HOL, NOR, S.AFRI, SUI, SWE, USA), Amikin (AUS, CAN, EIRE, S.AFRI, SUI, USA), Amoxidal (ARG), Amoxypen (FRG), Bacitracin (—), Bactramin (JPN), Bactrim (ARG, AUS, BEL, CAN, DEN, FRA, FRG, GBR, ITA, NOR, S.AFRI, SUI, SWE, USA), Biklin (ARG, DEN, FRG, JPN, SWE), Brulamycin (HUN), Ceclor (CAN, USA), Ccfro (JPN), Clamoxyl (BEL, ESP, FRA, FRG, HOL, JPN, SUI), Cloxapen (CAN, ITA, USA), Erythrocyn (AUS, CAN, FRG, S.AFRI, USA), Espectrin (BRA, HKG, MAL), Floxapen (AUS, BEL, GBR, HOL, ITA, NZL, S.AFRI, SUI), Fosfocin (FRA, ITA), Gantrisen (AUS, BEL, CAN, DEN, FRG, GBR, HOL, S.AFRI, SWE, USA), Garamycin (AUS, CAN, DEN, GBR, HOL, NOR, S.AFRI, SUI, USA), Keflex (AUS, CAN, DEN, GBR, JPN, NOR, S.AFRI, SUI, USA), Kefzol (AUS, BEL, CAN, DEN, FRA, GBR, HOL, S.AFRI, SUI, USA), Lemandine (ESP), Mandelamine (AUS, BEL, FRG, S.AFRI, SUI, USA), Mandokef (DEN, ESP, FRG, S.AFRI), Mandol (AUS, CAN, HOL, NZL, USA), Minocin (BEL, CAN, ESP, HOL, ITA, SUI, USA), Minomycin (AUS, JAP, S.AFRI), Nebcin(e) (AUS, CAN, S.AFRI, USA), Orbenin (AUS, BEL, CAN, ESP, GBR, HOL, ITA, S.AFRI, SUI), Oroxin (JPN), Panoral (FRG), Penbritin (ARG, AUS, BEL, CAN, HOL, S.AFRI, SUI, USA), Pentrex (S.AFRI), Purmycin (S.AFRI), Pyassan (HUN), Rondamycin (AUS, GBR, SUI, SWE, USA), Roscillin (IND), Semicillin (HUN), Taimoxin (JPN), Tobra (ARG), Totacillin (JPN), Ultramycin (CAN), Velocef (ARG, ESP, ITA), Veramina (ARG), Vibramycin (AUS, CAN, DEN, FRG, GBR, JPN, NOR, S.AFRI, SUI, USA).

17. Phenytoin and some other anticonvulsants

Celontin (AUS, BEL, CAN, ITA, S.AFRI, USA), Depakene (JPN, USA), Depakine (ITA), Dilantin (AUS, CAN, USA), Dilon (ARG), Epamin (ARG), Epanutin (BEL, ESP, FRG, GBR, HOL, NOR, S.AFRI, SUI, SWE), Gardenal (BEL, CAN, ESP, FRA, ITA, S.AFRI), Hermolepsin (SWE), Hydantol (JPN), Iktorivil (SWE), Majsolin (YUG), Mysoline (AUS, BEL, CAN, DEN, FRA, ITA, NOR, S.AFRI, SUI, USA), Neuracen (FRG), Nidrane (ARG, AUS, GBR), Ospolot (AUS, DEN, ESP, FRG, GBR, HOL, ITA, S.AFRI), Paradoine (AUS, BEL, CAN, FRA, USA), Peganone (AUS, DEN, NOR, SUI, SWE, USA), Phenobarbital (—), Prosoline (ISR), Rivotril (ARG, AUS, BEL, CAN, DEN, FRA, FRG, GBR, HOL, ITA, NOR, S.AFRI, USA), Tegretol (ARG, AUS, BEL, CAN, DEN, FRA, GBR, HOL, ITA, NOR, S.AFRI, SUI, USA), Timonil (FRG), Tridione (AUS, BEL, DEN,

116
Chapter 6
Uses and abuses
of drugs in sport:
the athlete's view

FRG, GBR, S.AFRI, USA), Zarontin (ARG, AUS, BEL, CAN, ESP, FRA, GBR, ITA, S.AFRI, USA).

18. Promethazine and other antihistamines

Actidil (AUS, CAN, DEN, ITA, S.AFRI), Actidilon (ARG, FRA), Allergex (S.AFRI), Alusas (JPN), Anthisan (AUS, DEN, GBR, NOR, S.AFRI), Antistin(e) (CAN, ESP, FRA, FRG, SUI), Astemizole (CAN), Atalis-D (JPN), Atarax (ARG, AUS, CAN, FRG, USA), Atosil (FRG), Avomine (AUS, S.AFRI), Azaron (HOL), Banistyl (AUS, S.AFRI), Bonpac (JPN), C-Meton-S (JPN), Chlorpheniramine (—), Chlor-Tripolon (CAN, USA), Clistin (ARG, AUS, ITA, USA), Dimetane (AUS, CAN, ESP, S.AFRI), Di-Paralene (AUS, BEL, FRA, ITA), Ebalin (FRG), Fabhistin (AUS, GBR, S.AFRI), Hismanal (CAN), Histalert (AUS, S.AFRI), Histantil (CAN), Histex (AUS), Histryl (AUS, BEL, S.AFRI), Homadamon (JPN), Idulamine (ARG), Ifrasarl (JPN), Incidal (HOL, ITA), Lecasol (JPN), Lenazine (S.AFRI), Migristene (ARG, BEL, FRA, FRG, JPN), Nuran (FRG), Omeril (FRG), Optimine (CAN, HOL, S.AFRI, USA), Periactin (ARG, BEL, CAN, S.AFRI), Peritol (HUN), Phenergan (AUS, BEL, CAN, FRA, S.AFRI, SUI), Polaronil (FRG), Prof-N-4 (ARG), Promaquid (CAN), Pyribenzamine (CAN), Pyrimetane (ARG), Reconin (JPN), Sacronal (JPN), Seldane (CAN), Tavegyl (ARG, BEL, HUN, S.AFRI, SUI), Tavist (CAN), Teldane (FRA), Trihistan (DEN, NOR, SUI), Triluden (CAN), Trimeton (ITA), Venen (JPN).

Beware

Use only plain preparations. Combinations often contain banned drugs like codeine, ephedrine, phenylpropanolamine, etc.

19. Purgatives (laxatives or cathartics)

Adjust (JPN), Alaxa (ITA), Anan (JPN), Bancon (ITA), Bekunis (FRG, JPN), Co-lace (CAN, USA), Dialose (USA), Dorbanex (GBR, SWE), Dulcolax (BEL, CAN, DEN, FRA, FRG, GBR, HOL, ITA, NOR, S.AFRI, SUI, SWE, USA), Eulaxan (FRG), Lunelax (SWE), Metamucil (CAN, GBR, HOL, USA), Milk of magnesia (—), Normalax (SWE), Senokot (AUS, BEL, CAN, ESP, FRA, GBR, USA).

20. Vaginal preparations

Betadine (AUS, CAN, ESP, FRA, GBR, HOL, S.AFRI, SUI, USA), Candeptin (CAN, S.AFRI, SWE), Deflamon (ITA), Empecid (ARG, JPN), Entizol (POL), Eparol (GBR), Flagyl (ARG, AUS, BEL, CAN, DEN, ESP, FRA, FRG, GBR, ITA, NOR, NZL, S.AFRI, SUI, SWE, USA), Floraquin (ARG, AUS, BEL), Gyno-Pevaryl (BEL, FRA, FRG,

117

*Chapter 6
Uses and abuses
of drugs in sport:
the athlete's view*

GBR, HOL, NOR, NZL, S.AFRI, SUI), Klion (HUN), Nida (JPN), Monistat (CAN, GBR, SUI, USA), Mycostatin (ARG, AUS, CAN, DEN, ESP, FRA, ITA, NOR, S.AFRI, SUI, USA), Pimafucin (AUS, BEL, DEN, FRG, GBR, HOL, ITA, NOR, S.AFRI, SUI), Vanobid (USA).

21. Vitamins and mineral preparations

Beware

All vitamins and minerals are permitted. Some so-called 'vitamins' preparations may contain banned drugs, such as psychomotor stimulants and anabolic steroids.

Part II: Generic names of preparations listed in Part I

1. Antacids and some other gastrointestinal agents like anti-diarrhoeals

Alginic acid
Aluminium glycinate
Aluminium hydroxide (dried)
Aluminium hodroxide–magnesium carbonate co-dried gel
Bismuth subsalicylate and methyl salicylate
Calcium carbonate
Dimethicone (activated)
Diphenoxylate hydrochloride
Hydrotalcite (aluminium magnesium hydroxide carbonate hydrate)
Hyoscyamine sulphate
Kaolin (hydrated aluminium silicate)
Loperamide hydrochloride
Magaldrate (hydrated magnesium aluminate)
Magnesium carbonate (light)
Mebeverine
Mepenzolate bromide
Neomycin sulphate
Proglumide
Sucralfate

2. Anti-asthmatic agents and anti-allergenic agents

Aminophylline
Beclomethasone Diproprionate*
Bitolterol*
Choline theophyllinate
Ipratropium bromide
Orciprenaline*

118

Chapter 6
Uses and abuses
of drugs in sport:
the athlete's view

Rimiterol*
Salbutamol*
Sodium Chromoglycate
Terbutaline*
Theophylline
*Note: the use of these substances is allowed by inhalation only.

3. Anti-nauseants and anti-emetic agents

Dimenhydrinate
Diphenidol
Hyoscine
Invert sugar
Meclozine

Metoclopramide
Prochlorperazine
Scopolamine
Triethylperazine
Trimethobenzamide

4. Anti-ulcer drugs

Burimamide
Carbenoxolane
Cimetidine

Metiamide
Metoclopramide
Ranitidine

5. Aspirin and similar analgesic (non-narcotic) and anti-inflammatory non-steroidal agents

Acetylcresotinic acid
Acetylsalicylic acid (aspirin)
Alclofenac
Aloxiprin
Aluminium aspirin
Azapropazone
Benorylate
Benzydamine
Bucolome
Bufexamac
Calcium
Carbaspirin
Diclofenac
Difenamizole
Diflunisal
Fenbufen

Fendosal
Floctafenine
Flufenamic acid
Glafenine
Ibuprofen
Indomethacin
Indoprofen
Ketoprofen
Mefenamic acid
Naproxen
Oxyphenbutazone
Paracetamol (acetaminophen)
Piroxicam
Sodium salicylate
Sulindac
Tolmetin

6. Contraceptives

Ethynodiol diacetate and ethinyloestradiol
Ethynodiol diacetate and mestranol
Lenonorgestrel and ethinyloestradiol
Lynoestrenol and ethinyloestradiol

Lynoestrenol and Mestranol
Norethisterone and ethinyloestradiol
Norethisterone and Mestranol

119
Chapter 6
Uses and abuses
of drugs in sport:
the athlete's view

7. Decongestants and nasal preparations

Beclomethasone
  dipropionate
Framycetin
Naphazoline

Oxymetazoline
Tetrahydrozoline
Xylometazoline

8. Expectorants and cough suppressants

Syrups

Bromhexine
Dextromethorphan
Guaiphenesin
Pholcodine

Suppositories

Cineol
Gaiacol
Morclofone

Tablets

Benzonatate
Bibenzonium
Bromhexine
Butamyrate citrate
Cloperastine
Dimemorfan
Zipeprol

9. Griseofulvin and other antifungal agents

Amphotericin
Chlormidazole
Clotrimazole
Flucytosine
Griseofulvin

Miconazole
Natamycin
Nystatin
Tinidazole
Tolnaftate

10. Haemorrhoidal preparations

Aluminium acetate
Benzocaine
Benzyl benzoate
Bismuth (oxide, subgallate)
Boric acid
Butyl aminobenzoate
Cinchocaine
Esculoside
Framycetin
Hexachlorophane

Hydrocortisone
Lignocaine
Neomycin
Peru Balsam
Polymyxin B sulphate
Pramoxine
Resorcine
Resorcinol
Zinc oxide

120
Chapter 6
Uses and abuses
of drugs in sport:
the athlete's view

11. Hypnotics, sedatives and tranquillisers

Acetylcarbromal
Amylobarbitone
Bromazepam
Butobarbitone
Carbromal
Chloral hydrate
Chlorpromazine hydrochloride
Chlordiazepoxide
Clorazepate dipotassium
Diazepam
Dichloralphenazone
Ethinamate
Flurazepam
Glutethimide
Haloperidol
Heptabarbitone

Hexobarbitone
Hexobarbitone and
  cyclobarbitone
Lorazepam
Meprobamate
Methaqualone
Methylphenobarbitone
Methyprylen
Nitrazepam
Oxazepam
Pentobarbitone
Phenobarbitone
Quinalbarbitone
Temazepam
Triazolam
Trifluoperazine

12. Insulin and other antidiabetic agents

Acetohexamide
Buformin
Carbutamide
Chlorpropamide
Glibenclamide
Glibornuride
Gliclazide

Glybuzole
Insulin
Metformin
Phenformin
Tolazamide
Tolbutamide

13. Muscle relaxants

Carisoprodol
Chlorphenesin
Cyclobenzaprine
Dantrolene
Meprobamate

Methocarbamol
Orphenadrine
Prydenol
Styramate
Tolperisone

14. Ointment, creams, lotions

Bacitracin
Calamine
Clioquinol
Dextranomer
Dimethicone

Diphenhydramine
Framycetin
Idoxuridine
Neomycin
Tretinoin

121

Chapter 6
Uses and abuses
of drugs in sport:
the athlete's view

15. Ophthalmic and otic preparations

Acetic acid
Antazoline
Antipyrine
Bacitracin
Benzocaine
Borate solution (neutral)
Chlorbutol
Dexamethasone
Idoxuridine
Naphazoline
Neomycin
Oxyquinoline
Phenazone
Pilocarpine
Polymyxin B sulphate
Sodium cromoglycate
Sulphacetamide sodium
Tetrahydrozoline
Triethanolamine polypeptide
  oleate condensate
Trypsin
Xylometazoline
Zine sulphate

SPORTS COUNCIL DOPING CONTROL IN SPORT
INTERNATIONAL OLYMPIC COMMITTEE
DOPING CLASSES AND METHODS: EXAMPLES

STIMULANTS e.g. amphetamine, cocaine, ephedrine and related compounds
NARCOTIC ANALGESICS e.g. codeine, morphine, pethidine and related compounds.
ANABOLIC STEROIDS e.g. nandrolone, stanozolol, testosterone and related compounds
BETA BLOCKERS e.g. acebutolol, atenolol, propranolol and related compounds
DIURETICS e.g. frusemide, hydrochlorothiazide, spironolactone, triamterine and related compounds
PEPTIDE HORMONES & ANALOGUES e.g. growth hormone, HCG, ACTH
BLOOD DOPING,
PHARMACOLOGICAL, CHEMICAL AND PHYSICAL MANIPULATION
Classes of drugs subject to certain restrictions
ALCOHOL, MARIJUANA (not prohibited but may be restricted)
LOCAL ANAESTHETICS, CORTICOSTEROIDS (except for approved treatments)

TREATMENT GUIDELINES:
EXAMPLES OF PERMITTED AND PROHIBITED SUBSTANCES
(based upon International Olympic Committee Doping Classes)

ASTHMA: ALLOWED – Terbutaline, Salbutamol, Ventolin, Intal, Becotide. N.B. Inhalers Only.
COUGH: ALLOWED – steam and menthol inhalations. Benylin Expectorant. All antibiotics.
BANNED – products containing codeine, ephedrines, phenylpropanolamine.
DIARRHOEA: ALLOWED – Dioralyte, Lomotil, Motilium.
BANNED – products containing codeine or morphine.
HAYFEVER: ALLOWED – Antihistamines, Triludan, Piriton, Histryll, Beconase, Otrivine, Opticrom eye drops.
BANNED – products containing ephedrine, pseudoephedrine.
HEADACHE: ALLOWED – Paracetamol, Aspirin, Anadin.
BANNED – Products containing codeine, dextropropoxyphene.
SORE THROAT: ALLOWED – Soluble paracetamol gargle.
VOMITING: ALLOWED – Dioralyte, Rehidrat, Maxolon.
WARNING: THE ABOVE ARE ONLY EXAMPLES OF SUBSTANCES CURRENTLY PERMITTED OR PROHIBITED.
IF IN DOUBT, CHECK WITH YOUR GOVERNING BODY OR THE SPORTS COUNCIL (01 388 1277).
REMEMBER – YOU ARE RESPONSIBLE   JULY 1989

Card issued to sports men and women summarizing substances banned by the IOC.
(From the Sports Council.)

122

*Chapter 6
Uses and abuses
of drugs in sport:
the athlete's view*

16. Penicillins and other antibiotics

Amikacin
Amoxycillin
Ampicillin
Bacitracin
Cefaclor
Cephalexin
Cephamandalate
Cephazoline
Cephradine
Cloxacillin
Co-Trimoxazole
Doxycycline

Erythromycin
Flucloxacillin
Fosfomycin
Gentamicin
Hexamine
Methacycline
Minocycline
Penicillin
Sulphafurazole
Tetracycline
Tobramycin

17. Phenytoin and some other anticonvulsants

Beclamide
Carbamazepine
Clonazepam
Ethosuximide
Ethotoin
Methsuximide
Paramethadione

Phenobarbitone
Phenytoin
Primidone
Sulthiame
Trixidone
Valproic acid

18. Promethazine and other antihistamines

Antazoline
Astemizole
Azatadine
Brompheniramine
Carbinoxamine
Chlorcyclizine
Chlorpheniramine
Clemastine
Cyproheptadine
Dexchlorpheniramine

Dimethothiazine
Diphenylpyraline
Homochlorcyclizine
Hydroxyzine
Mebhydrolin
Mepyramine
Promethazine
Terfenadine
Tripelennamine
Triprolidine

19. Purgatives (laxatives or cathartics)

Bisacodyl
Danthron
Docusate
Ispaghula Husk

Magnesium hydroxide
Phenolphtalol
Tinnevelly Senna Fruit

Yours sincerely,

Dr. T. Healey,
Consultant Radiologist

TH/RAG

15th August, 1990

Ruth Merrills,
Librarian,
B.D.G.H.

Dear Ruth,

a)   When you get back, give me a ring on 2729 and I will
return the expensive paperback on utricularia. In view of what
happened last time I do not want to leave so valuable a book lying
around on your desk.

b)   Could you obtain for me on loan via the BLL - The
Nightmare Season A.J. Mandel, 76 Random House, New York.

        Please obtain for me a zerox of Prokop L. (1970) The
Struggle of Doping and its' History. Journal of Sports Medicine
and Fitness <u>10</u> (1) 45-48.

Many thanks

123

*Chapter 6

Uses and abuses
of drugs in sport:
the athlete's view*

20. Vaginal preparations

Benzoyl metronidazole
Candicidin
Clotrimazole
Di-iodohydroxyquinoline
Econazole

Metronidazole
Miconazole
Natamycin
Nystalin

21. Vitamins and mineral preparations

Vitamins A, B, C, D, E, and others.

References

Anstiss T.J. (1989) Returning after injury — who makes the decision? *Coaching Focus* **11**, 7–8.

Buick E.J., Gledhill N., Froese A.B., Spriet L. & Meyers E.C. (1976) Effect of induced erythrocythaemia on aerobic work capacity. *Journal of Applied Physiology* **40**, 379–83.

Bullock W., White A. & Worthington J. (1968) The effects of anabolic steroids on amino acid incorporation by skeletal muscle ribosomes. *Biochemistry Journal* **108**, 417–25.

Donohue T. & Johnson N. (1986) *Foul Play — Drug Abuse in Sport*. Basil Blackwell, Oxford.

Gledhill N. (1982) Blood doping and related issues: a brief review. *Medicine, Science Sport and Exercise* **14**(3), 183–9.

Goodman A.G. & Gilman, A. *The Pharmacological Basis of Therapeutics*, 6th edn. Ballière Tindall, London.

Haupt H. & Rovere G. (1984) Anabolic steroids: a review of the literature. *American Journal of Sports Medicine* **12**(6), 469–84.

Heere L.P. (1988) Piroxicam in acute musculoskeletal disorders and sports injuries. *American Journal of Sports Medicine* **84**, 50–55.

Kruse P. (1986) Beta-blockade used in precision sports: effects on pistol shooting performance. *Journal of Applied Physiology* **61**(2), 417–20.

Kibble M. & Ross M. (1987) Drug review. *Clinical Pharmacy* **6**, 687.

MacIntyre J. (1987) Growth hormone and athletes. *Sports Medicine* **4**, 129–42.

Mandell A.J. (1976) The *Nightmare Season*. New York: Random House.

Mandell A.J. (1979) The Sunday syndrome: a unique pattern of amphetamine abuse indigenous to American professional football. *Clinical Toxicology* **15**(2), 225–32.

Medical news and perspectives (1987) *Journal of the American Medical Association* **257**(22), 3021–5.

Murray T. (1983) The coercive power of drugs in sport. *The Hastings Center Report*. New York, pp. 24–30.

Neff C. (1983) Caracas: A scandal and a warning. *Sports Illustrated* **59**, 18–19.

Pope G. & Katz D. (1988) Affective and psychotic symptoms in anabolic steroid users. *American Journal of Psychiatry* **145**(4), 487–90.

Prokop L. (1970) The struggle against doping and its history. *Journal of Sports Medicine and Physical Fitness* **10**(1), 45–8.

Roy S. & Irvin R. (1983) *Sports Medicine, Prevention, Evaluation, Management and Rehabilitation*. New Jersey: Prentice Hall.

Silverman F. (1984) Guaranteed aggression: The secret use of testosterone by Nazi troops. *Journal of the American Medical Association*, May, 129–31.

Silvester J. (1973) Anabolic steroids and the Munich Olympics. *Scholastic Coach* **43**, 90–2.

Taylor W. (1987) Synthetic anabolic–androgenic steroids: a plea for controlled substance status. *Physician and Sports Medicine* **15**(5), 140–50.

Thomson J.M., Stone J.A., Ginsburg A.D. & Hamilton P. (1983) The effects of blood reinfusion during prolonged, heavy exercise. *Canadian Journal of Applied Sports Science* **8**(2), 72–8.

Todd T. (1983) The steroid predicament. *Sports Illustrated* **59**, 63–77.

Todd T. (1987) Anabolic steroids: the gremlins of sport. *Journal of Sport History* **14**(1), 87–107.

7 The case against anabolic steroids

I. S. BENJAMIN

'He thought he saw a kangaroo that worked a coffee mill
He looked again and found it was a vegetable pill
Were I to swallow this he said I should be very ill'
From *Silvie and Bruno* by Lewis Caroll

The use of anabolic steroids to improve performance in sport has been known for 30 years, but has gained both momentum and notoriety during the last decade. General aspects of the use and abuse of drugs in sport have been discussed in a previous chapter (Chapter 6). This chapter will concentrate in detail on the history of developments in the use of anabolic and androgenic steroids, their desirable and undesirable effects, and the case against their use.

Biochemistry and physiology

Testosterone is the basic steroid molecule on which all of these compounds are based. It is secreted by interstitial cells of the testis in man, and is responsible for development of the male secondary sexual characteristics at puberty. Testosterone is metabolised in the liver to the less potent androsterone and dihydroepiandrosterone, which are conjugated and excreted in the urine. Testosterone was first successfully synthesised in 1935. In its native form it is ineffective when administered by mouth, largely because of hepatic metabolism. Numerous synthetic substances such as methyltestosterone, however, are effective as oral preparations.

The effects of these hormones are both androgenic and anabolic. Their androgenic effects in males include trophic actions on the activity of spermatozoa, as well as development of the accessory sexual organs. Exogenous androgens will obviate the deficiencies of pre-pubertal testicular underdevelopment, and will reverse the effects of post-pubertal castration. Endogenous testosterone is also largely responsible for the male emotional make-up.

The second group of activities is anabolic, promoting nitrogen retention and increased synthesis and deposition of protein in numerous tissues, especially in skeletal muscle. Since it is the anabolic effects which are sought by athletes, it is in the manifestation of undesirable androgenic effects that the weakness of these substances lies. Attempts have been made to produce related compounds in which anabolic activity is enhanced at the expense of androgenic

124

activity, but these have only been partially successful. Modification of the side-chains of the steroid molecule produces compounds
such as norethandrolone and methandrostenolone (Dianabol), compounds which possess both enhanced anabolic potency and oral
availability.

History of steroid use

In 1889 the French physiologist Brown-Séquard, believing old age
and its associated dwindling of sexual powers to be reversible by
agents contained in the testis, injected himself with crushed guinea-
pig testes. He reported to the Société Biologie in Paris that these
injections had proved effective, but his personal observations were
greeted with some hostility and scepticism. However, such is the
susceptibility of the public to this powerful suggestion that his
report laid open the way to Voronoff's celebrated xenotransplanta-
tion of monkey testis slices, which swept America and Europe
during the 1920s (Hamilton 1986).

Following the synthesis of testosterone in 1935 the substance
was said to have been used to enhance the aggressiveness of German
soldiers during World War II. If this account is not simply apocryphal, it was an interesting twist of fate which led to the use of these
steroids in the treatment of survivors of concentration camps at the
end of that war.

Probably the first use of anabolic steroids by atheletes was in the
1950s, when weight-lifters sought to increase strength and bulk by
the use of injectable synthetic testosterone. By the 1956 Olympics
in Melbourne, many athletes were using methandrostenolone (Dianabol), an oral steroid with a higher anabolic : androgenic ratio (Bierly
1987). At this time steroids had not yet been included on the list
of banned substances by the International Olympic Committee, a
move which did not take place until the 1976 Games in Montreal,
at which event six athletes were positive when tested for steroids.
Since that time the use of steroids has been detected in increasing
numbers of athletes, with disqualification of 15 athletes, and with-
drawals by several more, from the Pan-American Games in Caracas,
Venezuela, in 1983. In the 1984 Olympics in Los Angeles silver
medals were lost in the 10 000 m and wrestling events for the same
reason.

Spread from these high echelons of sporting achievement to the
American College Football scene was recognised in 1987. In this *that*
year the National Collegiate Athletic Association tested 720 football players at the end of the season, and suspended twenty-one who
tested positive. In 1988 the former British sprinter David Jenkins
was found guilty on charges of steroid trafficking in the USA, and
the scale of the problem became much more apparent. In the same
year at the Seoul Olympics in Korea the battle between the athletes

and the biochemists was brought to the newspaper headlines of the world by the stripping of Ben Johnson's gold medal in the 100 m event. By this stage there could be nobody with an interest in sport, medicine, law or ethics who was unaware of the phenomenon.

When it comes to estimating the scale of the problem, the matter becomes more complex. Informal surveys of athletes, particularly those in sports requiring either great bulk and strength or explosive power, have suggested that as many as 90% of those in serious training have used steroids at one time or another. Formal statistics are much less easy to achieve. A survey of amateur body-builders in a Scottish gymnasium was performed by McKillop (1987). Eight out of forty-one (19.5%) admitted to the use of drugs to enhance their performance, and most of these were anabolic steroids. All the users had taken combinations of drugs, and in no case had there been any medical supervision.

The same problem of gathering reliable statistics for what is a widely practised but illegal activity has also meant that any form of controlled trial for the use of steroids has been impossible. While some team physicians in the USA have said that they think steroid use is declining, one experienced observer stated that 'every professional football player I know takes them, with some position-related exceptions' (Wright 1987).

Do anabolic steroids work?

The evidence that anabolic steroids can in fact increase muscle mass and power is inconclusive. Lamb (1984) reviewed nineteen studies in which some form of control was available. Twelve of these studies showed that weight gains averaging 2.2 kg over a period of three to 12 weeks were attained by athletes taking methandrostenolone. While some of this gain may be due to increased fluid retention, there probably was also a substantial increase in lean body mass. In addition, approximately half of these controlled investigations showed that there was a progressive improvement in muscular strength when steroids were taken along with highly intensive weight-training. Athletes taking steroids typically achieved gains over those taking placebo which averaged 8 kg for single repetition maximum lifts in the bench-press and 11 kg in the squat.

An important physiological observation must be made in relation to these studies. Those athletes who gain a major beneficial effect from the use of anabolic steroids are invariably those already engaged in the most rigorous levels of physical training. The reason for this is that the anabolic effects of exogenous steroids are intrinsically very short-lived. Thus, little or no benefit may be gained by subjects in a neutral state of metabolism. However, intensively training athletes induce in themselves a persistent catabolic state, mediated by high levels of glucocorticoids resulting from increased

ACTH stimulation. A weight-lifter in intensive training may have difficulty in consuming enough protein (2–2.2 g/kg per day) to maintain positive nitrogen balance, and may thus be in a chronically catabolic state. It is the anticatabolic effect of steroids which may therefore allow these athletes to train at such intensive levels and still maintain the required protein anabolism (Haupt & Rovere 1984). Sadly, this message may not always reach susceptible young persons who may be tempted to try to achieve rapid results by pharmacology rather than by hard training.

Finally, it must be admitted that not all of the beneficial effects of anabolic steroids in training athletes are critically dependent on physiological changes. One of the principal effects reported by those using these drugs is increased physical tolerance to training and more rapid recovery from heavy training sessions. This may indeed be a physical effect, but may also have a strong psychological component. Moreover, the increased aggressiveness which is undoubtedly one of the effects of steroids may itself make a major contribution to the athlete's performance. The search for evidence from controlled trials for or against the physical effects of steroids is doomed to failure. Most clinical trials in medicine are aimed at demonstrating differences between groups of at least 10%. By contrast, an improvement in performance of only 1–2% may represent the margin between victory and defeat in international athletic events. It has been pointed out in a recent leading article that 'no negative trial is likely to be as convincing to athletes as Ben Johnson's performance in the Olympic 100 metre final' (BMJ 1988).

Undesirable effects of steroids

Cardiovascular system

Anabolic steroids cause fluid retention, which may in part account for the early weight gain during their use. Significant increases in blood pressure occur along with left ventricular hypertrophy. Changes in lipoproteins have been observed during several studies. In training athletes the ratio of low density to high density lipoproteins is reduced, and this is said to be one of the factors which lowers the risk of ischaemic heart disease in athletes. However, this relationship may be reversed by the use of anabolic steroids, by a ratio of almost four to one (Lenders *et al.* 1988). There has been one report of acute myocardial infarction in a 22-year-old world class weight-lifter who used anabolic steroids (McNutt *et al.* 1988).

Coagulation

Many steroids increase levels of clotting factors, particularly Factors V, X and prothrombin. In addition the drugs may induce polycythaemia and also have generalised oestrogenic effects. Increased coagulability increases the risk of arterial occlusion and there has been one case report of a stroke occurring in a 34-year-old body-builder (Frankle *et al.* 1988).

Male reproductive system

Testosterone and its analogues cause suppression of follicular-stimulating hormone and luteinising hormone. This will result in testicular atrophy, oligospermia and azoospermia. Gynaecomastia is a frequent finding, and one paper reported thirty-eight surgical procedures for this condition in body-builders (Aiache 1989). In addition, adenocarcinoma of the prostate has been reported in a 40-year-old bodybuilder (Roberts & Essenhigh 1986).

Female reproductive system

Uterine atrophy and menstrual irregularity are common, making pregnancy unlikely. However, if steroids are taken during pregnancy, pseudohermaphroditism or fetal death are both hazards. Amongst the secondary sexual changes in women, acne, deepening of the voice, facial hair and baldness, shrinkage of the breast and clitoral hypertrophy contribute to the rather unattractive features. Major stimulation of the sebaceous glands occurs in either sex (Kiraly *et al.* 1987).

Effects in children

Before closure of the epiphyseal plates, steroids will cause premature fusion with permanent stunting of growth. In adolescence, extreme virilisation may occur, along with gynaecomastia. Decreased sper-matogenesis and sterility occur, though these changes may be reversible. These effects are particularly worrying as the pressure to use anabolic steroids penetrates to younger age groups, with par-ticular influences having been noted in high school children in the USA (*Baltimore Evening Sun*, 8 June 1987). A survey carried out amongst high school athletes in the USA showed only minimal use of steroids (1% of 295 students) and amphetamines (2%). However, 32% of males and 13% of females believed that steroids were effec-tive, and 14% of males (but no females) said they would consider using these agents. There seemed to be little understanding in this group of the real hazards of steroids (Krowchuk *et al.* 1989).

Psychological effects

These include wild swings in mood and unpredictable aggressive behaviour. There have been reports of criminal activity resulting from these psychological disturbances. Changes in libido are also common, and may contribute to the impotence reported by some male athletes using steroids.

129
Chapter 7
The case against
anabolic steroids

Effects on the liver

Abnormal results of liver function tests are common, with increased transaminases, alkaline phosphatase, lactate dehydrogenase and bilirubin during administration. In severe cases a cholestatic hepatitis may occur. These changes are generally reversible on withdrawing the steroids, and have to be distinguished from the elevation of transaminases which may occur with intense weight-lifting alone.

Most of the hepatic side-effects of anabolic steroids have been reported in patients receiving these preparations for therapeutic purposes. Treatment with androgenic and anabolic steroids has proved effective in the management of Fanconi's anaemia, a rare genetic disorder resulting in pancytopaenia along with a number of growth disorders. The natural history of the disease is death from anaemia or sepsis within one or two years. Liver disease associated with such treatment was first reported in 1965 by Recant and Lacey and was followed in 1971 by a report from Bernstein *et al.* of both hepatoma and peliosis hepatis (a rare condition characterised by blood-filled cystic spaces within the liver) in a Fanconi patient under treatment. In a review article in 1983 Westaby *et al.* reported 33 cases of androgen-associated hepatic tumours, 14 being treated for Fanconi's anaemia and nineteen for other conditions. They added three cases of their own, all receiving therapeutic androgens. The range of liver lesions found in patients treated with anabolic steroids include generalised hyperplasia, hyperplastic nodules, liver cell adenoma, and hepatocellular carcinoma (Sweeney & Evans 1976). This suggests there may be a common mechanism for these abnormalities mediated by a stimulus to hepatocyte hyperplasia, although cholangiocarcinoma has also been reported with anabolic steroid therapy (Stromeyer *et al.* 1979).

All of these reports have been in patients receiving anabolic steroids for therapy. However, in 1984 Overly *et al.* reported the case of a 26-year-old body-builder who had taken a number of androgenic and anabolic steroids over a period of four years. He presented with weight loss and malaise, and was found to have a massive hepatic tumour with both cholangiocellular and hepatocellular elements, and with both intra-abdominal and pulmonary metastases. This important report was the first case of fatal hepatocellular disease in an athlete associated with androgenic steroid abuse. We have seen a similar case at Hammersmith Hospital.

Case report

David Singh was a 27-year-old body-builder who had taken intermittent courses of anabolic steroids (the preparations used are not
known) over several years. He presented to a District Hospital with
sudden onset of severe abdominal and left shoulder pain, which
initially improved but progressed to collapse and admission to hospital in a shocked state. Laparotomy was performed and 2 litres of
blood were found in the peritoneal cavity from spontaneous rupture
of the right liver. The abdomen was packed and the patient transferred to Hammersmith Hospital, where on arrival there were signs
of continued bleeding. Visceral angiography showed a diffusely abnormal circulation in the right liver with a tumour blush, and a
working diagnosis of spontaneous rupture of a hepatic adenoma
was made. Because there were signs of continued bleeding urgent
laparotomy was undertaken, and a rupture in the dome of the right
liver was found. There were several other nodules palpable in the
liver, and the whole texture of the organ was grossly abnormal,
friable and soft. Mobilization of the right liver was performed for a
hepatectomy, but it was found that the ruptured main tumour mass
involved the inferior vena cava, and despite all operative efforts
uncontrollable haemorrhage ended in death on the operating table.

At autopsy, examination of the resected right liver and the residual left liver revealed four nodules ranging from 5 to 40 mm in
diameter, the largest of these showing signs of extensive haemorrhage. The whole liver was the site of diffuse hepatocyte hyperplasia and peliosis hepatis. Histological examination showed that
the nodules were hepatocellular adenomas but the largest of these
showed histological evidence of malignant transformation (Creagh
et al. 1988).

A coroner's inquest returned a verdict which drew a cause and
effect association between the steroids and the ruptured liver which
led to this young man's death (Daily Telegraph, 1 July 1987), and
the coroner described the case as 'almost unique'.

Detection of drugs

Detection of drugs used to enhance sporting performance has become a new major industry. Workers at the Olympic Analytical
Laboratory in Los Angeles reported in 1987 that they had conducted
8000 tests for androgenic anabolic steroids over a three year period,
and found several hundred positive cases (Hatton & Catlin 1987).
The same authors noted that during the 1984 Los Angeles Olympic
Games almost 10000 analyses were performed during a 15-day
period, covering more than 200 different drugs and metabolites,
with only a 2% positivity rate (Catlin *et al.* 1987). Rosenbloom

and Sutton (1985) have pointed out that the drug testing facilities
used for the 1984 Olympics cost more to operate than the total
athletics budget of many countries.

131
Chapter 7
The case against
anabolic steroids

The scope and nature of drug testing in athletes has received
increasing attention during the last decade, and the publicity surrounding the Seoul Olympics in 1988 has sharpened both public and
medical attention on this topic (Cowart 1989). The need to set
detection levels at such a point that there are no false positives
may result in many athletes who are using drugs being able to beat
the testers readily. One example is the method used for detection
of testosterone abuse. This is detected by measurement of the ratio
of testosterone : epitestosterone in the urine. In normal men this
is between 1 : 1 and 1 : 2.5, and the level set by the International
Olympic Committee is 1 : 6. However, it is very easy to devise a
dosage of testosterone such that a ratio of 1 : 6 is never exceeded,
as proved in a trial of administration to military volunteers for six
weeks (Cowart 1989). The use of diuretics or masking agents has
become a covert biochemical science in direct competition with
advances in methods of detection, a fact which marks the determination of some athletes to beat the system, and clearly points
to a deliberate involvement of medical or paramedical persons in
promoting the use of drugs in sport.

The other problem is that anabolic steroids, unlike β-blockers
or short-term stimulants, are drugs primarily used during training
for sporting events rather than at the time of competition. Since oral
preparations are cleared from the body between two and 14 days
after withdrawal, and injectables after a month, it is not difficult
to use these agents during periods of intensive training and time
their use so as to avoid detection at competitions. Thus detection
would require random screening of athletes during training periods,
a procedure for which few national sporting bodies have either the
financial resources or the political will. Even were such testing to
take place, it is unlikely that it would extend into body-building
clubs, which remain largely immune because there are few competitions in which testing is carried out. This is in contrast to sports like
athletics, swimming and Olympic weight-lifting, in which the
Sports Council in this country spends £300 000 a year on its drug-
testing programme. Thus it remains difficult to see how elimination
of the use of anabolic steroids can be achieved by this form of
surveillance.

Is there a case against anabolic steroids?

Surprisingly, in the light of the above review, there is not unanimous
agreement that anabolic steroids should be banned. The ethical
issues are complex. Collier (1988) draws a parallel with use of the

oral contraceptive pill by female athletes to ensure that menstruation does not occur during an important event. He states that 'the long-term health hazards from the oral contraceptive in women seem rather better documented that those for anabolic steroids taken by men'. This remains a ~~fatuous~~ *valid* conclusion, because of the much wider database from which the evidence on the oral contraceptive pill can be drawn, and because the secrecy surrounding information on the use of steroids in sport effectively conceals the denominator of the equation. Charles Yesalis, an epidemiologist at Pennsylvania State University, stated that 'we don't know what the long-term effects of steroid use are. The evidence linking them to liver and heart problems is extremely weak' (Cowart 1987). Certainly, long-term controlled studies might be necessary in order to produce firm 'scientific' evidence for the side-effects of steroids, and for the reasons already noted it is unlikely that these will ever take place. Cowart (1987) reports on the proposal to perform such a study in football players and power-lifters, but the protocol as reported seems deficient in a number of respects, not least in the omission of any form of liver scanning. In commenting on this study, Yesalis states 'I think we would have picked it up anecdotally by now if there were excess deaths in a group of young, healthy men'. I believe that the 'anecdotal' evidence for the adverse effects of steroids is adequate, and the only question that remains is whether banning the use of such preparations is ethically mandatory.

The pressures on certain types of sports men and women to use steroids in their training are considerable. At international competitive levels in power sports the use of any performance-enhancing drug may provide that critical 1 or 2% difference between victory and defeat, and the degree of drive and motivation at this level of competition is enormously high. In relation to professional sport, the pressures are economic as well as emotional. As John Lombardo of the Cleveland Clinic remarked 'a professional football player who is more than six feet tall and weighs 210 lbs might not make it to the pro ranks, whereas if he were stronger and weighed 240 lbs he might make $200 000 a year. As long as they are in that type of situation they will continue to use steroids'.

Howard Connelly, the 1956 Olymic hammer champion, said in 1973 'the overwhelming majority of athletes I know would do anything and take anything short of killing themselves to improve athletic performance'. It does now appear that a sufficiently determined athlete need not stop short of suicide in an attempt to win. Arguably, this is a matter for individual choice, and cannot ethically be restricted. However, it is this author's opinion that the inevitable transmission of such pressures to other athletes, and particularly down to young aspiring sports men and women, is more than enough ethical justification for continuing the ban on their use. How one achieves this objective remains a much more difficult issue.

References

Aiache A. E. (1989) Surgical treatment of gynecomastia in the bodybuilder. *Plastic and Reconstructive Surgery* **83**, 61–6.

Baltimore Evening Sun (1987) Harmful steroids trickle down to younger bodybuilders. June 8, p. 1.

Bernstein M. S., Hunter R. L. & Yachnin S. (1971) Hepatoma and peliosis hepatis developing in a patient with Fanconi's disease. *NEJM* **284**, 1135–6.

Bierly J. R. (1987) Use of anabolic steroids by athletes. Do the risks outweigh the benefits? *Postgraduate Medicine* **82**, 67–74.

BMJ News (1988) Anabolic steroids: the power and the glory? *BMJ* **297**, 877.

Catlin D. H., Kammerer R. C., Hatton C. K., Sekera M. H. & Merdink J. L. (1987) Analytical chemistry at the Games of the XXIIIrd Olympiad in Los Angeles, 1984. *Clinical Chemistry* **33**, 319–27.

Collier J. (1988) Drugs in sport: a counsel of perfection thwarted by reality. *British Medical Journal* **296**, 520.

Cowart V. S. (1987) Study proposes to examine football players, power lifters for possible long-term sequelae from anabolic steroid use in 1970s competition. *Journal of the American Medical Association* **257**, 3021–5.

Cowart V. S. (1989) Athlete drug testing receiving more attention than ever before in history of competition. *Journal of the American Medical Association* **261**, 3510–6.

Creagh T. M., Rubin A. & Evans D. J. (1988) Hepatic tumours induced by anabolic steroids in an athlete. *Journal of Clinical Pathology* **41**, 441–3.

Daily Telegraph (1987) Steroids blamed for body-builder's death, July 1.

Frankle M. A., Eichberg R. & Zachariah S. B. (1988) Anabolic androgenic steroids and a stroke in an athlete: case report. *Archives of Physical Medicine and Metabolism* **69**, 632–3.

Hamilton D. (1986) *The Monkey Gland Affair*. London: Chato & Windus.

Hatton C. K. & Catlin D. H. (1987) Detection of androgenic anabolic steroids in urine. *Clinics in Laboratory Medicine* **7**, 655–68.

Haupt H. A. & Rovere G. D. (1984) Anabolic steroids: a review of the literature. *American Journal of Sports Medicine* **12**, 469–84.

Kiraly C. L., Alen M., Rahkila P. & Horsmanheimo M. (1987) Effect of androgenic and anabolic steroids on the sebaceous gland in power athletes. *Acta Dermato-Venereologica* **67**, 36–40.

Krowchuk D. P., Anglin T. M., Goodfellow D. B., Stancin T., Williams P. & Zimet G. D. (1989) High school athletes and the use of ergogenic aid. *American Journal of Diseases of Children* **143**, 486–9.

Lamb, D. R. (1984) Anabolic steroids in athletics: how well do they work and how dangerous are they? *American Journal of Sports Medicine* **12**, 31–8.

Lenders J. W., Demacker P. N., Vos J. A., Jansen P. L., Hoitsma A. J., Van-t-Laar A. & Thien T. (1988) Deleterious effects of anabolic steroids on serum lipoproteins, blood pressure, and liver function in amateur bodybuilders. *International Journal of Sports Medicine* **9**, 19–23.

Lombardo J. (1987). Medical news and perspectives. *Journal of the American Medical Association* **257**, 3025.

McKillop G. (1987) Drug abuse in bodybuilders in the West of Scotland. *Scottish Medical Journal* **32**, 39–41.

McNutt R. A., Ferenchick G. S., Kirlin P. C. & Hamlin N. J. (1988) Acute myocardial infarction in a 22 year old world class weight lifter using anabolic steroids. *American Journal of Cardiology* **62**, 164.

Overly W. L., Dankoff J. A., Wang B. K. & Singh U. D. (1984) Androgens and hepatocellular carcinoma in an athlete. *Annals of Internal Medicine* **100**, 158–9.

Recant L. & Lacey P. (1965) Fanconi's anemia and hepatic cirrhosis. *American Journal of Medicine* **39**, 464.

Roberts J. T. & Essenhigh D. M. (1986) Adenocarcinoma of prostate in 40 year old bodybuilder (letter). *Lancet* **2**, 742.

Rosenbloom D. & Sutton J. R. (1985) Drugs and exercise. *Medical Clinics of North America* **69**, 177–87.

Stromeyer F. W., Smith D. H. & Ishak K. G. (1979) Anabolic steroid therapy and intrahepatic cholangiocarcinoma. *Cancer* **43**, 440–3.

Sweeney E. C. & Evans D. J. (1976) Hepatic lesions in patients treated with synthetic anabolic steroids. *Journal of Clinical Pathology* **29**, 626–33.

Westaby S., Portmann B. & Williams R. (1983) Androgen-related primary hepatic tumours in non-Fanconi patients. *Cancer* **51**, 1947–52.

Wright H. A. J. (1987) Medical news and perspectives. *Journal of the American Medical Association* **257**, 3025.

8 Medical problems of transplant athletes

P. J. A. GRIFFIN

'It may be raining, but there's a rainbow above you'
From *Desparado* by The Eagles

Editor's introduction

There is perhaps no more dramatic example of the success of modern medicine than the patient who may participate in competitive sport following transplantation replacement of a failing vital organ. It must be recognised, however, that, although such patients have vastly improved the quality and quantity of their expected lifespan, their health and the continued function of their transplanted organ owe much to long-term medication with powerful drugs, which themselves may have significant side-effects. Therefore, although the patients' participation in sport is to be encouraged and is a tribute to their determination and their doctors' skill, many more medical problems than are seen in 'normal' athletes arise in this group of patients.

History of transplantation

The early history of organ transplants is closely linked with the developments of plastic surgery. Following early, very tenuous, reports from China concerning tissue transplantation and the transplantation of a leg by Cosmos and Damian, nothing really occurred until the late sixteenth century when Gasparo Tagliacozzi (1545–99) described a forearm skin flap to reconstruct a nose. John Hunter revived an interest in tissue transplantation, and throughout the eighteenth and nineteenth centuries advances in skin grafting were made.

Early in the twentieth century Alexis Carrel (1875–1944) developed the technique of suturing blood vessels and carried out experimental organ transplants. By the mid-twentieth century, immunological concepts of transplantation were beginning to be understood by the work of such people as Peter Medawar, Morten Simonsen, Rupert Billingham and many others.

Renal transplantation was carried out without immunosuppression in the 1940s for the treatment of reversible acute renal failure, and David Hume in Boston carried out nine transplants for chronic renal failure, one patient surviving for six months.

134

In 1958 the first attempts at immunosuppression, using whole-body irradiation, were attempted and then in the early 1960s three events took place which brought renal transplantation into the modern era. These were:

1 The development of tissue-typing methods.
2 The development of maintenance haemodialysis.
3 The discovery of 6-mercaptopurine and its derivative azathioprine as immunosuppressive agents.

In 1963 Thomas Starzel showed that adding steroids to azathioprine conferred improved immunosuppression and then in 1978 Sir Roy Calne in Cambridge reported the use and benefits of cyclosporin A in organ transplantation.

Organs transplanted

Any patient who has had a life-supporting organ transplant may compete in the Transplant Games. Thus any recipient of a kidney, liver, heart or heart and lung is eligible. Recipients of skin, corneas or pancreases alone are not eligible to compete.

Kidneys

Kidneys are transplanted heterotopically into either iliac fossa, the renal artery and vein being anastomosed to the iliac vessels and the ureter to the bladder.

Indication for transplantation is end-stage renal failure from any cause, the usual causes being chronic glomerulonephritis, chronic pyelonephritis/interstitial nephritis, polycystic disease and diabetes mellitus. Results in the order of 80% one-year graft survival are now regularly obtained, demonstrating the success of this form of treatment.

Liver

Orthotopic liver transplantation is performed for the treatment of end-stage liver failure (cirrhosis), primary liver malignancy or metabolic liver disorders.

Contraindications to transplantation include metastatic disease. Alcoholic cirrhosis and Australia (hepatitis B) antigenaemia are relative contraindications, as these patients tend to be less compliant.

Transplantation in children is particularly gratifying, 75% one-year graft survival being obtained when the age is less than 18 years.

Heart

Heart transplantation (orthotopic) is indicated for the treatment of advanced inoperable cardiac disease with functional disability.

Ideally patients should be less than 40 years of age with a history of cardiac disease of less than five years, with low pulmonary vascular resistance and minimal renal and hepatic dysfunction.

The types of heart disease amenable to this form of treatment include coronary artery disease, idiopathic cardiomyopathy, post-traumatic aneurysms, valve disease with cardiomyopathy, congenital heart disease and cardiac tumours.

Heart and lung

Heart-and-lung transplantation is performed for treating end-stage lung disease. By transplanting both organs as a 'unit' the anastamosis of the poorly vascularised bronchi is avoided, and only right atrial, aortic and tracheal suture lines are necessary. Although heart-and-lung transplantation is in its early days, successes are being obtained and patients with crippling lung diseases such as primary pulmonary hypertension, Eisenmonger's syndrome, cystic fibrosis, sarcoidosis, emphysema, bronchiectasis and histiocytosis X are being returned to a normal life style.

Benefits of organ transplantation

Although organ transplantation is relatively expensive and presents considerable risks, particularly with liver and cardiac transplantation, the benefits in the quality of life to the patient of a successful transplant are beyond dispute.

Patients who preoperatively are unable to climb stairs or even get out of a chair, due to crippling cardiac disease, are transformed following a successful heart transplant. Similarly patients who exist with the help of two or three dialyses a week return to a normal life after a successful kidney transplant. Such patients return to full-time employment or undergo successful pregnancy, and former athletes are able to return to their sport, turning in good performances on the track, in the field, in the swimming pool or on badminton and squash courts at the Transplant Games.

When considering the cost versus the benefits in kidney transplantation it has been estimated that the average cost of haemodialysis for a patient's lifetime exceeds the cost of the successful kidney transplant by £35 000. Even when the increased costs of cyclosporin are taken into consideration, the savings are considerable. Heart-and-lung and liver transplants are considerably more expensive per operation than are kidney transplants. However, it is worth remembering that, in contrast to kidney function, which can be sustained by artificial measures, there is no convenient or reliable treatment to support patients in end-stage heart, lung or liver failure. These operations therefore provide a life-saving element to the cost-versus-benefit equation, which, although difficult to evaluate in human terms, carries with it at the very least the possibility that the wage-earner could be restored to work.

Transplant Games

The concept of Transplant Games was the brainchild of the Portsmouth transplant surgeon, Mr Maurice Slapak. His idea was to promote the benefits of organ donation by showing that patients undergoing kidney transplantation could be returned to a normal life to such an extent that they are able to take part in competitive athletics.

The first-ever Transplant Games were held in Portsmouth in August 1978 and, following the success of these inaugural games, further games were held the next year, again in Portsmouth. Since 1978, when 99 kidney transplantees competed, British Transplant Games have been held every year, based on regional transplant centres. Birmingham, Manchester, Cardiff, Newcastle, Edinburgh, Liverpool and Exeter have all hosted the games, and over 400 heart, heart-and-lung, liver and kidney transplantees competed in 1987.

In 1980 the Transplant Olympic Association of Great Britain (TOAGB) was founded, the aims of which are:
1 To promote health and sporting activity in transplantees.
2 To promote the concept of organ donation.
3 To raise funds for transplant research.
It is under the auspices of the TOAGB that all British Transplant Games are now held.

World Transplant Games are also now held every two years. After the first two games in Portsmouth, where American, Canadian and various European transplantees all competed, international games have been staged in New York, Athens, Amsterdam and, most recently, Innsbruck.

At the games in Innsbruck in September 1987, the World Transplant Games Federation was founded, as the ruling body of all future international games.

The criteria to be fulfilled by any competitor is that he/she must have received a life-supporting organ transplant, the function of which is good and stable. Before the patient may compete in the British Transplant Games a certificate must be supplied giving details of graft function and general medical state (Table 8.1), and signed by his/her own physician or surgeon. This certificate is scrutinised by an official of the TOAGB. When a certificate is deemed to be inadequate the patient is checked medically before competing. An athlete may even be disallowed from competing if it is felt he/she is at risk.

Fortunately, due to the technical success of organ transplantation to date, most transplantees who present themselves as competitors have good graft function and have been adjudged fit to compete.

Table 8.1 Medical
certification

Date of transplant
Type of transplant
Haemoglobin (10 g/dl
Blood pressure (< 140/90)
Creatinine (for kidney transplantees (< 300 μmol/l)
Cardiac function (for cardiac transplantees)
Liver function (for liver transplantees)
Hepatitis B status
Diabetes
Visual acuity
Drugs

Table 8.2 Men's Gold
Medal winning
performances at the
Sixth World
Transplant Games,
Innsbruck, September
1987

100 m	11.18 sec
400 m	54.11 sec
1500 m	4 min 28.1 sec
5000 m	14 min 23.48 sec
Long jump	6.85 m
High jump	1.70 m
Ball throw	80.41 m
Shot put	10.61 m
4 × 100 m relay	46.23 sec
50 m freestyle	27.83 sec
100 m freestyle	1 min 03.44 sec
50 m breast stroke	37.84 sec
100 m breast stroke	1 min 24.26 sec
50 m back stroke	37.52 sec
50 m butterfly	30.98 sec
4 × 50 m freestyle relay	2 min 03.27 sec
4 × 50 m medley relay	2 min 21.76 sec

Excellent athletic performances are obtained, as demonstrated by
some of the Gold Medal performances at the Sixth World Transplant
Games in Innsbruck (Table 8.2).

Medical problems

Medical problems of the transplant athlete come under three broad
headings:
1 Problems related to chronic organ failure (native or transplanted).
2 Problems related to immunosuppression.
3 Acute sporting injuries.

Problems related to chronic organ failure

Renal failure

Under the heading of renal failure we are primarily concerned with
hypertension, anaemia and musculoskeletal disorders.

Hypertension is a common accompaniment of chronic renal
failure (CRF). The complications of uncontrolled hypertension are
well known and include myocardial infarction, cerebrovascular
accidents and exacerbation of renal failure. The importance of preventing hypertensive patients competing has been highlighted by a

patient who took part in the Amsterdam games with a blood pressure of 220/120. This patient became ill with headaches and vomiting after only moderate exertion in the initial competition. Blood pressure was easily controlled with minoxidil, but he was barred from competing further.

A greater tragedy was seen in Innsbruck when a German competitor competed with a blood pressure in the order of 240/120. He had a myocardial infarction overnight and was found dead the next morning. Such an incident would hopefully be prevented in the UK with our system of medical checks.

A late complication of kidney transplantation is renal artery stenosis. This may lead to further hypertension. In persistently hypertensive patients this should be excluded and treated before a transplantee may compete.

Anaemia is commonly seen in chronic renal failure. Apart from the feeling of lethargy, acute myocardial ischaemia may be seen. The adverse effects of anaemia were demonstrated in a British competitor at the international games in Athens, when she performed well below her best and was found to have a haemoglobin of 8.4 dl/l.

Renal osteodystrophy is well recognised as a long-term sequela of chronic haemodialysis. This can give rise to painful and pathologically weak bones. This was amply demonstrated by a transplantee at the 1987 British Transplant Games who sustained a fractured neck of the humerus while throwing a cricket ball.

Liver failure

The only significant long-term problem of the liver transplantee is long-standing bone disease due to osteoporosis, as a complication of cirrhosis.

Cardiac failure

As the patients offered cardiac transplantation are generally relatively young the procedure reverses any signs and symptoms of cardiac failure which were present preoperatively. The patients usually have not developed any secondary irreversible changes prior to transplant. Post-transplant, however, the occurrence of coronary artery atheroma may become a problem. The sequela of coronary narrowing is acute myocardial ischaemia, which could certainly be exacerbated by strenuous athletic activity. To exclude this, most heart transplantees undergo coronary angiography at two years post-transplant and yearly thereafter. A stress ECG should also be performed in the cardiac transplantee before he or she is allowed to compete, particularly as the transplanted heart is denervated and thus the athlete does not experience angina pain.

Problems related to immunosuppression

The problems of immunosuppressive therapy are similar in each group of transplantees. Three major drugs are used in immunosuppression, namely azathioprine, corticosteroids and cyclosporin. Each drug has its own specific side-effects in addition to their immunosuppressive action. All affect and reduce the activity of lymphocytes, the primary cell in the host-versus-graft immune response.

Cyclosporin seems to be more selective than azathioprine in its action on the lymphocyte. Azathioprine can in fact depress all bone-marrow elements — patients can become profoundly lymphopenic, neutropenic, thrombocytopenic and even anaemic. The side-effects of azathioprine include bone-marrow depression, megaloblastic erythropoesis, macrocytosis, cholestatic hepatic toxicity and, in the long term, an increased incidence of malignancy, particularly skin tumours and lymphoreticular tumours. Other complications include nausea, vomiting, pancreatitis, drug fever, skin rashes, myalgia and arthralgia.

Steroids have a multiplicity of side-effects, most of which are well known. These include sodium and fluid retention, hypertension, loss of muscle mass and weakness, osteoporosis, avascular necrosis of bone, peptic ulceration, pancreatitis, hirsutism, skin fragility, petechiae, headaches, Cushingoid features, suppression of growth in children, development of diabetes mellitus and cataracts. All of these complications may be seen in transplanted patients treated with corticosteroids.

Cyclosporin is the most modern of current immunosuppressive agents. It has the great advantage that it may be used without the concurrent use of steroids. Most side-effects appear to be dose-dependent and include hypertrichosis, nausea, hyperkalaemia, hypertension and liver dysfunction. The most important side-effect is that of renal impairment. In the long term it causes renal parenchymal vascular lesions with interstitial fibrosis and tubular loss. Deterioration in renal function and hypertension have been well demonstrated in cardiac transplantees with previous normal renal function.

General immunosuppressive-related problems become less frequent as time passes from the date of the transplant operation when immunosuppressive therapy is progressively reduced. However, the possibility of these complications occurring must always be considered when a transplant patient becomes ill. A further problem which can occur is that of opportunistic chest infection with such organisms as cytomegalovirus (CMV) and *Pneumocystitis carinii*, the severity of which can vary from mild to life-threatening. Another more common problem is that of herpes simplex infections (particularly labial), which fortunately are easily treated with acyclovir.

Sport injuries

As with any athlete, the transplantee is prone to sustain sporting injuries which can be brought on by inadequate training and/or failure to perform a warm-up procedure.

In those patients on steroids, where loss of muscle mass, weakness and osteoporosis may be present, the risk of acute musculo-skeletal injury is increased. Transplantees with known musculo-skeletal disorder must, therefore, be discouraged from competing in the more active and stressful events. Even the relatively 'tame' event of throwing the cricket ball can lead to fractures of pathological bones, as occurred in the 1987 British Transplant Games (fractured humerus).

The attending doctor

Clearly the doctor attending a team of transplant athletes, particularly a team which is going abroad, needs to be skilled in several ways. He needs to be able to treat:
1   acute sporting injuries,
2   minor every day ailments, e.g. coughs and colds, and
3   major medical problems related to immunosuppression and transplanted organs.

The team doctor needs to carry drugs and equipment to be able to treat acute sporting injuries, e.g. muscle and tendon tears and strains, and also for cuts and abrasions. Although I have never yet had to treat major injuries such as fractures, clearly equipment needs to be carried for the emergency treatment of such injuries. For the treatment of acute sprains I have found Movelat cream useful, and non-steroidal anti-inflammatory drugs are useful for the more chronic conditions. Very occasionally steroid injections for chronic tendinitis have proved useful. For the acute injury, however, nothing has proved more useful than rest, icepacks, compression and elevation (RICE).

The team doctor also needs to fulfil the role of general practitioner and needs to carry a supply of remedies for everyday ailments, such as headaches, coughs and colds, nausea, vomiting and diarrhoea. A supply of analgesics, antiemetics and antidyspeptic and antidiarrhoeal agents is needed.

Occasionally patients have developed chest or urinary infections while abroad, so a supply of antibiotics is necessary. I have also found it advantageous to carry a bronchodilator such as salbutamol.

The transplant patient does present special problems related to his or her immunosuppression. The patient's own supplies of immunosuppressive agents may be lost or stolen and therefore it is necessary for the doctor to carry a supply of prednisolone, azathioprine and cyclosporin. Although the chance of a rejection

Table 8.3 Drugs carried by British transplant team doctor

Cyclosporin	Frusemide
Azathioprine	Minoxidil
Prednisolone/Prednisol	Froben
Methylprednisolone	Movelat cream
Paracetamol	Depo-Medrone
Metaclopramide	Lignocaine
Imodium	Slow sodium
Asilone	Triominic
Salbutamol	Dressings, sutures, splints
Augmentin	Hypodermic needles, syringes

episode is very small, a supply of methylprednisolone should be carried. Hypertension may be a problem, especially in the renal transplant recipients; thus a supply of a potent antihypertensive agent is necessary. I have found minoxidil useful in a patient with a severe life-threatening hypertensive crisis.

In hot climates, such as Athens in 1982, where there is a problem of excessive sweating and salt loss, carrying supplies of salt tablets is useful.

In addition to the drugs carried (Table 8.3), a supply of sutures, local anaesthetics, dressings and splints should be carried in order to deal with minor injuries. 'Standard' medical equipment such as a sphygmomanometer, stethoscope and thermometer are also, of course, essential.

Ideally the team doctor should be a practitioner, with experience in transplant and sports medicine.

Should any major problem related to the transplant or immuno-suppression develop, then the athlete needs to be sent home to his or her own transplant unit.

Conclusion and recommendations

Undoubtedly organ transplantation is the cheapest and most effective way to treat end-stage organ failure; patients who exist on dialysis or are crippled with cardiac failure can be rehabilitated to a full and active life.

The benefits available through transplantation are clearly demonstrated by the number of transplantees who take up athletic activity following their operation, some of them achieving quite high standards of athletic excellence. Not only may transplantees compete well against each other, but there is at least one example of a world-class athlete having had a kidney transplant and then returning to top-class athletics.

The British team who were selected to compete in the Sixth World Transplant Games in Innsbruck, contained kidney, heart and heart-and-lung transplantees, performed with distinction, winning 25 Gold, 15 Silver and 18 Bronze Medals, and were awarded the prize for the top overall nation. All of these young transplantees demonstrated yet again the benefits of organ transplantation. However, before allowing these patients to compete in strenuous athletic activity we as doctors must be sure that they are fit to do so and unlikely to harm or injure themselves. As with exercise in the 'normal' person, physical exercise in the transplantee should be encouraged, as beneficial to their overall health. To what extent strenuous activity may be allowed, however, must be determined by the state of their cardiovascular system and also the adequacy of their graft function. We are asking for trouble if we allow an anaemic, hypertensive patient with chronic kidney graft rejection to compete in such strenuous events as the 100 m dash or the 1500 m.

I believe that the approach we in the UK have adopted before allowing patients to compete in the British Transplant Games is the right course of action. The Innsbruck disaster, in which the hypertensive German athlete died, serves to reinforce the necessity for an internationally accepted set of criteria permitting athletes to compete.

The criteria the Transplant Olympic Association of Great Britain laid down (Table 8.1) must be regarded as minimal medical requirements for the transplant athlete. Each patient's own medical adviser may consider more exhaustive examination and tests, e.g. X-rays and stress ECG may be necessary before permitting that patient to participate.

Despite the medical restrictions we place on our transplant athletes, the concept of the Transplant Games has many supporters amongst the patients who throng to the games in increasing numbers each year. It also gives encouragement to the dialysis patient, as exhibited to me by a young woman for whom I recently carried out a transplant. The first thing she said to me coming out of the anaesthetic after her operation was: 'Can I now compete in next year's Transplant Games?'

Apart from the patients themselves, I also believe the relatives of donors receive encouragement in knowing that some good has come out of the often futile death of their loved one.

Finally in my ten years of experience with transplant athletes I have become increasingly aware of the need to make sure they are medically fit, but having done so it has given me a great deal of satisfaction to help these patients return to a full and active life.

Acknowledgements

I would like to thank Mr Paul McMaster, Mr John Wallwork and Mrs Lyn Holt for their helpful comments concerning liver and heart transplantees, Mrs Tesni Williams and Ms Carolyn Morgan for their typing expertise, and finally all the transplant athletes I have come to know and respect over the last ten years.

Further reading

Calne R. Y., White D. J. G., Thiru S., Evans D. B., McMaster T., Dunn D. C., Craddock G. N., Pentlow B. D. & Rowles K. (1978) Cyclosporin A in patients receiving renal allografts from cadaver donors. *Lancet* **ii**, 1323–31.

Calne R. Y., Williams R., Lindop M., Farman J. V., Tolley M. E., Rolles K., MacDongall B., Neuberger J., Wyke R. J., Raftery A. T., Duffy T. J., Wight D. G. D. & White D. J. G. (1985) Improved survival after orthotopic liver grafting in Cambridge/Kings College Hospital series. *British Medical Journal* **290**, 49–52.

English T. A., Cooper D. K. C. & Cory-Pearce R. (1980) Recent experience with heart transplantation. *British Medical Journal* **281**, 699–702.

Hamilton D. (1982) A history of transplantation. In *Tissue Transplantation*, ed. P. J. Morris, pp. 1–14. Edinburgh: Churchill Livingstone.

Leader (1981) Liver transplantation comes of age. *British Medical Journal* **283**, 115–18.

McGregor C. G. A. & Jamieson S. W. (1985) Clinical heart and lung transplantation (leader). *British Medical Journal* **290**, 1682–3.

Penketh A., Higgenbottam T., Hakin M. & Wallwork J. (1987) Heart and lung transplantation in patients with end stage lung disease. *British Medical Journal* **295**, 311–4.

Sperryn P. N. (1983) *Sports and Medicine*. London: Butterworths.

Medico-legal problems of sport for the physically disabled 9

J. C. CHAWLA

'Possunt quia posse videntur' (They are able because they seem to be able)
From *The Aeniad* V. 231 by *Virgil*

For many years physically disabled people have shown an interest in sport, but it was not until after 1945 that sufficient interest was shown by doctors to provide facilities for their sporting activities. The Second World War left many people disabled and a major initiative was taken to provide facilities to enable them to overcome the handicaps which arose as a consequence of their disabilities. Following the passage of the Disabled Persons Employment Act in 1944, not only were there developments in the field of rehabilitation of the physically disabled but also there was a realisation of the importance of sport to the disabled. In 1944 Sir Ludwig Guttman introduced sporting activities as an essential part of medical treatment. He felt that, in a country where sport in one way or another is a part of the life of most people, it would be an omission to exclude this important pastime in the rehabilitation of spinally paralysed patients. In 1945 he published a work describing the effect of sport on these patients and felt that sporting activities not only enabled paraplegics or tetraplegics to overcome the boredom of hospital life, but also enabled them to develop physical and cardiorespiratory endurance.

At the Stoke Mandeville Centre sport was essentially used as a complement to the conventional methods of physiotherapy. In July 1948 the first Stoke Mandeville Teams for the Paralysed were founded and this event coincided with the Olympic Games in London. In 1952 the paraplegic games became international and this was followed by the first International Stoke Mandeville Games held outside the UK, which took place in Rome in 1960. The number of the participants increased from 16 in 1948 to 400 in 1960 representing 23 countries. The games were held soon after the Rome Olympics of 1960 in the Olympic Stadium.

The International Stoke Mandeville Games take place every year at the Stoke Mandeville sports ground and if possible during the Olympic year in the host country. The competitions are held under the Olympic rules. In 1980 the paraplegic Olympic Games in Holland were open to competitors other than those who had suffered spinal cord injury. The visually handicapped, amputees,

146
Chapter 9
Medico-legal
problems of sport
for the physically
disabled

victims of polio and people with physical disability due to cerebral palsy started to become involved as competitors.

Over the years, realisation that the recreational aspects of sport are as important as the peripatetic has led to the development of a wide range of activities, particularly outdoor and water sport. Further developments have taken place to provide facilities also for people with mental handicap (see Chapter 10).

The British Sports Association for the Disabled was founded in 1961 to assist with the development of sport for disabled people in England. Their headquarters were at Stoke Mandeville Hospital with regional offices throughout the country. Scotland and Wales have their own Sports Associations for the Disabled, whilst in Northern Ireland the Sports Council has a special committee which oversees sport for the disabled.

Therapeutic sporting activity leads to physical readjustment of patients with physical disability, by helping to develop strength, co-ordination and endurance. It instils self-discipline and competitive spirit and enables the newly physically disabled to regain integration within the community.

There are certain games such as archery, bowls, table tennis and snooker where the physically disabled are capable of competing alongside the able-bodied. It therefore allows the disabled to develop positive mental attitudes and to come to terms with their physical disability and achieve social reintegration.

Not only does sport produce psychological benefits, but it also enables the physically disabled to develop upper limb muscles to overcome the loss of function in the legs. For example, archery is an ideal sport for strengthening the arm and the trunk muscles and weight-lifting has become an accepted form of physiotherapy technique for development of muscles (Chawla *et al.* 1979).

Recreational sport

Recreational sport has resulted in a number of patients with psycho-depressive states achieving a resolution of this aspect of their disability (Bedbrook 1985). Recreational sport for the physically disabled is slowly increasing as is exemplified by the development of various facilities. In 1978 the Sports Council stated that sports buildings to which they gave grant aid had to provide recreational facilities for disabled people if they were to continue to qualify for aid. The guidelines were established by the Technical Unit of the Sports Council.

Types of sport

The following categories of sport are available for the physically disabled:

147

*Chapter 9
Medico-legal
problems of sport
for the physically
disabled*

1 Activities in which they may participate on equal terms, with little or no modification, e.g. bowls, archery and table tennis.
2 Existing sport which has been modified, e.g. wheelchair basketball.
3 Sports specially invented for the disabled, e.g. 'rollball' for visually handicapped people.

Competition

Increasing interest in sport has resulted in the development of competitive games such as the International Stoke Mandeville Games and the Para-Olympics. To enable people to compete in these games on equal terms, rules and classifications have been worked out for the individual sports. The disabled person is examined by a doctor or a member of the paramedical profession, e.g. physiotherapist, to be assessed according to his or her disability. The divisions have been established on the basis of disability. For example, in the spinal cord injuries, residual muscle function, sensory function, presence of spasticity, joint contractures and other factors including orthoses and arthrodeses are taken into consideration for classification.

Role of the medical profession

In general, disabled people are advised to consult their doctors before taking part in sporting activities. The doctor should assess the physical abilities of the person and also his or her cardiorespiratory function. He may be able to advise him or her on what precautions to take if precautions are indicated, e.g. caution should be applied in the epileptic who wishes to swim. The doctor should be aware of the implications of the disability of each individual patient and the handicaps that these may produce.

The general practitioner realistically can only advise in general terms. For specific information it is suggested that the disabled person be directed towards the appropriate specialist who will have a better comprehension of what is involved in the particular activity in which the patient is interested. In general terms, however, the doctor should be able to advise where strenuous activity is not advocated, for example, in patients with detachment of the retina. Precautions which are necessary for patients with heart disease, diabetes and other concurrent abnormalities should be treated on their merits.

The assessments of the physically disabled should also include the assessment of orthotic and prosthetic devices, and these should be frequently inspected and maintained.

The doctor who assumes the role of medical officer to a team involving paraplegic athletes has a responsibility for not only preventing the usual complications of their disability but also looking

148
Chapter 9
Medico-legal
problems of sport
for the physically
disabled

after various injuries which might result as a consequence of sporting activities. He also has an important role in educating those who are concerned with instructing and coaching the physically disabled. It is desirable that the doctor involved in assisting with competitive disabled sport should not only be involved in sports medicine but also be aware of the problems of physical disability.

The physically disabled undertake many sports within the constraints of their mobility. They will seek information and advice from their medical advisers, although it is realised that the advisers may not be fully aware of all the aspects of the sporting activity contemplated. It is to be hoped, however, that more medically qualified personnel will become involved with the sporting endeavours of the physically disabled in order that this expanding activity may be nurtured with greater safety for its participants and so that these praiseworthy ambitions of the disabled may be more readily realised.

References

Chawla J. C., Bar C., Creber I., Price J. & Andrews B. (1979) Techniques for improving the strength and fitness of spinal cord injured patients. *Paraplegia* **17**, 185–9.
Bedbrook G. M. (1985) Sport. In *Life-time Care of the Paralysed* Patient, ed. G. M. Bedbrook, pp. 214–6. London: Churchill Livingstone.

Suggested further reading

Guttman L. (1977) *Textbook of sport for the disabled.* University of St Lucia, Queensland: Queensland Press.
Thomson N. (ed.) (1984) *Sport and recreation provision for disabled people.* London: The Architectural Press.
Croucher N. (1981) *Outdoor pursuits for disabled people.* Cambridge: Woodhead Faulkner.

Mental handicap, sport and the law

10

G. RADHAKRISHNAN

'Let me win, but if I cannot win, let me be brave in the attempt'
(Oath of Special Olympians during opening ceremonies)

The last three decades have seen the care of the mentally handicapped move rapidly from large institutions into the wider community. Implicit in this process of 'normalisation' (Wolfensberger 1983) was the recognition that leisure and recreational facilities for the mentally handicapped would have to be developed and/or integrated with existing facilities. Since that time we have come a long way. Mentally handicapped people now regularly use community sporting and leisure facilities, wherein competitive standards are often reached. Excellence, however, is rare because of training and other problems.

In the context of sport and the mentally handicapped, the Special Olympics movement deserves special mention. From humble 'backyard' beginnings in 1968, under the auspices of the Joseph P. Kennedy Foundation, using volunteer high school students as coaches, the movement has grown to span the continents. Currently over a million people participate in the Special Olympics in the United States alone. Over 50 countries have Special Olympic programmes for mentally handicapped people. The movement believes that people with mental retardation benefit physically, mentally, socially and spiritually by training and competing in sport. Families and communities at large are strengthened and united with mentally handicapped people in an environment of equality, respect and acceptance (Cipriano 1980). 'In its purest form, Special Olympics has been a catalyst to help bring people with a mental handicap into the mainstream of life. It has encouraged families to recognise the abilities of their mentally handicapped loved ones, not reject them; it has inspired individuals from every walk of life to celebrate the unlimited potential of the human spirit by appreciating the skills, courage and joy expressed in the life of Special Olympians.' (From *The Meaning of the Special Olympics.*)

Benefits

Several studies have demonstrated that participation in sport improves physical well-being in the mentally handicapped (Hayden 1974; Rarick 1978), promotes a better image of self, at the same time increasing acceptance amongst peers, through a process of mutual interaction (Connolly 1984); other studies confirm the impression that sport has a positive effect on bodily competencies, and equally on emotional, mental and social competencies (Vermeer 1985). In a study in British Columbia, Tilley (1986) demonstrated that those mentally handicapped people who participated as Special Olympians showed a marked improvement with regard to physical fitness compared to mentally handicapped people who had not benefited from a training programme or participated in the Special Olympics. A further study indicates a considerable drop in absenteeism in a sheltered workshop amongst those who had participated in a physical exercise programme (Fraser & Stuart 1987).

Overall, participation in physical/sporting activities appears to benefit mentally handicapped individuals considerably. The benefits also appear to extend to their families and the wider community.

Barriers and restrictions

That there are barriers to participation is not in doubt. Perceived barriers may include parental interventions and an initial lack of motivation on the part of the mentally handicapped individual. For example: 'Bob's mother won't let him go swimming' (Bob is fit and 26). 'Jim has just started at our day centre. To get him involved we're taking him in our group jogging' (Jim is 63). 'Pat says he wants to take part in our voluntary group's rock-climbing course' (Pat is severely epileptic). 'Irene's not very good on her feet, so we've enrolled her in horse-riding' (Irene has Down's syndrome and upper motor neuron signs in her lower limbs). These are typical participation problems which may (or may not) be brought to the notice of the general practitioner or the community medical officer.

There are real barriers in addition: limited availability and access to facilities, bureaucratic inflexibilities to such issues as supervision, overtime, insurance and so on, veiled fears of 'catching something' and sometimes even undisguised prejudice.

There are few medical restrictions to mentally handicapped people participating in sport that cannot be overcome using a common-sense approach. It is essentially a matter of adapting a particular sport to an individual's handicap. Epilepsy affects approximately a quarter of the mentally handicapped population. As long as staff are aware of the situation and can provide close supervision, there is little reason to exclude epileptics from sporting activity. Similarly a large proportion of mentally handicapped individuals are on medication of one form or other. Again this does not prevent them from engaging in a full programme of sport.

Several conditions are associated with physical abnormalities in addition to the mental handicap. Of particular concern to the doctor in pre-activity assessment of the individual for suitability to participate would be the detection of cardiovascular pathology, which, apart from limiting physical activity, may be potentially dangerous. By way of example, one-third of patients with Turner's syndrome have congenital heart disease and renal anomalies, the commonest cardiac lesion being coarctation of the aorta. (Note, however, that mental handicap is not the rule in patients with this condition). In Down's syndrome incidence of congenital heart disease is at least 50%, in contrast to less than 1% in the general population. The commonest cardiac defect in Down's syndrome patients is an atrio-ventricular canal defect, which may be murmur-free. Heart failure in these patients may be attributed erroneously to developmental delay or hypotonia, to which these patients are prone. (Down's syndrome data are cited from Howells (1989).) It is imperative, therefore, that any mentally handicapped individual wishing to participate in sport receive a full medical examination. In case of doubt, a specialist opinion should be sought.

One problem currently causing widespread concern is atlanto-axial instability (subluxation in American literature) in patients with Down's syndrome. Described by Tishler & Martell (1965), symptoms include deterioration in walking and bladder control, neck pain and other neurological signs including hypertonicity, hyper-reflexia and clonus. Death may ensue following vigorous exercise causing hyperextension or severe flexion of the neck. Estimates of incidence vary widely from 2–3% (statement of the Chief Medical Officer, DHSS, 1986) to 37% (Fraser & Stuart 1987). No figures are available regarding the frequency of neurological symptoms or prognosis although Burke *et al.* (1985) point out that the condition may first present during adolescence with progressive instability and neurological deficits.

There has been much debate on both sides of the Atlantic regarding the best course of management. American and British views are widely divergent. The Americans advocate screening, treatment and follow-up as required, with free return to unrestricted participation (in Special Olympics) if they do not have atlantoaxial instability (Committee on Sports Medicine 1984). The British position on the other hand is 'that children with Down's syndrome and other skeletal dysplasias should not be encouraged to take part in any competitive sporting activity likely to throw considerable strain upon the cervical spine, particularly, for example, diving and judo' (British Orthopaedic Association 1985). Further controversy exists over appropriate treatment, with authorities divided over the efficacy of the operation of atlantoaxial fusion.

As a result of these uncertainties a wave of over-reaction swept over the country, when many local authorities stopped all forms of athletics for the mentally handicapped. A press statement by

Mencap (The Royal Society for Mentally Handicapped Children and Adults — the Society's view is outlined in Appendix 10.1) did nothing to allay these fears and it was left to the Chief Medical Officer, DHSS, to issue a statement (Appendix 10.2).

Our own position is that neither alarm nor total reassurance is justified. Radical curtailment of the physical education curriculum is probably not warranted, at least until further clinical and radiological evidence is available.

Informed consent

As may be expected this area throws up more questions than answers. Before attempting to relate the issue of informed consent to the mentally handicapped in the field of sport, it may be instructive to look at the origins of the concept. In their scholarly text, Faden & Beauchamp (1986) trace the history of informed consent to multiple disciplines, including health, law, special and behavioural sciences and moral philosophy. The most influential fields in recent years, however, have been moral philosophy and law.

Within moral theory, three principles, namely autonomy, beneficence and justice, underlie the concept of informed consent. Autonomy, from the Greek *autos* (self) and *nomos* (law), refers to personal self-governance: personal rule of the self by adequate understanding, while remaining free from controlling interferences by others and from personal limitations that prevent choice. A distinction is made between an autonomous person and autonomous choice, in that 'while autonomous persons can and do make non-autonomous choices through temporary constraints such as ignorance or coercion ... some persons who are not autonomous can and do occasionally muster the resources to make an autonomous choice under circumstances calling for informed consents and refusals'.

Beneficence, or the value of benefiting people, is sometimes regarded as the fundamental foundation in medical ethics; the celebrated maxim *primum non nocere* — 'above all do no harm' — is generally seen as the principle underpinning Hippocratic tradition. There exists much debate over such issues as to whom precisely the duties of beneficence are owed, to what extent the principle requires the benefactor to assume personal risk or inconvenience, and whether the principle generates moral duties (Faden & Beauchamp 1986). These arguments are outside the scope of this chapter.

As for justice, 'a person has been treated in accordance with this principle if treated according to what is fair, due or owed'. Appeals to justice alone may often present a confusing picture in any debate on informed consent since the appeal is not about a distinct principle but an amalgam of all three principles.

Within the legal tradition, informed consent is regarded as being based upon the moral principle of respect for autonomy. An over-simplification of the difference between law and moral philosophy would read as follows: 'The law's approach springs from a pragmatic theory. Although the patient is granted the right to consent or refuse, the focus is on the physician, who holds a duty, and who risks a liability by failure to fulfil that duty. Moral philosophy's approach springs from a principle of respect for autonomy that focuses on the patient or subject, who has a right to make an autonomous choice.' The liability referred to above is discharged or compensated, at least in civil law, by monetary damages. Not surprisingly, a degree of cynicism accompanies the law as a means of defining informed consent.

We can now turn our attention to whether informed consent applies in the context of voluntary participation in sport by the mentally handicapped. If one views sporting activity as a form of recreation, one could question the applicability of informed consent in this context. One could be accused of merely 'covering oneself', or simply being pedantic or indeed paternalistic, if one looked for an autonomously made decision, each time a mentally handicapped person wanted to have a good time! Several issues arise, however: suggestibility for example. Is participation truly voluntary? Does the individual really understand the risks involved, small as they are? Often the mentally handicapped person who seems overtly to understand simply has the ability to carry out linguistic conventions (the convention of communication being normally a two-way activity). There is also the possibility that the person is agreeing mainly to preserve 'face', this being the positive social value a person claims for himself in an encounter (Goffman, quoted by Fraser & Stuart 1987).

A further problem arises in that no guidelines exist that determine whether a parent or guardian can consent on behalf of a mentally handicapped adult (the position of mentally handicapped children is probably similar to children of normal abilities, in that parental informed consent would generally suffice (British Paediatric Association 1980; *Gillick* v. *West Norfolk and Wisbech AHA* [1985]; Royal College of Physicians 1986). A corollary of the above is that, since the term mental handicap envisages a spectrum of cognitive abilities from the near normal to profound handicap, there is no firm determining point beyond which an individual is able or unable to give consent. It may be possible to argue that, with the law as it stands at present, no other person is empowered to consent on behalf of an 'incompetent' mentally handicapped person. Such a view would automatically bar mentally handicapped persons from participating in activities intended to benefit themselves as individuals or as a group.

The following extract from a release statement issued by the

National Special Olympic Games 1989 illustrates some of these dilemmas: 'I, undersigned parent and/or legal guardian of athlete, hereby grant permission for the athlete to participate . . . On behalf of the athlete and myself, I acknowledge that the athlete will be using facilities at his/her own risk and I, on my own behalf, hereby release, discharge and indemnify Special Olympics . . . Signed parent/carer.'

In our institution, this document is automatically circulated to the responsible medical officer in charge of the care of a mentally handicapped resident desirous of participating in the Special Olympic Games, when his/her legal parent/carer cannot (for whatever reason) be contacted. We would suggest that, in constructing this document, the Special Olympic Games Committee assumes:

1   That no prospective participant is capable of giving informed consent.
2   That a parent/carer has the authority to consent on behalf of a mentally handicapped individual.
3   That where the legal parent/carer is not available, the responsible medical officer can adopt that role.

There are, of course, no easy answers. We would, however, suggest that the following points merit consideration:

1   An individual's ability to consent autonomously should, as far as possible, be assessed objectively. This may involve, for example, a five-question test with lie scores that indicate lack of understanding, positive bias to say yes, inability to express own intentions and so on.
2   An independent third party, or indeed a committee, checking on possible influences on decision-making and acquiescence for the wrong reasons.
3   Time and patience are essential; any explanations should be in language that will be understood.
4   It is desirable (although not legally necessary) to have the consent of parents or next of kin.
5   A form of court-appointed guardianship scheme may be a possible solution. Such schemes are in force in some states in America and Australia (Herr & Hayes, quoted by Gunn 1985) and are also envisaged in the United Nations Declaration on the Rights of Mentally Retarded Persons: 'Resolution 5. The mentally retarded person has a right to a qualified guardian when this is required to protect his personal well-being and interests.'

Appendix 10.1: Mencap's view

In the opinion of Mencap's medical advisory panel it is unwise to ignore the possible dangers of participation in certain sports by individuals with Down's syndrome who might have atlantoaxial instability. The lack of information on the true incidence of atlantoaxial instability in people with Down's syndrome and of the incidence of significant neurological disorder as a result are insufficient reasons not to take action.

Mencap supports the participation in sports activities by all people with Down's syndrome, but considers it essential for them to undergo X-ray examination to determine whether or not they could be at risk in certain sports because of atlantoaxial instability and endorses the Special Olympics (USA) recommendations that all athletes with Down's syndrome should:

1   be temporarily restricted from participating in high-risk activities until they have been examined by X-ray for atlantoaxial instability and the examination has shown them to be normal;

2   be permanently restricted from high-risk sports if they are diagnosed as having atlantoaxial instability;

3   have free return to unrestricted participation in all sports if they are found to have no evidence of atlantoaxial instability.

Advice on anaesthesia

Full clinical and radiological assessment of the cervical spine should be undertaken on people with Down's syndrome before they are given anaesthesia (Gallanaugh, S. C. (1985) *British Medical Journal* **291**, 116).

Appendix 10.2: Statement of the Chief Medical Officer, DHSS, May 1986

Perhaps 2 or 3% of people with Down's syndrome will have instability between the atlas and axis bones at the top of the neck, which can lead to pressure on the spinal cord and in exceptional circumstances to death. In some of these individuals, spinal cord compression develops slowly over a number of years, while, in others, accident or injury produces immediate damage. The question arose, therefore, whether, given this knowledge, the lives of people with Down's syndrome were being put at unreasonable risk, and in what way the risk should be limited. The Standing Medical Advisory Committee were asked to advise the Secretary of State on the matter, and I am writing now to let you know their views. The first thing to say is that at present only one case of injury to the neck and spinal cord during sporting activity has been reported in the world literature and that occurred during unsupervised trampolining to a girl already known to have nerve damage. Deaths have occurred, however, in a variety of other circumstances including car accidents involving whiplash injury, to which these individuals are more vulnerable. It is possible to identify the instability by X-ray from the age of 6 onwards and one response has been to suggest radiological investigation for all people with Down's syndrome.

Although this might be appropriate if there was an effective treatment available, current advice is that this is not so, and that it is not possible to stabilise the bones satisfactorily by surgery. The Standing Medical Advisory Committee therefore recommend the following compromise:

1 That people with Down's syndrome should continue to participate in a full range of daily activities including running, jumping and horse-riding.

2 Where more vigorous sporting activity such as diving or trampolining, which involves acute flexion of the neck, or violent contact sport, such as karate, is envisaged, the individual should first be X-rayed.

3 Where an instability is demonstrated, the individual should be medically examined. In the event that compression of the nervous system is demonstrated, consultant advice should be sought without delay. Where there is no evidence of compression, individuals should be encouraged to continue previous activities but be dissuaded from more vigorous activities such as diving or trampolining.

4 Care should be taken to support the body and head of a person with Down's syndrome when travelling by use of seat-belts and head-rests.

5 Because pressure on the spinal cord occasionally develops without any accident or injury, examination of the central nervous system should form an integral part of the medical examination of all people with Down's syndrome. On finding exaggerated knee jerks the doctor should arrange radiological investigation to exclude atlantoaxial instability.

6 At the time of a general anaesthetic or following a road traffic accident, particular attention should be paid to people with Down's syndrome because of the possibility of instability and its attendant complications.

References

British Orthopaedic Association (1985) *Atlanto-Axial Instability and Down's Syndrome — a Suitable Case for Screening.* London: Mencap National Centre.

British Paediatric Association (1980) Guidelines to aid ethical committees considering research involving children. *Archives of Diseases in Children* 55, 75–77.

Burke S., Graeme French H., Roberts J., Johnstone C., Whitecloud T. & Edmund J. (1985) Chronic atlanto-axial instability in Down's syndrome. *Journal of Bone and Joint Surgery* 6, 1356–60.

Cipriano R. E. (1980) *Reading in Special Olympics.* Connecticut: Special Learning Corporation.

Committee on Sports Medicine (1984) Atlanto-axial instability in Down's syndrome. *Paediatrics* 74 (1), 152–3.

Connolly, K. J. (1984) The assessment of motor performance in children. In *Malnutrition and Behaviour: Critical Assessment of Key Issues*, ed. J. Biozek & B. Schurch. Lausanne, Switzerland: Nestlé Foundation.

Faden R. R. & Beauchamp T. L. (1986) *A History and Theory of Informed Consent.* New York: Oxford University Press.

Fraser W. I. & Stuart R. A. (1987) Exercise and sport for mentally handicapped people. In *Exercise — Benefits, Limits and Adaptations*, ed. D. Macleod, R. Maughan, M.

Nimmo, T. Reilly & C. Williams. London: E. & F.N. Spon.

Gallanaugh S.C. (1985) *British Medical Journal* **291**, 116.

Gillick v. *West Norfolk and Wisbech AHA* [1985] 1 All ER 533.

Gunn M. (1985) The law and mental handicap. *Mental Handicap* **13**, 70–2.

Hayden F.J. (1974) Physical education and sport. In *Mental Retardation and Developmental Disabilities*, ed. J. Wortis. New York: Brunner, Mazel.

Howells G. (1989) Down's syndrome and the general practitioner. *Journal of the Royal College of General Practitioners* (in press).

Rarick G.L. (1978) The motor domain and its correlates. In *Educationally Handicapped Children*, ed. S. Lawrence, D. Rarick, A. Dobbins & D. Geoffrey. Broadhead, Englewood Cliff: Prentice-Hall.

Royal College of Physicians (1986) Research on healthy volunteers. *Journal of the Royal College of Physicians of London* **20** (4).

Tilley A. (1986) Physical fitness assessment of British Columbia Special Olympic Athletes. University of British Columbia. Cited by G. Zitnay. Washington: Kennedy Institute.

Tishler J. & Martell W. (1965) Dislocation of the Atlas in Mongolism: a preliminary report. *Radiology* **84**, 904–6.

Vermeer A. (1985) Sport for the mentally handicapped and Wolfensberger's concept of social role valorisation. Paper presented at the International Association for the Scientific Study of Mental Deficiency, New Delhi.

Wolfensberger, W. (1983) Social role valorisation: a proposed new term for the principle of normalisation. *Mental Retardation* **21**, 234–9.

11 Athletes at an overseas venue: the role of the team doctor

M. BOTTOMLEY

'"What matters it how far we go"
his scaly friend replied,
"there is another shore you know
upon the other side.
The further off from England,
the nearer is to France.
Then turn not pale beloved snail
but come and join the dance"'
From *Alice in Wonderland* by Lewis Caroll

It is a great privilege to be asked to be a team doctor whether it be for the local Rugby club or an Olympic team. As part of an international team one is also entrusted with a considerable responsibility, not only to keep the athletes going, but also to protect them against long-term harm that could, amongst other considerations, involve large sums of money in terms of potential earnings and sponsor's investment.*

*The doctor's responsibility is, however, primarily towards the individual team member as his 'patient'.

Sports Medicine is a speciality. There are now two Diploma examinations in the subject, that of the London Hospital being preceded by an academic year of full-time study, whilst the Diploma of the Society of Apothecaries can be taken following one of several part-time courses. Other Diploma examinations and courses are in the planning stage. Few official team Medical Officers are qualified in this way. Most have their grounding in the British Association of Sport and Medicine's one week residential introductory and advanced courses.* This may be topped up by attending such lectures and short courses as may crop up locally, together with reading articles and the few available textbooks. It is important to be interested in the problems peculiar to sport and to have a very real sympathy with the aims of the athlete. School or university doctors often develop an interest as an inevitable part of their job; others may have enjoyed success in sport themselves and have a particular empathy with sporting patients.

There is no career structure in sports medicine. For most it is a 'hobby' which just about pays for itself through sports injury clinics

*Further details about these courses can be obtained from the Education Officer, British Association of Sport and Medicine, c/o the London Sports Medicine Institute, St Bartholomew's Hospital, Charterhouse Square, London EC1M 6BQ.

159
*Chapter 11
Athletes at an
overseas venue:
the role of the
team doctor*

or, rarely, through a retainer paid by a club. Team doctors are not paid. Whilst it is true that reasonable expenses are claimable and all fares and accommodation are provided, most team doctors find that, in the long run, they are out of pocket. Absence from professional practice for prolonged periods of time during major championships is an inevitable demand which will draw heavily on holiday entitlement. Colleagues' co-operation to provide cover is an essential requirement. Drugs and treatments can be claimed as expenses, but more often than not it is the practice drug cupboard or the hospital that replenishes the team doctor's bag.

The team doctor, having been invited by the club or governing body of the sport in question, is acting as an agent of that club or body. There is no formal contract. The British Amateur Athletic Board, to which the author is a medical officer, relies largely on the goodwill of its medical officers, who are regarded as team officials. As such, they are covered by insurance for both personal ill health and for loss of personal property whilst abroad.

Athletes are very mobile people in many senses of the word, often competing and training all over Europe, if not the world. They are therefore exposed to a wide variety of medical opinion and will tend to seek out doctors whom they perceive as sympathetic to their needs, often being prepared to travel considerable distances. At every competition the organisers will have provided local medical and physiotherapy cover; at major competitions this may be supplemented by medical or paramedical services provided by equipment firms. Since the official team doctor is taken only on international representative trips and since there is no central system of record keeping, the medical care of athletes is likely to be haphazard and fragmentary.

The team doctor's role

The team doctor's job begins well before a trip. Although some of the team may be seasoned travellers there may well be others who are going abroad for the first time. Some kind of preparatory advice is always useful, both to remind the experienced and to inform the innocent.

The extent of the advice depends very much on the venue, but if travelling outside Europe recommendations on preparatory inoculations,[*] comfortable aircraft travel and minimising the effects of jet lag should be offered. Some advice on food hygiene may be appropriate as well as any special risks there may be in the area,

---

[*] Advice on inoculations is published regularly in various medical newspapers, notably *Pulse*, and in the DH booklets SA40 and SA41. Further information is in the book *Traveller's Health* by Richard Dawood, published by Oxford University Press. Specific advice on malaria requirements is obtainable from: 01–637 7921 (taped message, 24-hour service) or 01–637 0248 (Egypt, Morocco and Turkey only).

160

*Chapter 11
Athletes at an
overseas venue:
the role of the
team doctor*

e.g. rabies. Many athletes like to jog as part of their preparation and runners seem to have a magnetic attraction for dogs.

Weather and insect pests may be important. The athlete will probably have been briefed by his coach about climate, heat and humidity, but the doctor should be prepared to deal with any problems that may arise. If conditions are anticipated to be extreme it is hoped that the athlete has a chance to acclimatise.

A reminder about AIDS is not inappropriate in a situation where healthy young men and women from all parts of the world come together in an atmosphere of instant camaraderie (see Chapter 5).

Travelling as part of a large group will present logistic and organisational problems. The team doctor is always appreciated that bit more if he or she is willing to help. Such things as sorting out tickets, labelling luggage and negotiating with airline staff as to how the vaulters' poles can be handled or whether a javelin constitutes an offensive weapon are an inevitable part of any journey.

You may prefer to keep your medical bag as hand luggage or it may go into the hold. However, it is always as well to have some simple remedies to hand. The travel-sick may not have their favourite treatment, or the dysmenorrhoeic their pain-killer. Travel breeds headache and sleeplessness. Some paracetamol and a short-acting mild sedative* are therefore useful. It is important to ensure that your medical kit is available at times when it is required. You do tend to feel a bit inadequate if you have to confess that all your medical kit is locked away in the bowels of the aircraft.

*Opinions vary, but the author finds that temazepam is satisfactory; it is available as a 10 mg capsule. Loprazolam, lormetazepam and triazolam are similarly acting drugs.

Athletes are notoriously conservative about their diet and many will reject the very different foods that they are offered in, say, eastern Europe or Japan. Team doctors may well find that they are having to negotiate to try and provide more familiar foods and may even need to forage the local supermarket for supplies.

The team doctor is there to be available. It may at times seem that athletes are unreasonably demanding in their needs. If they want treatment, for whatever reason, they want it then and there so that their preparation schedule is not interrupted. In the opinion of the author, a competitor who has spent months or years training for an event does have a right to unlimited access to the team medical officer for treatment. It is important, therefore, that the team knows where you are at all times.

It is important also to remain 'one of the team' and thus it is essential not to appear aloof whilst at the same time maintaining professional detachment.

Accommodation overseas varies considerably. For the most part teams stay in good-quality hotels, which, at the more important events, may be designated as the competition village. For events such as the Olympics the accommodation may be purpose-built and used subsequently as housing stock for the host city.

It is unusual to have a separate treatment room where you are staying; neither is any equipment supplied. Your bed, or even, occasionally, the vanitory unit top, provides an examination or treatment couch. At major international events there may well be a medical centre in the village, which is usually staffed by the host country.

The organising committee will have made some provisions for medical care at the track, but it can be very variable, ranging from a couch in the corner of the dressing-room to a fully manned medical centre. Apart from the highly prestigious events, it is unusual to have any prior information as to what is available, so that a preliminary inspection of the arena is worth while. Even then it is unlikely that any responsible official will be available for advice so that the medical officer may have to wait until the technical meeting held by officials before the event to find out what medical facilities there are.

Ideally the organisers should have provided a track clearance team to transfer an injured athlete to the medical centre. An ambulance should also be available for evacuation to hospital where appropriate. The medical officer should know where the nearest hospital is and the facilities that they offer. In Japan, for instance, there can be difficulty in obtaining treatment at certain hospitals as a foreigner; it is necessary for the medical officer to be aware of the local rules. It is therefore important also to know where in the stadium the nearest phone is and how to use it, and to have some local currency handy.

At the best of times consultations will be relatively informal — in the hotel bedroom or a medical room at the stadium. Frequently, however, they can take place at the track side, in the bar or on the coach. Whilst it is generally better if privacy can be provided, one often finds in the gregarious atmosphere of a team that the patients are quite happy to be seen and treated in the midst of a crowd. This cannot always be taken for granted, however, and an alert eye must be kept open for those who really do prefer some privacy.

Athletes in general are a healthy group of people, but they are just as liable to minor illness as anyone else, and, indeed, may be more at risk than normally through being away from their normal environment. Certain more chronic diseases are not incompatible with sport at the highest level and athletes may be asthmatic, diabetic or even epileptic.

The health problems are mainly those familiar to any GP and the medical bag should reflect this. One important consideration is, however, that international athletes are subject to strict rules limiting the treatments they may have. The logic of these rules is not always immediately obvious but nevertheless the team medical officer should be totally familiar with the list of banned substances laid down by the sports governing body. In terms of day-to-day treatment, that principally means ephedrine and its derivatives, together

161

Chapter 11
Athletes at an
overseas venue:
the role of the
team doctor

162

Chapter 11
Athletes at an
overseas venue:
the role of the
team doctor

with codeine and caffeine, all present in many cold cures and pain-killers. Since these are sold widely over the counter the team doctor should insist that the athletes declare any treatments that they are having or have recently had.

There are, of course, problems related directly to sport. Injuries are common, but most of these are of a minor nature and affect soft tissues, often not amounting to more than localised stiffness. Whilst these injuries would pass unnoticed in the average individual, to an athlete performing at maximum physical effort they represent a source of serious anxiety or may even cause actual inhibition of function.

The physiotherapist is often the hardest-worked member of the team but simple massage should be well within the capabilities of the team doctor and it allows the physiotherapist to get on with more specialised treatments. The 'hands-on' experience is useful in many ways. Apart from the obvious relief to the athlete, it gives the doctor a real appreciation of what the athlete means when he describes a tight spot in a muscle. Often one can feel it relax as treatment is applied. It also helps in getting to know the athlete. The physiotherapy room often seems to be a social centre and chatting to the patients during treatment helps them to relax. A knowledge of some simple strapping techniques can also be useful.

Treatment is not necessarily aimed at helping the athlete to continue. There are certain situations where continued competiton will make matters worse. It is something that ought to be discussed with the athlete and perhaps also with the coach and team manager. The ultimate choice has to be that of the athlete, but the doctor should never be persuaded into treatment that allows the athlete to compete at the risk of worsening his or her condition. My own feeling is that local anaesthetics and local steroid injections are, as a general rule, best left at home, particularly as far as short trips are concerned.

The treatment that is given for anything other than minor problems may be looked on as 'first aid'. The aims of treatment are to prevent the condition getting worse and to establish a solid base for rehabilitation. Whilst in general terms rehabilitation is going to be along predictable lines, it is not fair on your colleagues who are going to do most of the work in getting the athlete better to commit them too specifically to a particular treatment.

Keeping comprehensive records is not easy. It is important, though, that you keep a record of your own management. This should include every patient that you see, which may include athletes of other countries who seek your help, since not all teams bring their own doctor. No standard form of record is available and it is probably easier to keep a diary or daybook from which information can be transferred to a more formal file if you wish. There are signs that, in the increasingly professional world of sport, medico-legal problems are cropping up and, without a record of your management, your position might be difficult to defend.*

One solution that has been suggested to the vexed problem of keeping a comprehensive record is that athletes are given their own case notes which they produce every time they are treated. Unless each doctor or physiotherapist keeps a duplicate of his or her own notes that would create enormous difficulties in the event of any dispute over treatment. A central record, held by the governing body, with appropriate notes being carried to a meeting and returned by a responsible official would be more satisfactory, but would involve considerable administrative costs.

163

*Chapter 11
Athletes at an
overseas venue:
the role of the
team doctor*

The professional relationship that exists between the team doctor and the athletes is akin to that of a factory medical officer* and its employees, although, when abroad, the function is extended since the doctor also has to act as the 'GP'. One of the problems in dealing with athletes is that doctors in general have a poor reputation in the treatment of sports-related problems. Many colleagues still take the view that they are self-limiting disorders that will eventually heal if they are not further provoked. Not only is this untrue but totally neglects the athlete's need for a speedy and total recovery.

*This being the case, the team doctor ought, in theory at least, to correspond with the athlete's own GP on returning home, notifying any treatment given, etc.

Referral of an injured athlete after a competition therefore raises a number of ethical problems. Advice to return to his or her own GP may well be rejected and ignored. If specialist help is necessary the GP may not know of an appropriate opinion. Physiotherapy is a vital ingredient in rehabilitation but by no means every physiotherapist is equipped to deal with the particular problems arising from sport.

The world of sports medicine is relatively small and those who work in it are generally known to each other and to the athletes. It is therefore likely that many athletes will refer themselves to an appropriate opinion, with or without the collusion of the team doctor, and the GP may well be bypassed. One of the great strengths of our system of medical care is that the GP remains at the heart of management and that specialists on the whole insist on GP referral whether it be through the NHS or privately. It is a great pity that the treatment of athletes undermines this principle but until sports medicine achieves a legitimate status this untidy situation is likely to persist.

The team doctor's bag is as idiosyncratic as general practice. In addition to emergency treatments for conditions like asthma, diabetes, severe pain or anaphylaxis it is useful to be able to deal with

*The Medical Protection Society provides legal advice and the opportunity to apply for indemnity against professional negligence for doctors all parts of the world except USA and Canada. When visiting North American or Canada, therefore, it would be prudent to establish with the organisers beforehand the extent of the legal cover which they would be prepared to provide.

164

*Chapter 11
Athletes at an
overseas venue:
the role of the
team doctor*

some of the simpler problems. The common cold, hay fever, indigestion, gastroenteritis, ear infections, cuts, blisters and bruises are all as common in athletes as in any other section of the population. In some countries insect bites can be a major problem, both from the irritation they cause and because of the risk of infection, so that some repellent cream and/or sprays may be helpful. If one sees simple physiotherapy as part of one's role, an assortment of strappings and various 'rubs' will also be useful.

The bag may well contain certain controlled drugs, such as pethidine. A Home Office licence, valid for the appropriate period, should be obtained before taking such drugs abroad in order to satisfy HM Customs, and clearance should be obtained in advance from the embassies of the countries to be visited. In practice customs officials tend to be tolerant towards teams and team doctors, which obviously implies a trust, and that should not be abused. Host countries usually provide someone to meet the team and guide them through the official channels. At large events the immigration and customs officials will often provide special clearance channels for the teams.

Particularly when visiting unfamiliar countries the author's own practice is to make a point of declaring the medical supplies carried. So far, over a period of ten years, bags have not been searched. It is nevertheless a good idea to have a list of the contents available to show to customs officers if necessary.

Athletic events are usually held in towns rather than villages and one can usually rely on there being somewhere locally to obtain medical supplies. It may be a salutary lesson as to how much drugs actually cost. It may be helpful to carry some form of proof of identity and also of medical qualification. It is also useful to carry a *National Formulary* since the brand name of many drugs varies from country to country and the generic name may be easier to identify.

All major competitions require selected athletes to provide a specimen of urine for testing for banned substances. One of the functions of a team doctor is to accompany the athlete through the procedure. The doctor is not just there for moral support but also as an observer to ensure that the test is properly explained to the athlete and properly carried out. It is at this point that the doctor can make sure that any drugs and their dosage taken by the athlete for treatment are declared. In the event of a subsequent disagreement, and in some countries athletes found positive have disputed the matter in court, the doctor could be a material witness.

Conclusions and recommendations

The successful team doctor must have the capacity to come out from behind his or her desk, and be able to deal sympathetically

165

*Chapter 11
Athletes at an
overseas venue:
the role of the
team doctor*

with a collection of individuals, all of whom have extremely strong personalities and who are, in various ways, fired up to a considerable degree. The multiple roles of physician, surgeon, occupational health adviser, counsellor, dietician and masseur/masseuse are largely familiar to a family doctor.

Away from familiar surroundings it is harder to practise the same high standards of professionalism as at home, but maintenance of standards is, if anything, even more important away from home. The present equivocal status of sports medicine in this country, together with the peripatetic habits of athletes, has led to different ethical standards in terms of referral, either back to the GP or on to the specialist.

There is no question that high levels of physical activity lead to physiological changes and patterns of illness and injury that are unfamiliar in the general practice of medicine. Sports medicine is a speciality. It is to be hoped that its present struggles lead it to a mature status where it is recognised as a speciality in its own right and can fit into the conventional framework of medicine. Until then the present unsatisfactory state, where athletes' medical care is fragmentary, uncoordinated and, unfortunately, sometimes contradictory, will continue.

Medical records are a vital part of satisfactory care. It is difficult away from the convenience of secretaries and a regular orderly existence to exercise the necessary discipline to keep proper records, but this effort must be made.

It is perhaps time that some attempt was made by the sports governing bodies to set up a central system of record-keeping. A medical records clerk with computer aid could easily maintain a file to which access would be given to certain authorised doctors, which would include the athletes own GPs. A print-out for each athlete in the team would be given to the team doctor and returned to the central file with any new information.* Athletes would be encouraged to notify the governing body whenever they received treatment, perhaps by means of a personal log-book into which any treating doctor would make an entry and which would be reviewed by the medical record clerk at regular intervals. There is no reason why confidentiality should be sacrificed.

To be asked to be a team doctor is a privilege; it is also great fun. Away from your protective, and perhaps inhibiting, screen of receptionists, nurses and the general environment of surgery or clinic, you are accepted as a friend as much as a doctor. It is a friendship that can, in time, cover the world.

---

*Such a system might be of considerable benefit to individual athletes, but could only function with their informed consent. Subject to the provisions of the Data Protection Act, the information contained about an individual on computerised records would have to be available to that individual on demand.

12 GP (primary care) sports clinics: benefits for patients and hazards to practitioners

P. L. THOMAS

'Myself when young did eagerly frequent
Doctor and Saint and heard great argument
About it and about: but ever more
Came out by the same door as in I went'
From the *Rubaiyat* by Omar Khayyam

'Injuries for all'

As leisure time increases with the increasing affluence of society the time spent taking part in sport also rises. The variety and complexity of sport generally available for the adult population has also grown.

With the increase in numbers participating in sport it follows that more sports injuries occur. Furthermore, the more an individual trains the greater is the likelihood of an injury being sustained.

Fortunately not all the results of increased sporting activities are detrimental and it is readily accepted that exercise, when taken regularly at a level to which an individual is accustomed, produces a beneficial effect on mental and physical well-being. It has been shown that women have healthier pregnancies with fewer complications and healthier babies if they take exercise regularly through pregnancy.

The injuries that do occur in the context of sport are no different from the ordinary soft tissue injuries which occur from other causes involving trauma, but each sport produces its own pattern of injuries. Just as the market-gardener may sustain 'brussel sprout wrist', the oarsman or oarswoman may develop tenosynovitis in the wrist extensors through inappropriate techniques, faulty equipment, exercising in cold weather or performing a training load to which he or she is not accustomed.

In the UK there is an increasing need for facilities which would provide a quick efficient service for sports men and women to enable them to receive appropriate advice, treatment and rehabilitation from a sympathetic clinician or therapist. While the National Health Service provides an excellent service for major injuries it is not always so well geared to provide such a comprehensive service for injuries which may not produce major morbidity but which may interfere with training and competition, and thus are of paramount importance to the athlete.

Provision of treatment facilities

There exist in the UK at present various levels of health care for injured sports people.

Untrained lay men and women assist at club level and, although possibly not qualified, may be known as the club physiotherapist. These individuals may be able to provide useful help in the treatment of minor self-limiting injuries.

Trained 'chartered' physiotherapists, who may work with a club or have a physiotherapy practice where injured athletes may be referred for treatment and advice, form a second layer of professional health care for injured sports men and women. Physiotherapists are encouraged not to attempt diagnosis or treatment without prior reference to a doctor. They receive appropriate training, however, and are well able to cope with many moderately severe sports injuries.

There now exist certain sports injury clinics, where patients are seen and assessed by a doctor with additional treatment facilities being provided by a chartered physiotherapist. These clinics may be referred to as 'primary care' sports clinics. The doctors are often general practitioners but do benefit from further training in sports medicine. The doctors and physiotherapists work as a team and should be able to cope with most sports medical problems and sports injuries which do not require referral for specialist treatment.

Referral centres for specialist problems exist as a hospital-based sports injury clinic, usually run by a hospital consultant with full and immediate access to back-up facilities for further investigations and operative procedures. It is, however, an unfortunate fact of life that the waiting lists for treatment of 'minor orthopaedic problems' may be unacceptably long for the athlete to wait for treatment. In these circumstances, unfortunately the only current alternative for the great majority of athletes is for them to seek treatment in a privately run hospital clinic.

A few clinics exist in the country where the athlete can not only receive advice, treatment and rehabilitation for injuries sustained but also have a full physiological profile undertaken on the same premises. The cost of equipping these specialist centres is very high and as a result the cost for the athlete may be prohibitive unless sponsored by the national governing body of a sport or by a professional club.

Primary care sports injury clinics

The scope of this chapter is to deal with the primary care sports injury clinics, where each patient is first seen by a doctor, with additional treatment provided by a chartered physiotherapist if this is required.

Objective

The aims of a primary care sports injury or sports medicine clinic must be to provide a service to the athlete which is accessible, produces a rapid recovery to full training or competition and is a service which he or she can afford.

Premises

The clinic will, of course, require premises from which to operate. It will need one or more doctors who have an interest in and an understanding of sports people's problems, in addition to one or more chartered physiotherapists who must also share the same interest and understanding. Equipment for diagnosis, treatment and ongoing rehabilitation will be required. All this costs money, and finance for the initial setting up of a clinic will have to be found, together with ways and means of maintaining the ongoing running costs.

It is unlikely that the Health Service will provide accommodation for a clinic as part of the NHS facilities although there are some clinics in the country which have been able to negotiate with a hospital for the use of their physiotherapy premises outside normal working hours, on agreed terms.

Sports and leisure centres are increasingly keen and willing to provide space for such clinics, either rent-free (as part of the service they provide to their clients), or at a rental which may or may not be fixed at a commercial rate. Other clinics have opened using the existing premises of a private physiotherapy clinic, or operating from one of the independent hospitals.

Staffing

Although it is possible to run a clinic single-handed, the author believes it to be preferable to have at least two doctors involved, so that holidays, study leave and illness are covered. Likewise, two or more physiotherapists are required if patients are to be treated promptly following consultation with the doctor. Alternatively an appointment system may be used, enabling a single physiotherapist to cope with the workload. The British Association of Sport and Medicine maintains a membership list of doctors and physiotherapists with an interest in sports medicine, and the Association of Chartered Physiotherapists in Sports Medicine also have a register. If difficulty arises in finding suitable physiotherapists, an advertisement placed in the *Physiotherapy Journal* will almost certainly produce a response from interested parties.

Equipment

The diagnostic equipment needed for the doctor need not involve a great deal of expense. An examination couch is of course essential, but most of the other equipment will usually be found in the general practitioner's emergency bag. The physiotherapist will require plinths, together with adequate floor space and mats. Weights, either free or fixed, are needed, together with wobble-boards for proprioceptive exercises. When starting up a clinic it is not absolutely necessary to purchase all the electromedical modalities of therapy available but an ultrasound machine for each physiotherapist would certainly be a priority. Strapping and tape and bandages should be available, and may be required in a number of patients in the first 48 hours following injury.

Costs

It is possible to set up a sports medicine clinic relatively inexpensively. Approximately £2000–3000 should be more than enough to cover the initial outlay. If the clinic is to be set up within a sports centre, the centre itself may fund the entire scheme and purchase the equipment which will be required by the doctors and physiotherapists. Likewise if the clinic were to be run from a private hospital it would seem probable that the company running the hospital would equip the clinic to the specifications of the staff who were going to work within it. The National Health Service is unlikely to provide any help unless you are fortunate enough to be allowed to use a physiotherapy department for either a nominal charge or an economic rent.

Fees

Staff involved in the running of the clinic, whether doctors, physiotherapists or receptionists, will naturally expect to receive renumeration for work undertaken. The daily running will have to be funded by the user, the injured athlete. As more clinics open up throughout the country it seems to have become more acceptable to the sports men and women themselves to pay for the advice and treatment they receive. Many people still except a free service, however, doubtless due to the fact that they have never had to pay for any medical service, other than dental or optical, within the context of the National Health Service.

The clinic launched and run by the author charges a set fee for a consultation with the doctor and a further fee to see the physiotherapist. The doctor and physiotherapist are paid a set percentage of the fees collected. The remainder goes towards the running costs of the clinic. In other clinics the medical staff may wish to receive a fixed sessional fee for working at the sports clinic or receive payments based on the number of patients that are seen depending on how the clinic is managed. If an independent hospital or large sports centre owns the clinic then the first alternative may be more appropriate but if the medical staff themselves are managing the running of the clinic the latter alternative is probably the more appropriate. If no patients attend, no expenses are incurred.

Running the clinic

At our clinic new patients are able to attend on two evenings per week and follow-up patients may attend on three nights. The clinic operates an open-access system with the agreement of the Local Medical Committee. Details of the scheme were submitted for their approval before the clinic opened.* The Committee were reassured that the patients' general practitioners would receive written notification of the consultations and recommended treatment regimes. The clinic has now been running for eight years and we have received no adverse comments regarding the system, even though, generally speaking, most doctors do not expect their patients to seek advice from us without being referred by themselves.

In our experience the doctor at the clinic is able to deal with 20% of the new cases without referring them on to the physiotherapists. Of the new patients, 50% only attend for one session, reflecting the nature of the clinic. The patients are given a diagnosis and receive advice on training, techniques and equipment, together with a programme of exercises which they can do at home, at the training venue, at school or at their place of work.

By holding the clinics in the evening both staff and patients are able to give and receive treatments without major interference to their normal work necessitating time lost in employment. By running an open-access system we are able to see patients quickly after an injury without them first having to go to their general practitioners and then having to rely on the vagaries of a waiting-list with subsequent further delays. The athlete is able to receive advice and treatment at the most crucial time within three to four days of the initial injury. Not by any means are all the cases seen in the clinic acute injuries and as the public becomes better informed of the treatment that we offer so the relative number of more chronic injuries seen in the clinic increases.

Records

Our sports injury clinic has made two changes in the medical record forms used so that information concerning types of injury, training

---

* Normally patients attending 'specialist' clinics (other than for sexually transmitted diseases) should have been referred by their GP. Failure to observe this rule could lead to accusations of unethical conduct. By notifying the LMC of the system and the patients' own GPs of the self-referral, however, the GP-run sports clinic should be able to demonstrate that it is not attempting to canvass for patients from neighbouring practices.

loads, age, sex and level of achievement can be reviewed at the end of the year. It is time-consuming going through each card by hand. Computerisation may in future assist in increasing the efficiency of record-keeping and also help with research.

The medical records have all been kept since the opening of our clinic some eight years ago, but only the three preceding years' notes are readily available in the filing cabinets with the receptionist. By allowing the patients to see and read their own records we can simplify the procedures for passing them on from receptionist to doctor and from doctor to physiotherapist via the patients themselves.*

Team approach

It is important that the sports clinic should have regular meetings for all the staff so that they can exchange information and ideas on who best to advise and treat the athletes. It is crucial that the staff work as a team, which includes doctors, physiotherapists and other therapists such as chiropodists and podiatrists, so that they can put forward a consistent approach to their patients. Many sports clinics are held during the evenings or at weekends and often involve considerable numbers of different personnel on a roster basis. A patient may therefore be treated by more than one therapist on successive consultations and it helps if the clinic has an agreed mode of practice for given types of injuries.

Further investigations

We are careful to refer back to their own general practitioners any patients whom we feel have attended with conditions inappropriate to the sports injury clinic.

Thus the need for laboratory investigations does not usually arise. X-ray investigations are, however, often necessary and we are fortunate in our area that we have open access to the X-ray departments in the local hospital. A patient is able to go directly to the X-ray department at a designated time with a referral card. The results are then sent back to the referring doctor at our clinic. The patients are now billed by the NHS X-ray department for the X-rays that have been taken.†

* Although it may be considered good practice to allow patients to have sight of their treatment records it should be remembered that the patient has no automatic right of access (unless the information is held on computer records). This is usually only of importance where the patient seeks redress for treatment perceived to be substandard — that is to say where medical negligence is alleged on the part of the doctor. In such circumstances the medical practitioner is advised to contact his protection organisation.

† It should be noted that, although such an arrangement is permissible by current standards of medical practice in the UK, there is no obligation for the local NHS hospital to release the X-rays to the clinic. Indeed, the hospital having been referred the 'patient' is under a legal obligation to 'provide all necessary medical cover'. Failure to diagnose and treat the patient adequately in these circumstances could therefore result in liability attaching to the Health Authority on behalf of its staff.

It is advisable, therefore, for those practitioners who wish to set up an 'X-ray service' for their sports injury patients at a local NHS hospital to make the necessary arrangements with the radiology department beforehand so that, ideally, films may be reported properly, and the patient referred back to the clinic — if possible with their films — for the appropriate treatment.

Prescribing

It is unusual for the patients seen in our clinic to require medication. By the time the patients present themselves the need for a short course of anti-inflammatory drugs has usually passed. If, however, they do require to have a course of anti-inflammatory pills we either give them a small quantity from supplies that we hold in stock or alternatively write out a private prescription. If any patients require longer-term medication we usually refer them back to their general practitioners so that they can undertake their patients' long-term care. In approximately 3% of the cases we will use injectable corticosteroids with or without local anaesthetics; the drugs themselves are paid for either by the patient or from the running costs of the clinic.

Referral

When a patient requires referral for specialist attention, for example if we have diagnosed a meniscus lesion in a knee, we write to the patient's general practitioner suggesting that he or she might consider referring them on for a consultant opinion.

More recently we have referred patients directly to consultants if they are going to be seen privately and have informed the general practitioner of our decision.*

Public awareness

One of the main drawbacks to starting up a new clinic arises from the problems associated with letting the lay person know that a clinic exists. In our case the local borough council encouraged us to start a clinic as did the Regional Sports Council.† The opening

---

*Either of these courses of action should be acceptable for most types of condition seen in the sports clinic. The former is the counsel of perfection but could be regarded as unnecessarily cumbersome for minor ailments. If the medical problem involved is more major, however, it would be wiser to err on the side of caution and refer the patient via his usual medical attendant, who will have had the benefit of the complete past history of the patient.

†Under the present GMC guidelines care must be exercised in any publicity used to attract patients. Paragraph 63 of the General Medical Councils' *Blue Book* ('Professional conduct and discipline; fitness to practice') states: 'Canvassing by a doctor for the purpose of obtaining patients, whether the doctor does this directly or through an agent or is associated with or employed by persons or organisations which canvass, is unethical and may lead to a charge of serious professional misconduct. The distribution of advertising material to members of the public, or advertising in the press or other media, with the intention of attracting prospective patients to a particular doctor or service, may be construed as canvassing on the part of the doctor or doctors to whose practice patients may be referred, or refer themselves, as a result of such canvassing.' Such constraints may be thought to be unnecessarily restrictive and perhaps even 'unfair'. They do, however, remain the guidelines in effect for the time being. Ethical guidelines relating to the acceptability of advertising for dentists have recently undergone radical change, and it may be that the same will occur for medical practice in the near future.

created a considerable amount of local interest and the local radio and television stations reported the opening of the clinic, as did the local press. As a result, within a few nights we had up to sixty people attending per night — which completely overwhelmed the staff. After the initial surge of interest we were left with the problem of maintaining a level of public awareness of our existance. Physiotherapists are now allowed to advertise but not able to claim any particular skill or expertise or to have any claims on special equipment. They are also able to notify local sports clubs and leisure centres of their times of opening and their charges. Doctors, however, remain constrained by the GMC from letting the public know of the existence of a clinic, even though many people ask why we cannot let them know where we are, our times of opening and our charges, etc. It seems unfair that private organisations such as BUPA hospitals or the AMI hospitals, some of whom run clinics and employ doctors, are allowed to advertise. The author believes we do a disservice to the public by not being allowed to advertise in the light of the fact that no such constraint is put on lay people who run so-called sports clinics or sports medicine clinics.

Chiropractors, non-medically qualified osteopaths and unregistered chiropodists have set themselves up and freely advertise in sports magazines and the local papers. It is only natural for the public to go to seek the opinion of these people when no choice of an alternative clinic with qualified staff is obviously available to them. Many of us with an interest in sports medicine would like at least to have the freedom to let people know we exist, where to find our clinics, at what times of the day we are open and what they can expect to pay. The Regional Sports Council has produced leaflets for clubs about our clinic, with none of the names of staff being mentioned, but whether this is acceptable in the eyes of the General Medical Council and ethically acceptable remains unclear.

The Sports Council of Great Britain, a Government-funded organisation, is keen to see more sports clinics set up, as they recognise that the National Health Service cannot and is unlikely to provide these kinds of facilities. The Sports Council also publishes details of all the clinics that it is aware of.

Postgraduate training

At present the training that doctors receive, both at medical school and as postgraduates, for the diagnosis and treatment of soft tissue injuries is inadequate. For example, few newly qualified doctors know the correct way to examine a shoulder joint or knee joint. There are ways in which a young doctor can receive further training in sports medicine but few courses are run by the National Health Service.

As a foundaton for the aspiring doctor a sound knowledge and understanding of soft tissue and orthopaedic medicine is essential. The Cyriax Foundation runs part-time and full-time courses of education on the subject. The Institute of Orthopaedic Medicine runs similar courses.

The London Hospital runs a three-term diploma course in sports medicine but the cost runs into several thousand pounds for tuition alone. Bursaries are available and further details of both the course and the bursaries are available from the Administrator to the Sports Medicine Course at the London Hospital Medical School.

The British Association of Sport and Medicine runs a one-week introductory course each year. At present the courses are held at the Lilleshall Hall National Sports Centre in Shropshire and details of the courses can be obtained by writing to the Education Officer, British Association of Sport and Medicine, c/o The London Sports Medicine Institute at St Bartholomew's Hospital in London. The British Association of Sport and Medicine is open to any under-graduate or graduate of medicine and publishes a journal four times a year. The journal publishes details of all the courses mentioned.

Although attending one of the courses will enable the physician to gain further knowledge in sports medicine, practical experience can be gained by an individual making enquiries with their local sports injury clinic or by offering their services to a local sports club or team. Most clubs are only too willing to accept the offer of help from an enthusiastic doctor and the experience gained will help if he or she has ambitions of looking after one of the national teams.

School sports day: medico-legal hazards for the school doctor 13

R. N. PALMER

'The better part of valour is discretion'
From *Henry IV* Part I by William Shakespeare

Mixed emotions are likely to be felt by the doctor who is approached to act as medical officer to the school sports day. The request may be posed quite casually and accepted with alacrity before the full implications sink in.

However casual the approach and whether or not some fee or other remuneration is offered, the doctor who accepts the invitation will, in law, be expected to perform his tasks with a reasonable standard of care. It is most unlikely that any formal contractual relationship will exist between the doctor and the school and even less likely that any formal relationship will exist between the doctor, the pupils and their devoted parents. It is important that this should not lull the doctor into a false sense of well-being and security, for the law of negligence is likely to apply, rather than the law of contract, should the doctor's ministrations to an injured child later form the subject-matter of a legal dispute.

A doctor who holds himself out to a patient as possessing medical expertise will be expected to achieve a reasonable standard of care in the conduct and execution of his professional duties. The legal test (the 'Bolam' test) is that the practitioner should achieve that degree of skill and expertise which is reasonably to be expected of competent colleagues of similar training and experience. Make no mistake: however cosy the relationship between the doctor and the headmaster/headmistress, this will not be known to the parents and pupils, who will be expecting the highest standards of excellence.

If one holds oneself out as having some particular skill or expertise (whether neurosurgeon, radiotherapist, sports injury specialist, etc.), then the law will expect the practitioner to achieve the standard relevant to that class of specialists and not necessarily the standard to be expected of the generalist. In the context of a school sports day, it might still be acceptable to bring to the task the skill of an ordinary family doctor but at many sporting events these days there can be little doubt that the practitioner will be expected to have specialist skills and to be judged accordingly. Much may depend upon the advice he gives, especially where professional sport is concerned.

176

*Chapter 13
School sports day:
medico-legal
hazards for the
school doctor*

It is unlikely, perhaps, that the doctor at the school sports day will face any profound ethical dilemmas nor are legal considerations likely to weigh heavily upon his mind. However, at least in those schools which continue to encourage boxing tournaments, the practitioner may have an ethical dilemma in deciding whether to offer his services and, if so, on the extent to which he wishes to have a say in the pre-tournament assessment of the prospective pugilists (see Chapter 18).

On the legal front, the doctor must take care to ensure that he is not negligent in the execution of his duties. At a practical level this duty is likely to translate itself into a duty to cope competently with illness and injury but also into a requirement to ensure that damage is limited by restraining the endeavours of well-meaning but over-enthusiastic amateurs. The most obvious way in which this is achieved is to ensure that, in cases of neck and back injuries, care is taken to avoid spinal cord injury. Careful attention to positioning of the injured patient and/or adequate splintage will help to ensure that an injury is not turned inadvertently into a tragedy by injudicious handling which leads to spinal cord damage.

Perhaps the other main area in which the doctor can be of assistance on sports day is in being on hand to cope with the fathers' races. Some fathers in sedentary occupations have their arms twisted by school teaching staff to participate in sudden exertions which their cardiovascular system may be ill-equipped to withstand. It is therefore as well for the doctor to attend the sports day with his medical bag well equipped with his stock-in-trade for dealing with sudden collapses in mature adult patients.

The wise doctor will also take some steps to check the state of the first-aid room, or at least the first-aid box available on the sports ground. This is likely, at the best of times, to be hopelessly ill-equipped and not to have been inspected critically since the last sports day. It is as well to check in advance that some person is deputed to ensure that the first-aid box is adequately stocked with dressings, bandages, splints, etc. There can be few spectacles more forlorn than the doctor who is in attendance upon a sick or injured patient whilst in possession of an ill-stocked bag and no means of dealing with the crisis except to turn to the assembled company of parents and dignitaries to request some bandaging, handkerchief for epistaxis or sticking-plaster for a cut.

There is perhaps one exception to the proposition that the doctor's main duty is to prevent others from doing irretrievable harm to those who are injured. This is the genuine first-aider who has been properly trained; such a person may indeed be far better equipped than the intrepid practitioner to deal with injury and to offer first aid.

Finally, the object of this short chapter has been to point out that medico-legal hazards face those who undertake to supply medical advice and treatment to schools with special reference to their sports activity. A modicum of forethought and a few elementary precautions will, however, serve to ensure that the experience is indeed pleasant and enjoyable rather than a possible source of costly tragedy.

For further information on the wider responsibilities of the school doctor, see Chapter 1.

177
Chapter 13
School sports day:
medico-legal
hazards for the
school doctor

14 Dental and facial damage in sport: risk management for general dental practitioners

R. W. KENDRICK

'What a word has escaped the barrier of thy teeth'
From the *Iliad* by Homer

Sports giving rise to dental and facial damage

Almost all sport can give rise to damage to teeth, mouth and face, though some sports, such as rugby, hockey, cricket and horse-riding, have been shown to be associated with a relatively high incidence of these injuries.

Dental or facial damage can occur due to contact with a club or stick, a ball, especially a hard ball, or another player's boot, fist or head. However, review of the literature would show that even such non-contact sports as tennis and walking have resulted in dental and facial injuries. In swimming, injuries result mostly from slipping on wet surfaces, but injuries due to diving or swimming into obstacles also occur. In horse-riding, particularly severe injuries are often seen, and these usually occur following falls from the horse or as a result of horse-kick injury. Cycling accidents can also lead to facial injuries, although most of these are not in the context of cycling as a sport.

Compton & Tubbs (1977) found that 7% (2128 patients) of patients attending the Birmingham Accident Hospital had injuries which had occurred during sport. La Cava in 1964, studying insurance claims for sporting injuries, found an annual average of 1.7% (8896 from 511 309) of those insured making a claim. Kramer in 1941 (quoted by Gelbier in 1966) found, in a study of 11 500 high school athletes enrolled in an Athletics Accident Benefit Plan, that there were 691 (6%) injuries requiring professional attention. Of these 159 were dental injuries. This represents 23% of those injuries and 1.43% of the total enrolled. Studies of the aetiology of maxillofacial injuries presenting to specialist units show that sporting injuries account for a range of 1.5% to 16.5% (Rowe & Williams 1985).

It should be recognised that there will be regional variations in the type of sport giving rise to injury. For example, Gaelic games are only played to any great extent in Ireland, and games such as bandy are native to the Soviet Union and Northern European countries.

178

A number of general principles can be considered in relation to prevention of dental and facial damage in all sports, and these will be discussed under the three main headings of interception, prevention and treatment.

179

Chapter 14
Dental and facial
damage in sport

Interception

It is important to recognise that, as well as, trauma, dental disease can affect a sports man's or woman's performance. Appropriate dental treatment may reduce problems in this regard and also the possibility of traumatic injury.

Interceptive treatment could really be considered as promoting general dental health and is not necessarily specifically related to sporting injuries. In relation to trauma, however, the special vulnerability of the incisor teeth needs to be considered. It has been shown in surveys that the correlation between the frequency and severity of fractures and the degree of protrusion of the incisor teeth is more than due to chance. Therefore, at the appropriate age, over-prominent incisor teeth are better corrected orthodontically to move these to a position where they are less likely to be traumatised, especially for those intending to continue participation in contact sport.

All players should be dentally fit. Team doctors and coaches should try to ensure that the players appreciate the need for this, especially just prior to a major competition or travelling to foreign countries. The loss of a player through being unfit due to dental problems, either from decay, apical abscess or infection around a troublesome wisdom tooth, is usually an avoidable problem. Severe dental pain often disturbs sleep despite treatment with large doses of analgesics, and this combination of pain and sleep deprivation will reduce the quality of performance or even prevent participation. Spreading dental infection or the removal of some wisdom teeth may require hospitalisation and the administration of a general anaesthetic, producing the need for a period of recovery. Wisdom teeth should not be removed during acute infection and therefore practitioners should make appropriate arrangements for sports men and women who have had a past history of dental sepsis. In this way treatment can be planned to minimise interference with training and competition schedules. The players should be made aware that it is impossible to obtain dental fitness through last-minute dental attention. Dental health requires ongoing and repeated attention to potential and established dental problems.

Prevention

The adage 'prevention is better than cure' may be profitably applied to dental and facial injuries. Prevention of such injuries should

180

Chapter 14
Dental and facial
damage in sport

ideally involve the governing bodies of the various sports, as well as individuals, parents, teachers and coaches.

It has been shown that the incidence of dental injuries is related not only to the type of sport but also to the age of the participant, the incidence decreasing with increasing age. It has been suggested that a learning process may be responsible for this trend, especially in certain sports such as horse-riding, swimming and golf. It is therefore important that adequate supervision is available, particularly for the beginner, where the combination of youthful enthusiasm and inexperience presents the greatest risk.

In the prevention of dental and facial injuries the use of mouth-guards and face-masks has been shown to be effective.

The mouth-guard, mouth-protector or gum-shield is appropriate equipment to be worn by all players participating in contact sports, and is compulsory in American football and boxing. However, to be effective, a mouth-guard must fulfil certain criteria:

1   It must fit accurately and should occlude evenly with the lower teeth and not 'prop' the occlusion.
2   It should have sufficient retention not to drop out during play, with the mouth open or as a result of a tackle.
3   It must be comfortable.
4   It must allow for normal breathing and as normal speech as possible.
5   It should cover the attached mucoperiosteum but not impinge on the soft tissue reflections of the mouth.
6   It must be made of a sufficiently resilient material to absorb the forces applied in both vertical and horizontal directions.
7   It must be large enough not to be inhaled or swallowed.
8   It must be easily made at an economic cost.
9   It should be capable of being kept clean and hygienic, with a surface texture acceptable to the wearer.

There are two main forms of the mouth-guard, either the proprietary, over-the-counter type, or custom-made.

Proprietary mouth-guards may be a simple channel of a moderately flexible plastic which corresponds to the outline of the average dental arch. One of this type may be softened in hot water and adapted to conform to the subject's teeth. These adapt relatively poorly, however, and are not recommended. Other proprietary mouth-guards are modified by infilling or loading the channel with a silicone material which adapts closely to the teeth and soft tissue while in its viscous state. This then 'cures' to provide a material which helps to absorb the shock of a blow and to stabilise the mouth-guard to an acceptable degree. These are, however, not suitable for markedly irregular or protruding teeth.

The custom-made mouth-guard requires the services of a dental surgeon and a dental technician, as it is made to models of the subject's mouth and teeth. It is usually made out of a heat-cured

181

Chapter 14
Dental and facial
damage in sport

silicone rubber or sheets of polyvinyl–polyethylene plastic which are vacuum-formed to models of the mouth and teeth. They are suitable for all cases and fulfil all the above criteria, but are, of necessity, more expensive than proprietary mouth-guards.

Individuals who are fitted with crown and bridge work, especially in the anterior part of the mouth, should be advised to wear a mouth-guard in contact sport. Players who have removable appliances should be instructed to remove these. A mouth-guard for these players should be constructed to cover the edentulous areas and the remaining teeth.

During orthodontic treatment a looser-fitting mouth-guard may have to be accepted so as to avoid prevention of planned tooth movements, and also to circumvent the need for frequent remakes of the mouth-guard.

Mouth-guards not only prevent dental damage but also help to reduce the incidence of soft tissue injuries and fractured jaws. Davies *et al.* (1977), in their survey, found that 45% of club rugby players had experienced a dental injury while playing, but none of these had been wearing a mouth-guard.

Mouth-guards also help to absorb some of the forces applied when the jaw is struck, especially when the clenched teeth position is adopted. This reduces the forces transmitted to the temporomandibular joints, skull and brain, and therefore helps to reduce the severity and incidence of acute and chronic brain damage.

In economic terms the value of a mouth-guard is well illustrated when it is realised that it costs approximately 5–10% of the cost of a porcelain crown for an anterior tooth.

Face-masks, if correctly designed and worn, are effective in preventing damage to the face and teeth, and, if extended to cover the skull, provide excellent protection for this area. However, they must fit accurately and be adequately retained. The helmet type of face-mask which incorporates facial and cranial coverage is preferable. The face-masks should not be solely supported on the facial bones as this type transmits the forces directly to the structures it is supposed to protect. Many goalkeepers in field- and ice-hockey have an additional extension to the helmet type of face-mask with a flap of padded material coming down from the mask to cover the otherwise unprotected throat and larynx. In sports such as cycling and horse-riding, helmets which include face or chin protection help to reduce dental and facial injuries and are recommended.

The Bureau of Dental Health Education of the American Dental Association estimated, in 1973, that, since the introduction of mandatory wearing of face-masks and mouth-guards for American footballers, 100 000 oral injuries had been prevented annually.

Governing bodies of sports have a responsibility for the prevention of accidents. They should advise or legislate within the rules of the game for players to be allowed to, or required to, wear ap-

182
Chapter 14
Dental and facial
damage in sport

propriate protective equipment. The example of American football illustrates dramatically the benefits to health which may accrue. Rules governing the type and condition of the sporting equipment used are important, and this would include such diverse items as sticks, helmets, goalposts, pitch surface and surrounds. It is the responsibility of the playing officials, referees, umpires and linesmen, etc. to check equipment before the players take the field. Match officials should order a removal of equipment that may have become dangerous through damage during play. Coaches and managers should be encouraged to ensure that players have maintained their sports equipment in a safe condition and that they make full use of protective equipment that is available.

Rules outlawing interpersonal violence are essential and must be strictly applied. Clearly this is an area which is and should be controlled by referees and disciplinary committees of the respective sports.

Treatment

While damage to the teeth, jaws and soft tissues may produce spectacular injuries, it must always be remembered that the general condition of the patient is of vital importance. Control of the airway, control of bleeding and assessment of the level of consciousness must still take priority, as with any accident victim.

Damage can occur to the hard tissues, i.e. teeth and bones, and to the soft tissues.

The extent of damage that occurs to the teeth from a direct blow can vary from no displacement of the tooth, to partial loss of tooth substance, to complete avulsion of the tooth from its socket. The tooth that has been traumatised with no loss of tooth substance can, however, suffer damage to its nerve and blood supply and may subsequently die. In cases where this has occurred the patient should be warned, and the vitality of the tooth monitored by the practitioner and appropriate radiographs taken when indicated. Root treatment and/or crowning may be required at a later date.

In young children, deciduous teeth which have been displaced usually require little treatment unless they are interfering with the bite or subsequently become infected. If the displaced teeth are interfering with the normal occlusion, then they need to be either repositioned or extracted. It is worth warning the parents that the permanent tooth may be displaced or damaged (dilacerated) by the trauma, but a 'wait and see' policy can only be adopted.

Damage to the permanent teeth should be actively treated. This treatment is based on Ellis's classification and a summary is shown in Table 14.1.

Fractures or displacement of the teeth may not always be obvious unless careful examination is undertaken. This is particularly so in

183

*Chapter 14
Dental and facial
damage in sport*

the vertically split tooth as seen in the premolar and molar regions, which may only be diagnosed with careful probing of the cusps of the teeth when acute pain will be produced. Fractured or displaced teeth may lead to a part or the whole of a tooth being embedded in the soft tissues of the lips or mouth, and therefore any laceration associated with damaged teeth should be carefully explored or X-rayed for this complication. Another rare complication is the inhalation or ingestion of a tooth or a tooth fragment. Should there be any suspicion that this has occurred, the appropriate chest and/or abdominal X-ray should be taken.

Damage to the soft tissues of the mouth and lips may or may not require suturing. The generous blood supply in this region means that healing is usually rapid and seldom complicated by infection. Minor abrasions or splits of the inside of the lips will often heal themselves without recourse to suturing. However, where the gingival margin has been displaced this should be accurately sewn back into position. In all cases of intraoral wounds instruction should be given with regard to oral hygiene to prevent secondary infection. Careful use of the toothbrush is mandatory, supplemented with hot saline mouthwashes or chlorhexidine mouth rinses as indicated.

Lacerations of the skin require careful cleaning and closure. A tattooed or stepped scar is very difficult to correct subsequently. Accurate suturing is especially important where the wound involves the vermilion border of the lip.

Damage to the bone of the jaw may involve the supporting alveolar bone of the teeth, in fractures of the jaw or cheek-bones. Fractures of the maxilla are relatively rare in sports injuries. Fractures of the cheek-bone and mandible, however, show a much higher incidence in contact sports. These may not be associated

Classification	Injury to tooth	Treatment notes
Class I	Enamel chipping only	Smooth enamel, ? composite restoration
Class II	Coronal fracture involving enamel and dentine only	Cover exposed dentine, e.g. $Ca(OH)_2$ ± temporary crown
Class III	Coronal fracture exposing pulp	If root has an open apex, carry out pulpotomy and cover with $Ca(OH)_2$ and zinc oxide/eugenol dressing. If apex closed extirpate pulp and root-fill
Class IV	Root fracture ± coronal fracture	Depends on the position of the fracture. Apical third fracture may require root extirpation ± splinting. Other fractures generally indicate extraction
Class V	Displaced tooth	If sufficient periodontal support, reinsert at the earliest opportunity and consider splinting, e.g. wiring or acid-etch to adjacent teeth. Minimum handling of root surface is important

Table 14.1 Treatment of damage to permanent teeth, based on Ellis's classification

Source: Poswillo *et al.* (1986), p. 13.

184

Chapter 14
Dental and facial
damage in sport

with displacement or marked symptoms, but their diagnosis is important as further trauma before healing is complete can lead to marked displacement and complications. It is therefore important following a blow to the face or teeth that the appropriate X-rays should be taken to exclude such fractures. This may even apply after a blow to a tooth with no apparent loss of tooth substance. This emphasises the point that it is important to make a thorough examination of the patient who has been injured.

Treatment follows the usual pattern of interdental and, where necessary, intermaxillary wiring for alveolar and mandibular fractures. Fractures of the middle third of the face (maxilla and zygoma) usually require referral to the appropriate hospital specialist.

It is usual to suggest a period of six weeks before recommencing playing after a simple zygomatic or mandibular fracture. In complex or comminuted fractures it may be necessary to advise the patient to avoid contact sports completely until solid clinical union has been obtained. This may be in excess of 12 weeks.

Conclusions and recommendations

Facial and dental damage can occur in almost all sports. The number and severity of these injuries can be reduced with the appropriate use of protective equipment and through legislators and officials framing and enforcing appropriate rules.

Patients who may be, or have been, involved in a sporting injury may present some legal pitfalls for the practitioner. These may arise from a failure to adequately warn or inform a patient of possible risks or complications, e.g. failure to warn a patient that a traumatised tooth may give rise to problems at a later date, or to advise a patient to wear a mouth-guard after crown and bridge work. Patients who wear removable appliances should be warned to take these out prior to participating in contact sports, or in situations where oral or facial damage is a possibility. Other problems may arise through failure to diagnose a split tooth, tooth fragments becoming embedded in the soft tissues, or an inhaled or ingested tooth. Failure to take appropriate X-rays may lead to an indefensible medico-legal position.

References

Compton B. & Tubbs N. (1977) A survey of sports injuries in Birmingham. *British Journal of Sports Medicine* **11**, 12–15.

Davies R. M., Bradley D., Hale R. W., Laird W. R. E. & Thomas P. D. (1977) The prevalence of dental injuries in rugby players and their attitude to mouthguard. *British Journal of Sports Medicine* **11**, 72–4.

Gelbier S. (1966) The use and construction of mouth and tooth protectors for contact sports. *British Dental Journal* **120**, 533–7.

185

*Chapter 14
Dental and facial
damage in sport*

La Cava G. (1964) The prevention of accidents caused by sport. *Journal of Sport Medicine and Physical Fitness* **4**, 221–8.

Poswillo D., Babajews A., Bailey M. & Foster M. (1986) *Dental, Oral and Maxillofacial Surgery.* London: William Heinemann Medical Books.

Rowe N. L. & Williams J. L. (eds) (1985) *Maxillofacial Injuries.* Edinburgh: Churchill Livingstone.

Vincent-Townend J. R. L. & Langdon J. G. (1985) Appendix. In *Maxillofacial Injuries,* vol. 2, ed. N. L. Rowe & J. L. Williams, pp. 999–1014. Edinburgh: Churchhill Livingstone.

Further reading

Blonstein J. L. & Cutler R. (1977) Mouth and jaw protection in contact sports. *British Journal of Sports Medicine* **11**, 75–7.

Hill C. M. & Mason D. A. (1985) Dental and facial injuries following sports accidents: a study of 130 patients. *British Journal of Oral and Maxillofacial Surgery* **23**, 268–74.

Jarvin S. (1980) On the causes of traumatic dental injuries with reference to sports accidents in a sample of Finnish children. *Acta Odontologica Scandinavica* **38**, 151–4.

Rontal E., Rontal M., Wilson K. & Barclay C. (1977) Facial injuries in hockey players. *Laryngoscope* **87**, 884–94.

Sane J. & Ylipaavalniemi P. (1987) Maxillofacial and dental soccer injuries in Finland. *British Journal of Oral and Maxillofacial Surgery* **25**, 383–90.

15 The Firearms Act and mental health

R. R. H. SHIPWAY AND J. C. TAYLOR

15.1: Recent amendments in the law

R. R. H. SHIPWAY

'*Arma Virumque Cano*' (I sing of arms and man)   *opening words*
From *The Aeniad* V. 1 by *Virgil*

On 2 December 1987 the Home Secretary announced a full package of proposals for tightening the law on control of firearms, which are now contained in a White Paper, and include the prohibition of certain weapons, raising some into a higher classification, and a safe-keeping requirement for shotguns. The new firearms proposals came in the wake of a series of tragedies involving the use of high-powered and sophisticated weapons and it may be considered by some that a review of firearms legislation was long overdue.

The Firearms Act 1968 consolidated various Acts extending from the first Firearms Act of 1920, before which there was effectively no specific control of firearms. The Criminal Justice Act 1967 was to provide for a series of graded controls over the acquisition and possession of various types of firearms. Prohibited weapons included automatic weapons, such as machine-guns, and weapons designed for the discharge of noxious substances. Special authority from the Secretary of State is required for their manufacture, sale, acquisition or possession, and authority is only issued after careful enquiries by the police. Private individuals are not normally authorised to possess them. A firearms certificate issued by the Chief Officer of Police is required for the acquisition or possession of rifles, pistols, short-barrelled shotguns, and especially dangerous high-powered air weapons. The police must be satisfied that the applicant for a certificate has good reason for wanting the weapon, that he is fit to be entrusted with it, and that public safety will not be endangered.

A shotgun certificate is required for the acquisition or possession of long-barrelled shotguns — those with a barrel of 24 inches or more in length. A shotgun certificate can be refused by the Chief Officer of Police if he considers that the public safety or the peace will be endangered if the certificate is granted. A certificate authorises the possession of an unlimited number of shotguns and there is no condition requiring safe-keeping. In addition, most shotgun ammunition is not controlled.

Substantial maximum penalties are laid down in the present legislation for firearms offences such as possession with intent to endanger life and use of firearms to resist arrest. These carry life imprisonment, and possession whilst committing an offence and carrying a firearm or imitation firearm with intent to commit an indictable offence or resist arrest carry a maximum penalty of 14 years. Carrying a loaded firearm in a public place carries five years' imprisonment.

The Government now proposes:

1 to prohibit a range of weapons, including self-loading and pump-action rifles, burst-fire weapons, self-loading or pump-action short-barrelled smooth-bore guns;

2 to include normal-length (24 inches or over) pump-action and self-loading shotguns under Firearms Act control;

3 to enable Chief Officers of Police to refuse to issue a shotgun certificate if they are satisfied that the applicant does not have a good reason for possessing a shotgun. It is not intended to impose an obligation in every case to show a good reason because, in the majority of cases, this will be readily apparent;

4 to require Chief Officers of Police to be satisfied, before granting a shotgun certificate, that the applicant can be permitted to possess a shotgun without danger to the public safety or the peace;

5 to prohibit the movement of the weapon into the less strictly controlled category by means of conversion;

6 to take powers to require a firearm or shotgun certificate to bear a photograph of the applicant;

7 to require shotgun owners to have regard to the safe-keeping of their shotguns;

8 to require shotguns to be listed on a shotgun certificate and disposals to be notified to the police;

9 to make the purchase of shotgun ammunition subject to production of a valid shotgun certificate;

10 to hold a firearms amnesty in 1988 timed to coincide with the introduction of the new controls;

11 to remove the foreign visitors' exemption from shotgun certificate requirements in the 1968 Act and to replace it with a tightly drawn permit system;

12 to put beyond doubt that devices known as 'stun guns' are prohibited weapons;

13 to ensure that only legitimate firearms dealers will receive authorisation by confining the status to those who can establish that dealing in firearms is a substantial commercial or business activity. To require dealers to retain their register for a minimum of five years after the date of the last entry which will provide a detailed record of transactions over the last five years. Where a firearms dealer ceases to trade, for whatever reason, he will be required to surrender the register;

14 to improve the control of gun clubs by giving the Secretary of State specific powers to approve both rifle and pistol clubs. They will have to be run by fit and proper persons, be properly constituted and have access to an approved firing range. Approval to be renewed every six years;

15 to make provision for the Royal Ulster Constabulary to exercise greater control over the movements of firearms from England, Wales and Scotland to Northern Ireland;

16 to regularise the position of certain museums holding collections.

The most significant proposals will enable Chief Officers of Police to refuse to issue a shotgun certificate if they are satisfied that the applicant does not have a good reason for possessing a shotgun. The firearms or shotgun certificate will have to bear a photograph of the applicant and shotguns will also be required to be listed on the shotgun certificate, with disposals having to be notified to the police. The purchase of shotgun ammunition is to be made subject to production of a valid shotgun certificate.

The new provisions also ensure that only legitimate firearms dealers will receive authorisation by confining this status to those who can establish that dealing in firearms is a substantial commercial or business activity. And, where a firearms dealer ceases to trade, for whatever reason, he or she will be required to surrender the register, which he or she must retain for a minimum period of five years after the date of the last entry.

The control of gun clubs is also to be improved by giving the Secretary of State specific power to approve both rifle and pistol clubs, to be run by fit and proper persons with access to an approved firing range, the approval having to be renewed every six years.

The Home Secretary commented that an attempt was made to strike a balance between the protection of rights and interests of legitimate users and the assurance of public safety. It is intended to provide shooters with a solid basis for continuing their sport whilst strengthening safeguards for the public.

15.2: Firearms certificates and the role of the doctor

J.C. TAYLOR

'Is the nightmare black or are the windows painted?'
From *Madman Across The Water* by Bernie Taupin

Editor's introduction

The legitimate requirement of farmers and sports men and women to own and use firearms has been brought into question by the apparent ease with which criminal elements of society and the mentally unstable can legally, although inappropriately, possess high-powered guns. This obviously undesirable situation has been recognised by the police, who are aware of increases in armed crime in recent years. The tragic events of Hungerford in 1987 have raised these anxieties further and doubtless have been the stimulus for the Home Secretary's proposals to tighten the regulations outlined in 15.1.

Dr John Taylor, a forensic psychiatrist, reviews the role of the doctor in helping to ensure safe certification of licence holders by attempting to identify the features that may be seen in individuals seeking a firearms certificate for whom possession of a gun would be entirely inappropriate and against the public interest. Some ethical dilemmas which may face the general practitioner directly or indirectly involved are also discussed.

A substantial proportion of the adult population in the UK enjoys the use of firearms. At the end of December 1986, there were on issue over 160 000 firearms certificates and more than 840 000 shot-gun certificates. As a shotgun certificate enabled, until the reform of the law (see 15.1), the holder to own as many of these weapons as he chooses, the actual number of shotguns in the country has been estimated at about 2 million. Different sorts of firearms may be used in a variety of settings. Rifles and pistols are generally confined to target shooting in clubs but some rifles may be used for activities such as deerstalking or vermin control. Shotguns may be used in such pastimes as clay pigeon shooting, game shooting (especially birds), and their use is also widespread in keeping down vermin.

Control over the ownership and use of firearms has been felt necessary for the prevention of death and injury to people, either in domestic disputes or in the course of organised crime. Although most people nowadays would probably take it for granted that strict firearms control legislation is necessary and desirable, it is a relatively recent innovation and a complete reversal of previous policy. During the Boer War, the British Government had been very impressed by the performance put up by the Dutch farmers against the British Army. It was felt that, if England were ever under threat, it would be useful if the population were proficient in the use of firearms. Indeed, in 1900, the Prime Minister, Lord Salisbury, said that he would 'laud the day when there was a rifle in every cottage in England'. Prior to 1920, there was very little in the way of legislation. The Gun Licences Act of 1870 required anyone wishing to use a gun other than at home to purchase a licence from the Post Office. This was strictly a revenue measure. The Pistols Act of 1903 prohibited the retail sale of pistols to those under the age of 18 years and required other purchasers to produce either a gun licence or a game licence, or reasonable proof that they were householders intending to use the pistol at home.

In 1920, the Firearms Act was passed, which established that framework of controls still in use. This complete reversal in policy was put through as a crime prevention measure, although at the time there was very little such activity. During the period of 1911–13, firearms were involved in an average of 45 crimes of all types per year and, during the period of 1915–17, the average had fallen to 15 cases per year. However, the real reason for this legislation, as recently released Cabinet papers have revealed, was that the Government was extremely concerned about the possibility of an armed Bolshevik-style revolution in Britain. Sir Eric Geddes, a minister in the government, feared 'a revolutionary outbreak in Glasgow, Liverpool or London in the early spring, when a definite attempt may be made to seize the reins of Government. It is not inconceivable that a dramatic and successful *coup d'état* in some large centre of population might win the support of the unthinking mass of labour' (PRO CAB 25/20). There were insufficient police to deal with the anticipated troubles and the Army, after demobilisation of conscripts, would be insufficient as well. In such a climate, the Prime Minister had been told in Cabinet that 'a Bill is needed to license persons to bear arms. This has been useful in Ireland because the authorities knew who was possessed of arms.' The Act was passed in the same year and made possession of a rifle or pistol dependent on a certificate issued by Chief Constables, who were given wide powers of discretion. Shotguns were excluded. There was further legislation in the 1930s and the 1960s, the 1968 Firearms Act being the basis of present-day legislation.

It is interesting to compare the general situation relating to firearms in the UK and that in the USA, where half of all households have guns and one in five has a hand-gun, and where there are now approximately 130 million guns in circulation. In the US more than 20% of all robberies and 65% of all homicides are committed using firearms. In 1982, firearms killed 33 000 Americans: 1756 of these deaths were classed as unintentional, 16 575 as suicide, 13 841 as homicides, 276 as legal intervention and 540 of undetermined intent (National Centre for Health Statistics). Firearms are the second leading cause of death in the USA for ages 15–34, with motor vehicles in first place, and, for ages 30–54, firearms generate as many deaths as motor-vehicle accidents. A study of death-rates from the Aarhus region of Denmark compared with north-eastern Ohio showed that the rate for all assaultive injuries treated in hospitals was almost the same. The Danish homicide rate, on the other hand, was only one-fifth the rate for Ohio (1.4 versus 7.2 per 100 000). The discrepancy is largely explained by two facts. First, firearm injuries have an extremely high case-fatality rate (15 times the rate for knife assaults in the Danish study) and, secondly, private ownership of guns in Denmark is much more restricted than in the USA.

In the USA there is a particular problem over the possession of hand-guns. These account for about one-quarter of the privately owned firearms but are involved in three-quarters of all gun killings. In the big cities, hand-guns account for more than 80% of gun killings and virtually all gun robberies. Although the most commonly given reasons for owning a hand-gun in the USA is self-protection at home, their possession may create more problems than it solves. A study in Detroit found that more people died in one year from hand-gun accidents alone than were killed by robbers or burglars in four and a half years.

In the UK, the situation is very different. In 1977, there were 29 homicides in which firearms were involved. This constitutes about 6% of all homicides in England and Wales for the same period and actually represents a slight drop in the rate compared with 1969. In about half the homicides, long-barrelled shotguns were used and pistols accounted for the other half. There were only three cases of homicide involving the use of sawn-off shotguns or rifles.

As regards non-fatal injuries in the UK in 1977, the vast majority were caused by airguns. There were more than 2000 injuries caused by airguns as compared with 256 injuries from all other types of firearms.

It is commonly asserted that the dangerous use of firearms in offences of violence is escalating rapidly. This cannot be answered by looking at the criminal statistics of one year only, but over a period of time. On the basis of the data in Table 15.1, it would be difficult to sustain the conclusion that firearms use in dangerous crime is increasing independently of the general increase in dangerous and violent criminal behaviour. As regards armed robbery, the trend appears to be moving away from the use of hand-guns to the use of sawn-off shotguns. It should be noted, however, that either sort of weapon would not be difficult to obtain by a determined criminal. There are vast numbers of shotguns in the country and hand-guns are relatively easily obtainable by smuggling them in

Table 15.1 Criminal statistics 1975–8

	1975	1976	1977	1978
Homicide	515	565	484	532
Attempted murder, serious woundings	4898	4383	4576	4689
Robbery	11311	11611	13730	13150
Total	16724	16559	18790	18371
Firearms used in the above crimes				
Homicide	46 (8.93%)	45 (7.96%)	29 (5.99%)	40 (7.52%)
Attempted murder	296 (6.04%)	227 (5.18%)	230 (5.03%)	239 (5.09%)
Robbery	949 (8.39%)	1068 (9.20%)	1234 (8.99%)	996 (7.57%)
Total	1291	1340	1493	1275

from countries such as Belgium, where they can be bought over the counter.

Overall, it would seem that the use of firearms in serious crime in the UK should not be regarded as excessive or alarming and, in so far as firearms use in crime can be said to be increasing, it is doing so only as a function of the reasonably slow increase in serious crimes of violence.

Although the 1968 Firearms Act was amended in 1988, the general thrust of the legislation remains unchanged. The Act recognises two categories of weapons; those that require firearms certificates under Part 1 of the Act, and shotguns. Part 1 weapons include rifles, pistols and certain high-velocity air rifles. Each firearms certificate lists the make, serial number and calibre of each weapon, as well as stating where the firearm must be kept and where it must be used; it also details the amount of ammunition the certificate holder may buy and hold at any one time for each calibre of weapon. Firearms certificates have to be renewed every three years. All pistols and most rifles may be used for target shooting only, and then by members of an approved club. The club's ranges are inspected by the Army, who determine what sort of calibre weapons may be used at that particular range. In some instances, rifles may be used in other circumstances, such as deerstalking or vermin control, but, in these cases, as in all Part 1 weapons, the individual has to show that he has a legitimate need for this type of firearm.

In order to obtain a firearms certificate, the individual would have to show his legitimate need for the particular weapon and to give the name of his gun club, as well as supplying a character reference from a doctor, minister of religion or MP. Most gun clubs require a probationary period of at least six months in order to get to know the individual and assess his suitability for membership. The local police then check with the secretary of the gun club and with the character referee. If the individual wishes to keep his weapon at home, the local police firearms officer visits the premises and lays down the conditions of security that must be met. If all the requirements are in order, the application is processed by the Metropolitan Police, who check whether or not the individual has a criminal record. Some people are banned from legally possessing firearms. Anyone who has served a prison sentence of three years or more is banned for life. Anyone who has served a sentence of between three months and three years is banned for five years. Nobody under the age of 17 years may buy a firearm and young people are also subject to a variety of special regulations. When all factors have been taken into account, the Chief Constable of the country may then issue a firearms certificate.

The law relating to shotguns is somewhat different. All shotguns with barrés less than 24 inches (60.96 cm) long are now prohibited weapons for private individuals. In applying for a shotgun licence, the individual does not have to show a need to own the weapons but now has to have a police-approved secure place to keep them and, as with Part 1 weapons, has to provide a character reference. In future, as shotgun certificates are renewed, the information on those certificates will be more detailed.

From time to time doctors may face some problems in relation to their patients and the use of firearms. There are some people who, by reason of a medical disorder, would be unsuitable to handle lethal weapons. These disorders may include alcohol and drug abuse, organic brain disorder, major functional mental illness such as schizophrenia, manic depressive disorder or depression and well-established personality disorder, where there is a history of impulsive and/or violent physical behaviour. Before issuing a character reference, it is therefore important that the doctor actually knows the person well over a reasonable period, rather than for instance merely having them on their patient list for some time.

If the police contact a medical practitioner and inform him that a patient has applied for a firearms certificate and has given his or her name for a character reference, but the doctor is aware of the sort of problem outlined above, he can decline to give the reference. The police would then refuse to issue the certificate and are not obliged to give their reasons for so doing. In a case where a person indicates to the practitioner that he would like to give the doctor as a character reference, but the doctor deems him unsuitable, he should discuss with the person his reasons and try and persuade him not to go ahead with the application. The person may indicate that he will use another referee instead. The doctor is then faced with a dilemma between his duty of confidentiality to his patient and the risk to the general public. In these circumstances, the doctor should examine all aspects of the case extremely carefully before contacting the local firearms officer and expressing the view that it would not be in the interests of the public safety for the person to possess a firearm. In cases of doubt the doctor should contact his medical protection organisation for discussion and advice.

Occasionally, it may occur that a doctor has a patient who he is aware is in possession of a firearms certificate and later develops some problem such as depression. In such circumstances, if the practitioner feels that the problem may be of a temporary nature, he could discuss the risks with the patient and suggest lodging the weapon with a registered dealer for safekeeping. Again, if the patient refuses and in all the particular circumstances the practitioner feels that there is a serious risk to his patient, the patient's family or the public, he may then have recourse to contacting the firearms officer. Each case, however, would have to be judged on its merits.

The use of firearms for recreational use is widespread in the UK and is in the main well regulated and poses few problems, despite a few well-publicised recent tragedies. It is incumbent, however, on practitioners issuing character references to give the matter the serious consideration that it deserves. In cases where the practitioner is in doubt or feels that the person may be a risk to himself or others, advice should be sought before overriding the duty of confidentiality owed to the patient by the doctor.

Part II: Specific sports

Medical hazards of equestrian pursuits

16

M. ALLEN

'The best thing for the inside of a man is the outside of a horse'
Nineteenth century proverb

Introduction

The close relationship between equestrian pursuits and injury has
been recognised ever since man became involved with the horse,
and it was in the ancient writings of Persia that the first records of
this fact were noted in the form of a saying in the literature of the
time: 'The grave yawns for the horseman.' What was true then is
equally true now, the only difference being that in ancient Persia
there was no coroner to inquire into a disaster and no claim against
the practitioner of medicine.* Indeed, then the only forfeit operative
was instant death to the court physician if the patient was of sufficient importance and died! How different today — we live in an increasingly litigious society: legal advice is sought by many if they
feel that there is the slightest hint of negligence or carelessness
on the part of either the purveyor of a service at an event or the
organiser of such an event. Legal aid is used in the context of
leisure activities just as much as in the context of employment, thus
opening the prospect of litigation even further.

No longer is it acceptable for a token medical officer to be
quietly positioned in the corner of a hospitality tent, imbibing his
fee in port after a generous lunch, equipped only with his inherent
skill and a stethoscope.†

Since each type of equestrian event presents a particular type of
problem and consequently produces needs which may be additional
to the central core requirements, we must consider and describe the
main types of equestrian activities.

1 Horse-racing. This involves six types of racing, as follows:

(a) flat racing;

---

* The penalties for medical mistakes of the ancients varied, e.g. writings of the
Hammurabi, *circa* 1800 BC: 'if a doctor operates on a man with a severe wound with a
bronze lancet and causes the man's death or opens an abscess in the eye of a man with
a bronze lancet and destroys the man's eye they shall cut off his fingers'.

† Drinking while on duty is to be deplored in any branch of medicine on the grounds
that it is unprofessional. It may therefore attract the unwelcome attention of the
General Medical Council, but more importantly, because of its adverse effects on
mental concentration and perception, it may alter clinical judgement, resulting in
poor treatment. This will lead to the possibility of legal liability in negligence.
    In any case the acts of a drunken doctor are virtually impossible to defend in
court!

(b) national hunt racing — where obstacles, small such as hurdles and large such as fences, are to be jumped;

(c) point-to-point racing — a totally amateur variation of steeple-chasing;

(d) Arab racing — flat racing confined to Arab horses;

(e) trotting — mainly an American and Continental sport which does occur in certain UK centres, but which only has a very small number of drivers involved;

(f) quarter-horse racing — flat racing confined to American-bred quarter-horses.

2   Show jumping.

3   Eventing, consisting of three elements: dressage, show jumping and cross-country riding.

4   Polo.

5   Other, for example:

(a) pony club riding;

(b) team cross-country chasing;

(c) long-distance riding.

In each of these events there is a marked element of risk and falls are common.

The degree of medical cover afforded to the activities outlined above depends very much on the policy of the controlling body of the specific sport. It varies from the very sophisticated in horse-racing under the rules of racing, to the almost non-existent in certain local shows and events.*

Until recently there had been little or no formal medical cover provided for any of the activities outside polo and horse-racing, and even in horse-race trotting there are no structured rules. However, with the advent of the Medical Equestrian Association, organising bodies have been made aware of the need to have experienced medical officers who are properly equipped, with adequate back-up facilities, such as ambulances with a four-wheel drive cross-country capability and similar vehicles to carry the medical officers to the scene of the accident. It is of no use to have a medical officer and ambulance in one field if the accident happens two fields away and neither the ambulance nor the medical officer can get there because of the fences and/or mud.

On the other hand, the Hurlingham Club (the governing body of polo) and the Jockey Club (the governing body of flat, national hunt and point-to-point racing) have taken an extremely realistic view of

---

* The responsibility for providing cover rests primarily with those organising the particular event, and there may be guidelines provided by the sport's governing body. Once the doctor has been approached and agrees to provide medical cover, however, the responsibility rests with the doctor for drawing to the attention of the organisers any deficiencies of the medical facilities. For Jockey Club regulations regarding accidents to riders and provisions for medical attention on racecourses, see Appendix 16.1.

their medical responsibilities. They have laid down specific instructions for the provision of medical cover at events under their control which, unless fulfilled, result in the event being cancelled or postponed until such time as the prescribed criteria can be met.

Common riding injuries

Incidence

The incidence of injury varies with each particular branch of the sport. However, some generalisations can be made from figures already in our possession. We know, for example, that, over a two-year period in an area where intense racehorse training took place with some 4000 people employed and with a horse population of 2250, some 622 people were injured to such a degree that attendance at hospital was necessary. This gives an average of six cases per week (Edixhoven *et al.* 1981).

We also know that in the general population riding injuries occur more frequently in school holidays, especially Easter, and most frequently amongst young adolescent females.

However, the collection of statistics in horse-related incidents is very poor. No accurate figures are available from the DHSS; indeed, there is no codification for horse-related injuries in accident and emergency departments. Individual governing bodies vary very considerably in their attitude towards the collection of accident statistics. The British Horse Society, in conjunction with the Medical Equestrian Association, is currently trying to remedy this omission, but at the present time the only comprehensive statistics on riding injuries are those kept by the Jockey Club.

It is from these figures that we know that one in every ten rides over obstacles results in a fall and of these falls 3% result in injuries, the main ones being:

Limb fractures   60%
Concussion   34%

In flat racing the injury rate is 42% per fall (in other words 14 times greater than in steeplechasing) but with only 60 falls for every 32 500 runners, i.e. approximately one fall per 5500 rides. The injuries here are mainly fractures of limbs, concussion and soft tissue injury.

Mechanism of injury

The mechanism of injury is as follows:

Falls from the horse   45%
Kicks by the horse to the rider   33%
Bites by the horse or blows with its head   10%
Falls with the horse and entrapment beneath   7%

It is important to be aware of the kinetics involved with a moving horse and the salient features which one should remember are:

1   a horse weighs 500 kg (approximately);
2   the rider falls 2–3 m;
3   the horse, and thus the rider, is frequently moving at a speed of up to 65 km per hour;
4   the force developed from a kick by a horse's hoof can be in excess of 300 joules.

It is therefore self-evident that quite large forces are commonly involved in horse-riding accidents.

Types of injury

A classification of the types of injury that are associated with horse-riding will be of value to those involved in providing medical cover, since it will serve to alert the medical officer to the appropriate action to be taken and to the equipment to have at hand.

1   Nervous system.
(a) Concussion resulting in unconsciousness.
(b) Fractures of the spine with spinal cord damage (both actual and potential).
(c) Cervical whiplash injury resulting in post-traumatic head injury syndrome
2   Locomotor system.
(a) Fractures of all long bones — simple, comminuted and compound; may be complicated by damage to vessels.
(b) Soft tissue haematoma.
(c) Sprains and ligamentous injuries.
3   Thorax.
(a) Fractures of the ribs.
(b) Pneumothorax.
4   Abdomen.
(a) Kidney damage leading to haematuria and/or less of renal function.
(b) Rupture of liver/spleen with consequent intraperitoneal haemorrhage: possible life-threatening hypovolaemia.

Role of equestrian medical officer

The role of the equestrian medical officer faced with such severe injuries is to preserve life by effecting a stabilisation of the condition of the patient, and to alleviate suffering by judicious use of analgesia.

There is no place for heroic intervention in the field — such action nearly always ends in disaster. The stabilised patient should be transferred to a prearranged designated hospital or specialist centre for definitive treatment. The duties of the doctor in the field are really to ensure that basic equipment is available to retrieve the casualty safely, alleviate pain, ensure adequate splintage and, above all, to maintain a satisfactory airway. Here it is important to remember that one has only 180 seconds to ensure that an obstructed airway is made patent again and thus, above all else, the medical officer must arrange:

1 Satisfactory access for himself and ambulances to all parts of the arena, no matter how large this may be.

2 Efficient evacuation to the nearest district general hospital with an operational accident and emergency department, the availability of which should be established in advance of the event.

It is clear, therefore, that specialised skill is required of the equestrian medical officer to be able to deal adequately with the primary care of serious, life-threatening and unstable injuries. Training in accident and emergency medicine and/or trauma surgery would be ideal, but as a minimum requirement the practitioner should be able to deal confidently with the injuries described above.

The responsibility of providing equipment (with the exception of emergency drugs) rests with the organisers of the event. The doctor, however, may be consulted for his recommendations. The equipment that will be required is as follows:

1 Stretchers. Undoubtedly the scoop stretcher is mandatory at equestrian events for it allows safe retrieval of spinal and pelvic injuries. 'Scoop', as the name implies, is a stretcher which opens out at both the head and foot end and is so designed as to allow one to slide it under the patient and scoop up the injured person, locking the stretcher at the head and foot end before moving.

There has been a recent development in the introduction of the Jordan/Donway lifting frame. The frame is placed over the patient and slats introduced under the patient which are attached to the frame, thus allowing a steady and even lift.

2 Splints. The Donway Traction splint for fractures of the femur and the Emtech Vacuum splint for limb fractures are absolutely essential. Inflatable splints carry the risk of over-inflation from which soft tissue and vascular damage has been reported. The Donway Traction splint is an updated form of 'Thomas splint', which uses a pneumatic principle rather than an ankle windlass. The Emtech Vacuum splint works on the principle that the splint moulds itself to the injured limb as air is withdrawn (rather than pumped in). This therefore abolishes any hazard from over-inflation.

3 Airways of varying size, e.g. Gudel sizes 1, 2 and 3.

4 Suction and resuscitation equipment (see Appendix 16.1). The type and choice can easily be left to the individual, but Laerdal and Ambu provide a very good range, easily packed and remarkably transportable.

5 Ambulances, fully equipped to front-line standard — as provided

* Controlled drug
register requirements
should be observed if
opiates or other
controlled drugs are
used. NB: Keep the
black bag in a safe
place: controlled drugs
should be kept locked-
up at all times.

by the local health authority ambulance service, St John Ambulance Brigade or Red Cross Society.

6   Drugs. Each medical officer will have his/her own particular preferences. The following generic groups, however, should be included:

(a) analgesics — both non-opiate and opiate;*

(b) antihistamines;

(c) antiemetics;

(d) hydrocortisone.

7   Mini-tracheostomy kit. The possession of a mini-tracheostomy kit and knowledge of how to use it is essential.

Indications for use:

(a) obstructed airway;

(b) deeply unconscious patient ± cervical fracture to provide intermittent positive-pressure ventilation.

Technique: stretching the skin laterally between the finger and thumb of the left hand, a small vertical incision is made over the skin of the cricothyroid membrane and the minitrach plus introducer is pushed through this into the trachea.

8   Infusion fluids. The provision of infusion fluids in the form of plasma expanders, together with suitable intravenous cannulae and giving sets are essential for the primary management of severe haemorrhage.

The responsibility for provision of such equipment is something of a 'grey area': should the medical officer provide it or should the organiser? It is suggested it should perhaps be a joint exercise between the two — the medical officer will often have easier access to the equipment and the organiser can provide the necessary finance.

Prevention: medical advice to organisers

The medical officer has a duty to give general advice to the organisers of an event. Initially he/she should insist that correct BSI standard headwear is worn by all competitors. Advice must be given about obtaining access to jumps and all parts of the course. The doctor must clearly state the number of four-wheel drive cross-country vehicles and ambulances required to give adequate access and provide full cover. The medical officer must reconnoitre the course with the organisers of the event before the actual day and produce a medical operational plan so that the organisers, colleagues and ambulance staff can all be fully briefed. Finally the nearest general district hospital with an operational accident and emergency department should be notified of the impending event, and their co-operation sought.

The equestrian medical officer should be aware that competitors taking part in an event who are known to be insulin-dependent diabetics or who are diagnosed epileptics present potential difficulties in the management of their injuries in the event of an accident. Whilst these conditions are not absolute contraindications to participation in competition, the increased susceptibility in epilepsy to the effects of head injuries should be remembered, as should the dangers of fluctuation in blood sugar in insulin-dependent diabetics possibly causing falls and certainly complicating treatment.*

Conclusions and recommendations

From the foregoing it should be obvious that the responsibility of the doctor at an equestrian event is not just 'to be there' for moral support. He or she is an active participant in the event, and should be in total readiness at any time to deal with an incident, be it concussion, a fractured thoracic spine, internal bleeding, or just a physically exhausted competitor.

The doctor concerned should be fully aware of the responsibilities attaching to the post of equestrian medical officer. If the facilities provided do not come up to expectations or the arrangements are in any way inadequate, the doctor should have no hesitation in declining to undertake the task. It is better to say 'no' before the event rather than to have to explain to the coroner's court how you tried to do your best with what was provided. Likewise an action in negligence may be indefensible because the splints for treatment of a fracture were unavailable or the retrieval of a spinal injury without a scoop stretcher was attempted.

Above all, remember to keep good notes on what you recommend and also on the reply you receive.

Appendix 16.1: Accidents to riders and provisions for medical attention at racecourses (From Jockey Club General Instruction No. 12.1)

Minimum requirements for medical arrangements on racecourses

1 Medical staff.

(a) Racecourse medical officers (RMOs). There shall be at least two doctors on duty at all flat, steeplechase and hurdle race meetings, with additional doctors at the discretion of the Racecourse Executive for the larger race meetings.

(b) Nurses. One qualified (SRN and SEN or BRCS/SJAB equivalently

---

* The medical officer has a clinical responsibility to the riders to advise and treat as the need arises, but is engaged primarily as an agent of the race organisers. If, therefore, a conflict of duties arises, the prime responsibility with respect to fitness to ride rests with the organisers, who are in turn advised by the medical officers. This illustrates the difference between the doctor/patient relationship that exists between a GP and his patient and that pertaining to doctors engaged by a body such as those organising an equestrian event.

qualified) nurse shall be on duty in the medical room by arrangement of the senior racecourse medical officer. At larger meetings, additional trained nurses should be provided from one of the voluntary bodies.

(c) First-aid personnel. First-aid personnel must be available for all enclosures.

In all steeplechases and hurdle races, there shall be one first-aid person to each fence or flight of hurdles, except in the event of two fences or hurdle flights being very close together where both can be covered by one person. Where policemen holding the necessary qualification are employed as first-aid personnel, they must be used for that purpose solely, and not for usual police duty.

In the event of a shortage of trained first-aid personnel, provision should be made for a suitable vehicle to be available, with a medical officer positioned to cover those parts of the course not manned by first-aid personnel, with a mobile team at his/her disposal, which he/she can direct to best advantage.

2 Equipment.

(a) Medical room. To contain at least one screened bed, with necessary blankets. The room must also have adequate heating and lighting and an adequate supply of hot water, with access to toilet facilities.

(b) Medical accessories Donway and Emtech splintage systems, stretchers, blankets, and such medical supplies as are required for the rendering of first-aid must be available and the senior racecourse medical officer will be responsible for ensuring that adequate medical equipment is provided.

(c) Ambulances. At least two ambulances must be present and available from 45 minutes before the commencement of racing until 15 minutes after the last race. All ambulances must be equipped with a scoop and a York style stretcher, oxygen and airway equipment, and blankets. A scoop stretcher must always be available in the ambulance or other vehicle used to transport the RMO to a seriously injured casualty. Should it be necessary to evacuate the casualty to hospital during the hours of racing, another ambulance should be summoned from the nearest depot to remove the casualty or replace the ambulance used.

In dealing with a seriously or very seriously injured jockey, the RMO should pay particular attention to the following points.

(i) The casualty should remain on and be examined on the initial recovery stretcher before a decision regarding his/her disposal is made.

(ii) If the causalty is seriously injured and in the RMO's opinion his/her clinical condition warrants it, the casualty should be evacuated immediately to hospital in the recovery ambulance without transfer to another ambulance. If the RMO makes such a decision, he/she should inform the clerk of the course of his/

her decision so that provisions for a relief ambulance can be made. In such instances, relief ambulance vehicles equipped with a scoop stretcher may be used, e.g. four-wheel drive Land Rovers, Subarus, etc., until the arrival of the relieving ambulance.

(d) Field posts. The first aid personnel stationed at steeple chase fences and hurdle flights shall be provided with flags to be waved when the services of a doctor or an ambulance are required, as follows:

(i) white flag — ambulance required;

(ii) red and white chequered — doctor required.

They shall also be provided with a carrying sheet, a stretcher (conforming to British Standards Institute specification) blankets, and small pack pillows. Shelters erected at intervals on the race-course for the use during inclement weather of first-aid personnel stationed in the country and as stores for their equipment, are a desirable addition where possible.

(e) First-aid posts. First-aid posts will be provided. These should be accessible for all enclosures and must be manned during the hours that the racecourse is open to the public until such time as they are closed after the last race at the direction of the senior racecourse medical officer. These posts should be equipped with medical supplies, bed, stretchers, and blankets. The first-aid posts should be clearly indicated by a flag or red cross with a notice to show how further medical assistance can be obtained (e.g. position of medical room and how to get there) and the location of the nearest telephone on the internal racecourse circuit.

(f) First-aid boxes. First-aid boxes will be positioned in the stable guard's office and hostel canteen kitchen. The contents must be adequate for the number of personnel served and be up to the standards laid down by the *Health & Safety (First Aid) Regulations* (1981) which came into force on 1st July 1982 and fully described in *First aid at Work* Health & Safety Service Booklet HS(R)11 (ISBN 0 11.883446.0). The boxes must be inspected regularly by the senior racecourse medical officer and an initialled record be kept of the dates of inspection.

3 Standing orders and deployment of medical resources.

Written orders will be prepared for the detailed deployment of the medical resources at each course. Copies of these orders will be in the possession of the clerk of the course and all RMOs. They will consist of the Jockey Club Instruction (JCI) 12.1 together with a copy of the Medical Resources Deployment Plan, a copy of which will be available in the weighing room, medical room and all first-aid posts. The standing orders and Medical Resources Deployment Plan will detail the deployment of RMOs and ambulances as below:

(a) Flat racing. One RMO and one ambulance must be at each starting stalls' start or in such a position that they can respond very rapidly to any incident occurring at the start. Furthermore their disposition should be such that they are also available to follow the field after the start.

(b) National hunt racing.

(i) One RMO (more on larger courses) must follow the runners around the course.

(ii) If no track or access for (i) above is available, one RMO must be sited at a position on the track enabling him/her to reach any seriously injured rider as quickly as possible.

(iii) Transport to facilitate (i) and (ii) above. Four-wheel drive vehicles must be provided where necessary.

Duties and responsibilities

1 Clerk of the course.
The clerk is responsible for providing the necessary accommodation — ambulance, first-aid personnel and necessary equipment for the medical room apart from those items which are the responsibility of the senior medical officer, and for field and first-aid posts. He or she will arrange for the most efficient methods of communication between the following: doctor, medical room, course manager, weighing room, ambulance. Communications will include such transport as is necessary to enable the doctor to carry out his/her duties. He or she is responsible for providing the necessary written orders to ensure that all medical arrangements function smoothly and efficiently. The clerk must ensure that an ambulance can reach casualties on any part of the course in any weather, and that facilities are available for towing the ambulance. He or she must ensure that the senior uniformed police officer has been told what the medical arrangements are, and has been instructed to inform his officers accordingly so that they can assist the public when necessary. The clerk will inform the chief inspector of RSS Ltd of the medical arrangements so that the latter and his staff can be of assistance when necessary. The clerk must ensure that the senior racecourse medical officer alerts the hospital, which he/she regards as being most suitable for receiving casualties, that there is a race meeting to be held that day.

The clerk must instruct the declarations clerk as to the procedure in regard to riders' medical record books. The clerk of the course will direct all riders by notice to the declarations clerk and arrange a suitable place where riders who require examination before riding can be seen by the medical officer responsible for duties in connection with medical record books.

The clerk of the course will arrange that a notice is placed in a prominent position in the weighing room notifying all riders, amateur and professional, that they must report to the medical officer on every occasion immediately after they have met with a fall or an accident.

The clerk will be responsible for ensuring that all RMOs have a copy of JCI 12.1, together with the operative Medical Resource Deployment Plan in their possession. He or she will immediately inform the stewards' secretary if the medical officer advises him/her before racing that the ambulances are not present.

2 Racecourse medical officer.

The senior doctor at the course must:

(a) satisfy himself that the medical arrangements are suitable, and will then report to the clerk of the course not later than one hour before the time of the first race on each race day;

(b) (i) be responsible for briefing all the first-aid personnel before racing of their duties and positions on the course, and

(ii) inform the clerk of the course 30 minutes before the first race if there is a shortage of first-aid personnel and it has been necessary to take action under 1(c) (p.204) para 3 of this instruction or if the statutory number of ambulances (two) have failed to arrive;

(c) make himself known before the commencement of racing to the clerk of the scales in the weighing room;

(d) arrange for a RMO to report to the weighing room after every race, at a position to be designated by the clerk of the course to deal with any incidents and report to the clerk of the scales any such incidents involving medical suspension of jockeys;

(e) report to the clerk of the course before leaving after the last race, and consult with him/her before any medical facilities are withdrawn;

(f) ensure that all medical staff are acquainted with their duties, that the ambulances have reported, and that the method of communication to the ambulances in the event of their being required is quick and efficient and known to the ambulance drivers;

(g) watch racing from the stewards' or officials box during races and be in communication with the clerk of the course to ensure the most rapid and efficient retrieval of injured jockeys.

Note. The RMO's primary responsibility is to the licensed personnel, racecourse technical services (RTS) staff (including stalls handlers) and racecourse staff. The RMO is *not* expected to attend members of the public except in cases of extreme emergency — and even then not to the detriment of his primary medical responsibility as detailed above.

At all race meetings a racecourse medical officer shall be responsible for duties in connection with riders' medical record books. He must be in attendance from one hour before racing starts and will be stationed at a place appointed by the clerk of the course.

3 Ambulance drivers.

The ambulance drivers will be in allotted positions which afford a ready means of proceeding rapidly to any portion of the course. The ambulance drivers will not leave the course after racing until permission has been received from the senior medical officer. The ambulance drivers must remain with their ambulances during the period of racing and must be alert for messages and signals calling for their assistance. They must ensure that at all times during the running of a race that their vehicles are in a state of readiness to move immediately on receipt of instructions to do so. The ambulance drivers must have trained assistants.

4 First-aid personnel.

Having been briefed in their duties and deployment by the RMO, they will be on duty throughout the hours of racing, and for half an hour before the first race, and may not leave until instructed by the medical officer after the last race. They must know how to get the doctor quickly (use of telephone or of the broadcast system). They must know the locality of the nearest ambulance depot, so that extra ambulances can be summoned when required by the course doctor.

Medical officer's reports

Procedure to be followed in all flat races, steeple chases and hurdle races

The medical officer will examine every rider who falls in a race.

1 In the case of both professional and amateur riders, the medical officer will enter on the sheet headed Medical Officers Report the name of the race, the name of the rider and particulars of the injuries sustained. If a rider who has fallen is unhurt, an entry to that effect must be made. In cases where the rider is told not to ride again before being passed fit to do so by a doctor an entry must be made in *red ink*. Should any rider come to the meeting without his medical record book and be told not to ride again before being passed fit to do so these facts must also be recorded in *red ink* on the report.

2 In cases where a professional rider licensed by the stewards of the Jockey Club have sustained injury which will, in the medical officer's opinion, result in a claim on the Compensation Fund for Jockeys, an accident insurance claim form must be given to the jockey or his representative and this fact must be recorded in *red ink* on the report. This certificate must be completed by the jockey's own medical attendant, and not by the medical officer on the course.

3 In the event of a professional or amateur rider sustaining injuries which necessitate his being removed from the course, the address to which he is removed must be stated on the medical officer's report and in the rider's medical record book and recorded in *red ink*.

4 When a rider, professional or amateur, who has been injured at a previous meeting has been told by the medical officer of that meeting that he must not ride again that day or before being medically examined, he will report to the medical officer of the course where he next intends to ride. He will produce his medical record book for the relevant entry to be made in it. The medical officer will in all cases make an entry on the medical officer's report as to the result of his examination. If the rider is still unfit the entry must be in *red ink*.

5 The medical officer's report must be handed to the clerk of the course who will forward it to the secretary, The Compensation Fund for Jockeys, The Racecourse, Newbury, Berks RG14 7NZ (telephone: Newbury (0635) 45707).

Note. Riding work and schooling. The racecourse medical officer must inform any rider who has been suspended from riding on medical grounds that he is also suspended from riding work and schooling.

Medical confidentiality

Information regarding the details of injuries sustained by riders are confidential between the RMO and his patients, i.e. the injured persons, and their disclosure in detail would be a breach of medical etiquette.

It will not be permitted for riders to sign a form of indemnity granting racecourse medical officers or racecourse officials the authority to divulge the medical condition of injured jockeys. It therefore follows that the presence in the medical room of persons other than the injured person, the nurses and medical personnel breaches this confidentiality and the necessary measures to exclude these persons from the medical room should be a matter for consultation and action between the senior racecourse medical officer and the clerk of the course.

Notwithstanding the above paragraph there are likely to be occasions when in the interest of good public relations practice it will be advisable to make a general statement about the overall clinical state of the injured. Such a statement should follow the guidelines of accepted medical practice in respect of the release of information regarding incidents affecting public figures involved in sporting events.

Reference

Edixhoven P., Sinha S.C. & Dandy D.J. (1981) Injury. *British Journal of Accident Surgery* **12**, 279.

17 Combat sports: common injuries and their treatment

G. R. MᶜLATCHIE

'We live in a freakish world, a vicious world. People like to see blood.'
Mohammed Ali

There are three main groups of combat sports, all of which have their origins in actual combat:
1 Predominantly punching sports, e.g. boxing, karate.
2 Predominantly grappling and throwing, e.g. aikido, judo, ju-jitsu, wrestling.
3 Weaponry, e.g. fencing, kendo, use of weapons in karate.

Boxing

Historical background

In 1100 BC Epeus won by a knock-out over Euryalus. The prize was a mule and the fighters assailed each other with their fists enclosed in cesti — leather gloves impregnated with metal studs. They wore head protection in the form of leather helmets and the only absolute rule was that the victor should not kill his opponent.

Boxing eventually became so popular that even the storming of the Bastille in 1789 was relegated to the back pages of English newspapers because of a clash with an important fight. It remained so until the end of the Second World War, since when it has given way to other sports. There are still, however, around 7000 bouts each year in the UK. The first recorded British champion was in the late seventeenth century, when eye-gouging was legitimate. These contests then gave way to the bare-fist fights and subsequently the modern sport.

Philosophy of injury

The sport has been dominated by the 'no pain, no gain' philosophy. This is the concept that it is impossible to improve unless extreme physical commitment is involved and that injuries (especially head injuries) can be ignored; the former is probably true, but the latter certainly false. However, it is fair to say that this attitude has been eroded in recent years.

An adherence to this philosophy, however tenuous, will of course present difficulties for the attending doctor, whose primary duty is to preserve the health interests of his patients (the boxers). In philosophical terms this would mean that a fight should be stopped as soon as a fighter has a bleeding nose or a facial laceration. In practice, however, only specific injuries will lead to the fight being stopped.

211

*Chapter 17
Combat sports:
common injuries
and their
treatment*

Specific injuries

The main target of attack (the head) and the instruments of attack (the hands) are the most common sites of injury. Injury to other sites is uncommon.

Head injuries

Head injury is the most serious boxing-related injury. When death occurs from an acute head injury it is nearly always due to intra-cranial bleeding, with subdural haemorrhage into one of the middle cranial fossae being the most common post-mortem finding. Such bleeds are thought to be due to prolonged battering, with bleeding from the dural emissary veins (Green 1978). The punch-drunk syndrome (traumatic encephalopathy) was first described by Martland in 1928 and since that time medical supervision has become mandatory. Regular medical examinations of professional boxers, including electroencephalography, are now carried out and, if a boxer has been knocked out, a minimum period of four weeks must elapse before he can take part in further bouts.

The onset of traumatic encephalopathy is insidious and initial clinical signs are difficult to detect but when fully developed the deterioration of the boxer can best be observed in the ring. His movements become slowed, he stands in a broad base and, with impaired reflexes, he is less able to avoid a blow. At a later stage he appears to be drunk, with emotional lability, slurred speech and loss of social control. The memory and intellect become impaired. Pathologically there is progressive cerebral ventricular dilatation with diffuse cerebellar and cerebral neuronal degeneration. These changes can particularly affect the temporal lobes. Repeated minor trauma is thought to be the cause (Roberts 1970).

Injuries to the eye and orbit

The commonest injuries are periorbital lacerations or abrasions from punches and head-butting, although gloves themselves can result in abrasion or laceration of the cornea. Most small abrasions of the cornea heal in two to three days. Such minor injuries require only the wearing of an eye pad for a few days. Lacerations of the skin require approximation of the edges, which is best achieved by sutures or Steristrips. In this way a broad scar is prevented. These

212

*Chapter 17
Combat sports:
common injuries
and their
treatment*

are liable to break down again if further traumatised and it is well known that many boxers have a 'cut' problem. Some have even required special surgical techniques to obtain a good repair.

Serious eye injury is rare but retinal detachment, paralytic diplopia and optic atrophy have all been reported (Doggart 1965; Rugg-Gunn 1965). Where serious eye injury is suspected or visual impairment is present, the patient must be referred promptly to an ophthalmic surgeon.

Other facial injuries

Nosebleeds and nasal fractures or dislocation of the nasal septum are fairly common. These result in the characteristic 'boxer's nose', with considerable cosmetic deformity. Fractures of the mandible and facial bones also occur but they are unusual. Haematoma of the pinna leads to 'cauliflower ear' and is best treated by early aspiration and the injection of proteolytic enzymes, such as hyaluronidase, to allow resolution.

Hand injuries

Hand injuries can be prevented by ensuring that correct punching techniques are taught. Glove design with the thumb in a different compartment makes injury to this digit more likely. More recent designs of gloves, however, have incorporated a flange so that a blow to the thumb will be deflected. Fracture or fracture dislocation to the base of the first metacarpal is a fairly common injury (Montanoro & Francone 1966). These injuries require manipulative reduction and occasionally surgical treatment because they are unstable. The necks of the second and fifth metacarpal bones are the next most commonly fractured. They should be reduced and immobilised for three to four weeks in a dorsal slab.

The early detection of cerebral damage in boxers

Although the long-term effects of severe brain damage, both physical and psychological, are well recognised, it is often not appreciated that even minor head injuries with brief periods of post-traumatic amnesia can be associated with permanent impairment of psychological function. After such minor head injuries, a 'post-traumatic' syndrome consisting of headaches, irritability and difficulties with concentration may develop, symptoms which can take months to resolve. Where recurrent head injury may occur, such as in boxing, then the risk of cumulative damage develops and further trauma will produce greater psychological impairment (Gronwall & Wrightson 1974, 1975). To date, two sports, boxing and steeplechasing, have been implicated in cases of cumulative brain damage and there have been anecdotal reports of cerebral damage in many other sports men and women (Foster & Leiguarda 1976). Quite recently a high incidence of electroencephalographic disturbance, most probably due to neuronal damage as a result of repeated trauma, has been noted in active Norwegian football players and there is a considerable increase in the incidence of electroencephalographic disturbances in former football players. These changes are due to repeated blows to the head as a result of heading the football (Tysvaer & Storli 1987).

Cumulative damage can only be prevented by making sports officials and participants aware of the risks of continuing active participation following head injury. In combat sports, such as boxing and karate, sprung or padded flooring can reduce the incidence of secondary head injuries which can occur when a fighter falls to the floor as the result of a blow and then strikes his head on the canvas. The use of adequate headgear in boxing has reduced the number of knock-outs in Czechoslovakia but paradoxically, whereas a knock-out will stop the fight, protective headgear may simply allow a partially incapacitated fighter to continue the bout, sustaining multiple minor traumatic cerebral injuries producing the inevitable risk of cumulative brain damage (Lindsay et al. 1980).

The evidence of brain damage in professional boxers is conclusive but there is now also strong evidence that a degree of brain damage may occur in active amateur boxers.

In the search for the most sensitive method of detecting abnormal cerebral function and established brain damage, a Finnish study included neuropsychometry, clinical examination and EEG and found them to be equally sensitive (Kaste et al. 1982). The CT scan was rarely abnormal, but this is not surprising as CT scanning only detects severe degrees of damage reflected in gross anatomical changes that occur in the well-recognised abnormalities seen in professional boxers. A normal brain scan, therefore, does not exclude significant brain damage and so should not be used as the sole method of detection. The best method of detecting neurological abnormalities and possible brain damage is neuropsychometry. In one study (McLatchie et al. 1987), where boxers' neuropsychological performances were compared with a control group, it was noted that in some tests the boxers were significantly poorer than the controls. EEG abnormalities were also twice those of the normal population. In the young population with less mature brains the EEG is more likely to be abnormal. Therefore, although EEG does detect abnormalities they are not always necessarily due to brain damage and a single EEG, therefore, is not the best method of diagnosing damage. On the other hand, a series of EEGs showing an emerging abnormality would be of significance.* In conclusion a combination of neuropsychometry, clinical examination and serial EEG is the only satisfactory method for detecting early cerebral

213
*Chapter 17
Combat sports:
common injuries
and their
treatment*

*Doctors who are asked to assess boxers for fitness to fight should refer the patients for these tests unless they are competent to provide these services themselves.

214

Chapter 17
Combat sports:
common injuries
and their
treatment

damage in boxers. These fighters should then be advised to reduce the number of fights or to stop boxing altogether.

Karate

Historical background

In modern Japanese karate means 'empty-handed'. In its simplest sense this implies unarmed combat or fighting without the assistance of weapons. On a deeper philosophical level it implies infinity of self-discipline and religious conviction.

Although the origins of karate can be traced to China it is said to owe its development to the Ryukyu islanders who, when overrun by the Kyshu in 1609, circumvented the veto which banned weapons of any kind by devising an efficient empty-handed form of combat. This was so effective that a trained exponent could punch through the bamboo armour of his oppressors with his hardened fists or dismount horsemen with high-jumping kicks.

Karate is a very popular martial art and is currently practised in the UK by approximately 60 000 people.

Philosophy of injury

To understand attitudes to injury in karate one must consider the concept of 'bushido'.

Bushido is the code of honour and conduct which the Samurai warriors of feudal Japan were required to observe. Disciples of this philosophy offer absolute loyalty to immediate superiors and subject themselves to unquestioning obedience. The Samurai warrior had to be prepared to fight and die without the slightest hesitation, to be oblivious to pain and to have no fear of death. Clearly these warriors made daunting adversaries. The acceptance of pain as a necessary part of advancement is one reason why there was initially a very high injury rate in the sport of Japanese karate. Fortunately this principle has been gradually eroded, on grounds of common sense.

Forces in karate

The 'secret' of the karate blow is the concentration of the body's energy into a small area on the target. In a straight punch 3000 Newtons/cm^2 of force are generated by a good standard karateka. More force is required to break wood than concrete, which may seem surprising but wood is more elastic than concrete and therefore absorbs much of the energy applied to it.

However, all karate exponents know that wood is easier to break than concrete. In the collision between hand and target, only part of the kinetic energy of the hand is transferred to the target — the remainder is retained in the hand and causes pain. Wood will absorb most of the hand's kinetic energy but concrete obstinately refuses at least half of it; hence, perhaps not surprisingly, concrete is more likely to produce pain and damage to the hand than is wood when an attempt is made to break slabs of equivalent thickness.

Provided the force of collision is directed along the lines of stress in the bone no fracture will occur. Bone is tougher than wood or concrete, by virtue of its lamellar structure but it is important that the forces involved are directed along the lines of force.

215
Chapter 17
Combat sports:
common injuries
and their
treatment

Forms of sport karate

There are three forms of sport karate (McLatchie 1976; McLatchie *et al.* (1980):

1 Traditional karate. In this form the attacker makes his attack at full speed but withdraws his blows just before they reach the target. Fine judgement is required.

2 Semi-contact karate. This is a further development of the above theme. Some areas of the body, such as the testicles and face, are exempt from attack, but full contact is allowed to the head with the feet and to the trunk with the hands and feet.

3 Full-contact karate. In this sport blows of unmitigated force are directed against the target area of the opponent, i.e. the head and trunk.

Serious injury

There are four possible sites of injury (McLatchie 1976, 1981, 1982; McLatchie *et al.* 1980):

1 Craniofacial and cervical injuries.

2 Injuries to the trunk.

3 Injuries to the limbs.

4 Nerve injuries.

Craniofacial and cervical injuries

Lacerations, abrasions, nosebleeds and black eyes are all common and should only cause withdrawal from the contest when bleeding is persistent or vision becomes impaired due to periorbital swelling. Steristrip or sutures to minor lacerations and adrenaline packs for serious nosebleeds are effective methods of treatment. Nasal fracture is fairly common, and karateka can often present with features of boxer's nose. Fracture of the malar bone is also fairly frequent and is recognised by a depression on the affected side of the face and infraorbital paraesthesia due to nerve entrapment.

Head injuries are also common, concussion and skull fractures

216

*Chapter 17
Combat sports:
common injuries
and their
treatment*

being the most worrying. Both can be caused by uncontrolled blows or by the occiput striking a hard floor after a fall. Therefore, padded flooring is essential at all competitions. Cervical injury occurs rarely although cervical dislocation has resulted when spinning kicks have been used. Many associations have now outlawed these dangerous techniques.

Injuries to the trunk

The pleura can be damaged from direct blows, resulting in pneumothorax secondary to rib fracture.

The abdominal viscera are also vulnerable. Hepatic, splenic and renal rupture have all been reported, as has acute traumatic pancreatitis. Probably the commonest injury is 'winding' due to a blow to the solar plexus (the coeliac plexus). In most cases recovery is rapid, within 30–90 seconds.

Blows to the testes due to uncontrolled kicks are painful and force retirement from the competition. Protection is afforded by the use of a proper groin guard.

Injuries to the limbs

As in boxing the hand is one of the commonest sites of injury. The fingers can be dislocated by attempts to parry blows. Toes can be dislocated from defective blocking of kicks. Fractures to the bones of the upper and lower limbs are sometimes seen, and should be treated on their individual merits.

Thumb injuries are common. Both 'gamekeeper's thumb' and 'karate thumb' occur, as well as 'Bennett's fracture dislocation'. In gamekeeper's thumb the ulnar collateral ligament is avulsed from the base of the proximal phalanx with a wedge of bone. In karate thumb the radial collateral ligament is affected. Gamekeeper's thumb requires surgical fixation since it is potentially unstable. However, karate thumb can be treated conservatively. In karateka who harden their fists on padded wooden boards traumatic bursitis over the heads of the second and third matacarpal bones is commonly seen (puncher's knuckle).

Fascial compartment compression of the leg and quadriceps haematoma are a serious group of injuries caused by low hard kicks to the shins and thighs in order to weaken the opponent. Severe bruising of the large muscles of the thighs can be a source of chronic pain if there is subsequent calcification of the haematoma with the formation of myositis ossificans. Traumatic anterior tibial compartment syndrome (fascial compartment compression) can present as a surgical emergency requiring fasciotomy. The use of ice-packs with elevation and bandaging of the affected limb can considerably relieve pain and reduce swelling. Withdrawal from the competition in these situations is mandatory.

217
Chapter 17
Combat sports:
common injuries
and their
treatment

Knee injuries are also quite common. In performing a technique such as the 'roundhouse kick' there is a degree of rotation on a fixed tibia and this can produce tears of the menisci in a similar mechanism to that of football injuries. The injury to the menisci thus caused may be severe enough to necessitate subsequent menisectomy.

Nerve injuries

The peripheral nerves most often affected are:
1   The radial nerve. Injuries to the radial nerve may be associated with a fracture of the humerus and require surgical repair but most are traumatic neuropraxias from kicks to the mid-part of the upper arm. Historically, kicks to this region prevented an armed man from gripping or wielding his weapon, and indicate considerable astuteness of clinical observation in the early exponents of the art.
2   The ulnar nerve. This is most often injured from kicks to the elbow. Another site of injury to the nerve is the hand. It may affect those fighters who toughen their hands on hard objects. One unfortunate student presented to his doctor with wasting of all the muscles on the hypothenar eminence due to traumatic apraxia of the deep branch of the ulnar nerve.
3   The superficial peroneal nerve. This nerve is often injured during sweeping manoeuvres. The patient will complain of tingling and weakness of eversion of the foot. Symptoms usually settle in hours but may persist for several weeks.

Reduction in incidence of injury

Tables 17.1–4 present salient features from the Scottish Karate Injury Register over the ten-year period 1974–83. This relates only to injuries sustained in traditional karate, which is by far the most popular of the three types (McLatchie 1979).

Table 17.1 Injuries to the head and neck

Injury	Number of cases		
	1974–6	1977–9	1980–3
Epistaxis	91	17	20
Facial lacerations	110	33	15
Periorbital laceration	51	5	2
Head Injury (PTA/concussion) (Skull fracture)	170	83	45
Blows to the trachea	23	4	5
Cervical dislocation (C6/C7)	1	0	0
Maxillary sinus rupture (with pneumatocele)	2	1	0
Mandibular fracture	7	0	1
Malar fracture	8	2	1
Total	463	145	89

Table 17.2 Injuries to the trunk

Injury	Number of cases		
	1974–6	1977–9	1980–3
Rib fracture	35	22	16
Pneumothorax	15	3	2
Blows to solar plexus	185	115	70
Blows to testes	43	12	15
Splenic rupture	2	2	0
Acute traumatic pancreatitis	0	1	0
Total	280	155	103

Table 17.3 Injuries to the limbs

Injury	Number of cases		
	1974–6	1977–9	1980–3
Fractures	97	13	15
Karate thumb	27	5	4
Gamekeeper's thumb	15	5	3
Traumatic neuropraxia	27	5	7
Anterior tibial compartment syndrome	2	2	1
Retropatellar pain	35	21	18
Meniscus symptoms	80	52	32
Total	283	103	80

Table 17.4 Injuries in karate — change in incidence over ten years, 13 566 contests

	1974–6	1977–9	1980–3
Total injuries	931	403	272
Number of contests	4003	3449	6114
Incidence	1 per 4 contests	1 per 8.5 contests	1 per 22 contests

Three separate periods of study were undertaken. After the first three-year period preventive measures introduced included the use of protective clothing in the form of gum-shields, groin guards, knuckle pads, shin guards and foot pads as well as the introduction of padded flooring (McLatchie 1986a). Three years later a national campaign in the UK was launched, the aim being to educate referees and participants to the risk of injuries, including means of prevention and immediate management. Further measures taken during these periods were the introduction of equivalent weight classes (except in team events) and the banning of dangerous techniques. The other recommendation was that there should be statutory medical control at all competitions where more than 20 participants took part.

219

Chapter 17
Combat sports:
common injuries
and their
treatment

It is apparent that the incidence of injury fell from one per four contests in 1974–6 to one per eight contests in 1977–9. Following this period the injury rate dropped further to one per 22 contests in major competitions in Scotland.

From this study of 13 566 karate contests we may conclude that, even in a combat sport, injury can be reduced considerably by the avoidance of dangerous techniques and provision of adequate medical attention. More importantly, the introduction of preventive measures in the form of protective clothing and coach and participant education does not appear to have adversely affected performance. This is adequately borne out by the fact that Scotland won four European championships during that ten-year period and that Great Britain during the same time won the world championship on four occasions.

The introduction of weight classes at major national competitions and the outlawing of dangerous techniques have also reduced the incidence of injury. Use of padded flooring is another means of prevention of injury in combat sports, and has been extremely successful in reducing the number of head injuries which hitherto occurred in falls on to concrete flooring.

In karate, if a fighter is concussed he or she should not fight again for at least three or four weeks. If there are symptoms of the post-traumatic syndrome he or she should not return to sport until they have resolved completely. Any fighter who has suffered a head injury severe enough to cause a coma or who has had a neurosurgical procedure should be advised to give up combat sports altogether.

Grappling and throwing sports (McLatchie 1981, 1982)

Judo

Judo, 'the way of gentleness', has been popular in Britain for more than 30 years. It is an Olympic sport and an effective method of self-defence. It is not a martial art but was invented in the mid-1860s by a Japanese college professor, Dr Jigaro Kano. He made a detailed study of the many ancient fighting forms of the orient and, realising that each fighting school saw their concept as superior to all others, he synthesised all he had learned and called the art judo, the gentle way. He argued that the most efficient way of fighting was to use intellect, personal ability and the mistakes of one's opponents. Thus if an attacker threw a punch the defender would throw the attacker using his or her attacker's own momentum.

Judo involves rapidly changing one's centre of gravity to perform throws as well as the use of ground work and locks against joints to maintain an opponent in a helpless position. Strangles, chokes and

220
*Chapter 17
Combat sports:
common injuries
and their
treatment*

locks against the joints are characteristic of ground work and so it is not surprising that injuries may involve many of the joints of the limbs and the neck.

Aikido

The Japanese martial art involves the redirection of an attacker's energy with grappling and striking. It also involves some use of weapons. Approximately 1300 people practise the art in Britain.

Ju-jitsu

This is a Japanese martial art of uncertain origin which involves throws, locks and holds with ancillary strikes to weaken or divert the attention of an opponent whilst the grappling technique is applied, the object being to gain a submission. The art developed in several areas independently and therefore several schools of style exist today. There are around 2250 practitioners in the UK.

Particular injuries

Strangles and chokes can compress the carotid arteries and produce unconsciousness. In all events episodes of unconsciousness should be treated as if they were minor head injuries and a lay-off period is encouraged. Recently a top-class judoka has sustained a cervical dislocation resulting in quadriplegia. This is a rare injury but emphasises the inevitable risks of the application of strangle-holds or throws in a strangle position. For neck injuries in children, see Chapter 10.

The most commonly injured joints are the shoulders, elbows and fingers in the form of dislocation or sprains and these are treated along standard lines. Mat burns, grazes and bruises are common. Serious abdominal injury is rare.

Injury situations

Most injuries happen when:
1 A breakfall is poorly executed.
2 A limb lock is over enthusiastically applied or not submitted to.
3 A choke or strangle is applied for too long.

The wrist, elbow and head are the sites most frequently injured after ineffective breakfalls. Prevention lies in the use of adequate warm-up and frequent falling practice. If an injury to a major joint does occur the affected limb should be supported gently either with broad bandages lightly applied or with pillows and sandbags until transfer to hospital is available.

221
*Chapter 17
Combat sports:
common injuries
and their
treatment*

Injuries particular to children (McLatchie 1981)

Judo is extremely popular amongst children. One of the common injuries is 'pulled elbow'. In this condition the radial head is pulled out of its annular ligament. This produces symptoms of immediate pain and tenderness over the radial head associated with almost complete limitation of pronation and supination. The treatment is simple: firm alternate pronation and supination with the elbow held at a right angle allows the radial head to click back into position. Post-traumatic sequelae are rare.

Wrestling

Wrestling is one of the oldest sports in the world and probably the most widespread. In Egypt, it was already a highly organised sport (around 3000 BC), with complicated rules and protocol as is witnessed by some 4000 holds and throws inscribed on the walls of tombs of Ben-y-Hassam.

Numerous fabled contests are reported in antiquity: Ulysses and Ajax wrestled at the funeral games before the walls of Troy. Rustam killed Sohrab, his son, before the King of Afghanistan. In the fourteenth century when the Turkish tribes made raids into Europe, two men wrestled for three days without decision and then died, not surprisingly, of exhaustion. In recognition of their efforts a three-day wrestling tournament has been held each year on the site ever since.

Many cultures measure courage by wrestling ability and several eastern countries send only wrestling teams to the Olympic Games. Indeed, in the Turkish language the word for hero and wrestler is the same — *pehlivan*.

In Britain there are three types of wrestling:
1 Olympic or freestyle.
2 Graeco-Roman.
3 Professional.

The fighters must have well-cut nails and short hair and be of equivalent weight. No jewellery is permitted. In freestyle wrestling any fair hold is allowed. In Graeco-Roman style wrestling holds below the waist are forbidden and trips or throws using the legs are also illegal.

All-in professional wrestling is a spectacular sport where no holds are barred — save direct chokes. The forearm and the flat of the hand are permitted as instruments of attack. However, apparently extremely violent injury and death are rare. In the last 40 years there have been few deaths — mainly due to heart attacks or head injuries after falling out of the ring.

Professional wrestling seems to provide a high degree of safety for the wrestlers as well as crowd satisfaction — especially for female fans.

222
*Chapter 17
Combat sports:
common injuries
and their
treatment*

Serious injury

The well-known hazard of wrestling is cervical injury. This can occur if one contestant falls heavily on his opponent when he is 'bridging'. Strict adherence to the rules is therefore vital if these injuries are to be avoided and it is illegal to jump upon a wrestler who is bridging.

As in boxing and karate, fractures and fracture dislocations of the metacarpophalangeal joints of the thumb are common and these require surgical intervention to produce a stable joint.

Chronic injuries

Common sites for 'chronic' injury are the knees and the shoulders. Meniscal and ligamentous injuries occur and are often a source of persistent trouble. Shoulder pain is usually the result of innumerable minor muscle sprains. Wrestlers with chronic knee pain may present with effusions, ligamentous laxity and limitation of movement.

In Japan sumo wrestlers present with an interesting range of injuries. This is a professional sport. The participants are reared from a young age in establishments known as stables, to prepare them for their sport. They eat a particularly high fat diet and their training is intensive. Their hands become subjected to repeated trauma against padded posts. As a result stiffness of the metacarpophalangeal joints and proximal phalangeal joints of the fingers and thumbs occur. These men are also said to present with a punch-drunk type syndrome in later life due to the repeated concussions from butting each other in competitions. Many are also reported to be partially sighted. They have short lives, usually dying in their mid-40s from heart disease related to their high fat intake.

Grazes, facial cuts and mat burns are all extremely common in all types of wrestling. Of these, mat burns can be very painful and if wrestling continues the burned area should be carefully covered to protect it. Grazes and facial cuts respond to simple first-aid measures but, if extensive, admission to hospital may be required.

Prevention of injury

Neck strength is essential. All trainee wrestlers must begin by practising gentle bridging exercises. As expertise increases kick-over bridging and bridging with weights can be practised. During the souplesse and salto techniques some wrestlers land on their foreheads in the bridged position. This demands immense muscular strength and training. Such a forehead landing should not be attempted by novices and it may be better for them to rotate out so that their full weight and that of their opponent do not stress the cervical vertebrae.

223

*Chapter 17
Combat sports:
common injuries
and their
treatment*

Neck-strengthening exercises are also an important part of injury prevention. Effective strengthening can be achieved by using weights, shoulder shrugging and pulling exercises, keeping the weight as close as possible to the body.

Contestants in all combat sports should keep their hair short so that there is no impairment of vision. Pre-fight medical examination and rest periods after head injury are mandatory and the doctor present must decide whether a man can continue after injury.

In freestyle and Graeco-Roman wrestling no hold is allowed which will cause a man to submit because of pain. No strangleholds against the joint's normal movement are permitted.

Weaponry (McLatchie 1982)

Fencing and kendo are combat sports in which the original sword is replaced by an épée or shi-ai respectively. Both sports have long histories but since they make use of protective equipment serious injury is rare and does not require further detailed discussion. The commonest problem encountered is bruising, usually to the chest and upper arms, and these are rarely troublesome in the long term.

Deaths resulting from kendo accidents have been secondary to eye injuries. In each incident the shi-ai shattered and bamboo splinters penetrated the face-guards and eye socket. One victim of such an accident died from intracranial bleeding, another from infection. This underlines the importance of ensuring that protective equipment is in good condition and emphasises the need for frequent inspection and care of weapons.

Use of weapons in karate (McLatchie 1982)

One extension of karate is the use of oriental farming instruments as weapons. These have also become popular as instruments of attack in urban violence. Whilst learning the use of these weapons in class, strict control and slow repetitive movements are necessary before mastery can be achieved. Many inexperienced weapon users find the weapon more dangerous to themselves than to any imaginary opponent.

Recommendations for doctors attending sports competitions

It is recommended that a doctor, preferably one who is interested in sports injuries and sports medicine, should be in attendance at combat sports competitions. Further, on many occasions it is also possible to have representatives from the Red Cross, St John or St Andrew's ambulance services in attendance, provided that these voluntary bodies are given prior notice.

224

Chapter 17
Combat sports:
common injuries
and their
treatment

Responsibilities of the doctor (McLatchie 1986b)

The doctor may be asked to examine competitors before the competition if required by the rules of the sport. This is necessary in boxing and usually in international competitions involving karate, judo, aikido and wrestling. Fighting areas should be inspected to ensure that adequate flooring is in use. In boxing the ring should be sprung and in judo, wrestling and karate padded flooring should be used since head injury is a common sequel to falls on hard floors.*

The doctor should also treat any minor injuries received, such as lacerations and sprains, but should refer the more serious injuries to hospital for further examination and treatment. He should also be able to advise the referees, where requested, as to the fitness of competitors to continue in a competition. In sports such as karate he should be able to discuss the potential danger of various techniques when dubious points are under discussion. It is obvious, therefore, that the doctor attending such competitions should know his sport well.

Injuries which exclude further participation

1 Fractures.
2 Head injuries which have resulted in disorientation, amnesia or unconsciousness.
3 Ocular injuries where sight is impaired. This would include periorbital injuries and depends upon examination.
4 Certain cases of testicular injury where recovery is not rapid and scrotal haematomata are present.

Protective clothing

This should be used as permitted by the governing body and should be inspected by the officials of the sport concerned. The doctor should, however, note that in some karate and judo competitions competitors may have the habit of wearing jewellery such as earrings in pierced ears. It is mandatory that all jewellery be removed before any competition takes place.

Fitness to compete

1 Following a knock-out, a period of at least four weeks should elapse before any further competition takes place. Training, but no sparring, is permitted.

---

*If the doctor is unhappy about any of the arrangements for the contest, e.g. inadequate flooring or unsatisfactory medical equipment, etc., or if after examination one of the contestants is judged unfit to take part, his or her misgivings should be made known to the officials of the tournament.

225

*Chapter 17
Combat sports:
common injuries
and their
treatment*

2   When there is a serious eye or ear injury, return to competition should be dictated by expert opinion, e.g. an ophthalmic or ENT specialist. In such a case the competitor will be required to produce evidence of his fitness to compete in the form of a discharge letter from the specialist concerned.

3   Following bony injuries to the face, nose or hands the time away from training and competition will depend on the extent of the injury, and return to competition will be subject to further medical examination. Three to six weeks will be the norm for these types of injury.

Management of sports men or women with acute head injuries

Medical attendants to contact sports must be fully conversant with the diagnosis, assessment and acute management of head injuries and this is especially so in combat sports. The most important clinical manifestation of head injuries is alteration of the conscious level, which may be observed as a knock-out, a period of post-traumatic amnesia with automatism, or a fluctuating level of consciousness deteriorating to coma at a variable rate. Where there is clear-cut loss of consciousness or obvious deterioration in conscious level, management is relatively straightforward, and is discussed below.

The difficulty arises when a player who has received a head injury apparently recovers fully and is able to speak, but on closer examination is found to have a degree of post-traumatic amnesia or is mildly disorientated. All such competitors should be encouraged to leave the combat area and indeed in sport karate sometimes have been sent off by the referees for their own safety. The mildly concussed individual is more liable to sustain a second head injury or to develop secondary brain damage from an intracranial haematoma.

For the more seriously injured player, with regard to head injury, the crucial question is whether admission to hospital is required. If the patient experiences a period of an altered level of consciousness even if he is walking and talking, it is essential for a skull X-ray to be performed in order to identify the small number of patients who have sustained a skull fracture. Lacerations and haematomata must be carefully examined and the possibility of depressed fracture should be entertained.

Table 17.5 The Glasgow Coma Scale

Eye opening		Motor response		Verbal response	
Spontaneous	4	Obeys commands	6	Orientated	5
To speech	3	Localizes pain	5	Confused	4
To pain	2	Normal flexion	4	Inappropriate words	3
Nil	1	Abnormal flexion	3	Incomprehensible sounds	2
		Extension	2	Nil	1
		Nil	1		

226

*Chapter 17
Combat sports:
common injuries
and their
treatment*

The Glasgow Coma Scale (Table 17.5) permits a ready means of assessing, recording and displaying level of consciousness. It tabulates in a scaled form the functions of eye opening, best verbal response and best motor response. Its simple terms provide an objective descriptive standard for patients with head injuries. For patients who have sustained injuries serious enough to warrant referral to hospital, Glasgow Coma Scale observations should be commenced and recorded as soon as possible.

If there is prolonged unconsciousness the patient should be placed in the coma position, or alternatively nursed supine only if aspiration equipment is available. The airway must be cleared and maintained during transport. In less serious cases of head injury the player should be advised to refrain from eating or drinking for 12 hours and alcohol should be specifically prohibited. Following assessment, suitable arrangements with relatives, friends or club officials are necessary to ensure a journey home and adequate subsequent observation thereafter. If any focal neurological signs develop or if vomiting or persistent headaches are present further medical aid should be sought. These instructions can be given to the accompanying person on a printed card.

Common injuries of combat sports and their treatment

The injuries commonly seen in exponents of this group of sports are: blisters, friction burns, lacerations and haematomata.

Each of these conditions should be treated on its merits according to the principles described below. As a general rule blisters and friction burns may be treated by the doctor attending the event, whilst lacerations and haematomata all generally require referral to a local accident and emergency department. Clinical assessment of the severity of the condition will be the final determining factor.

Blisters are caused by shearing forces on the skin, usually of the hands and feet and are commonly seen in judoka and karateka. The fluid should be aseptically aspirated or drained* as often as it accumulates and the roof of the blister left intact. It acts as a 'biological dressing' and allows healing to occur more rapidly. The area should then be covered with barrier cream or a dressing to prevent further damage.

*If aseptic conditions cannot be guaranteed at the 'ringside', the patient must be referred to an accident and emergency department where this service can be provided.

Mat burns are generated by friction and are commonly seen in wrestlers and judoka. The affected area should be immediately cooled with tap-water or an ice-pack. Unless extensive, when hospital care is needed, this and an analgesic are all that is required.

Lacerations

Lacerations of the face are especially common in karate and boxing, usually in the periorbital region. The edges should be carefully ap-

227

Chapter 17
Combat sports:
common injuries
and their
treatment

proximated with sutures, after thorough cleaning, and using aseptic technique. Thus infection and excessive scarring are avoided.

Haematomata may collect following injuries to the soft tissues of the limbs, particularly the thighs, and around the eye. If the collection is large it should be aspirated under aseptic conditions. Haematomata affecting the lower leg can lead to compartment syndromes unless treated promptly. All combat sports men and women should be encouraged to have full tetanus immunisation. For adults, booster doses of a tetanus vaccine are recommended at five-yearly intervals.

The abuse of drugs in combat sports

Anabolic steroids

In Britain the use of steroids has been outlawed by the governing body of combat sport. Detection techniques are becoming more accurate, but there is evidence that the use of anabolic steroids amongst the strength combat sportsmen may be increasing. Anecdotally, the athlete on steroids is less susceptible to fatigue and injury and both aggression and confidence in training are increased. Doctors should play no part in aiding or abetting the administration of these drugs. It is important to be aware of their side-effects.

In the prepubertal male accelerated epiphyseal calcification producing diminished height has been reported as well as gynaecomastia and acne. Ironically it is arguably the least serious side-effect, namely acne, that users find most unacceptable. After puberty adult sexual function may be altered because of the suppression of pituitary luteinising hormone with resultant diminution in the production of endogenous testosterone resulting in reduced spermatogenesis. Alteration of liver function, cholestatic jaundice, abnormal thyroid function tests and changes in plasma proteins have also been observed in sports men and women using anabolic steroids.

Such drugs taken in their oral preparation are hepatotoxic if ingested over a prolonged period of time and are associated with primary liver cancers. Hyperinsulinism has also been reported, which has now been identified as a significant factor in the development of atherosclerosis, especially of the coronary arteries. Abnormal glucose tolerance may also occur, leading to diabetes mellitus.

It is now standard practice at international meetings to randomly test athletes for steroid drug abuse. Any fighter who is found to have taken such drugs to assist performance is guilty of cheating and he will be banned from competition.

Conclusions and recommendations

Much has been done to make these potentially dangerous sports safer but much still needs to be done. There is considerable poten-

228

*Chapter 17
Combat sports:
common injuries
and their
treatment*

tial for further prevention of injuries in combat sports. This would involve action for change in the philosophy of the referees, to stop the competition at earlier stages to prevent a partially injured competitor becoming seriously injured. Action by the governing bodies of the sports is required to alter the rules to ensure that safer practices and equipment are adopted by players and officials, both in competition and in training. The accurate gathering of injury statistics and monitoring of potential injury situations is also an important new development which should receive further attention in order that the gains in safety already made should be consolidated.

Medical recommendations for reduction of injuries

1 A medical certificate of fitness to compete should be presented to the official before a contest as a prerequisite to entry.

2 Each fighter should carry a fight record in which previous performances and injuries are recorded.

3 A doctor should be present at all competitions.

4 Following an injury to the eye, ear or head the competitor must be examined medically before fighting again. A minimum of four weeks should elapse before fighting after a head injury (knock-out, post-traumatic amnesia).

5 Equivalent weight classes should be encouraged. Ideally no fighter should outweigh his opponent by more than 3.5 kg.

6 Referees and instructors should be encouraged to learn first-aid.

7 The governing body should issue a summary of the rules of the sport. They should be freely available to all members of the association.

8 Before competitions a summary of the rules should be announced.

9 Suitable protective equipment must be worn as specifically recommended by the governing body in liaison with the medical officer to the sport.

References

Doggart J. H. & Rugg-Gunn A. (1965) Eye injuries. In *Medical Aspects of Boxing*, ed. A. L. Bass, J. L. Blonstein, R. D. James & J. G. P. Williams, pp. 3–19. Oxford: Pergamon Press.

Foster, J. B. & Leiguarda R. (1976) Brain damage in national hunt jockeys. *Lancet* **i**, 981.

Green M. A. (1978) Injury and sudden death in sport. In *The Pathology of Violent Injury*, ed. J. K. Mason, pp. 255–77. London: Edward Arnold.

Gronwall D. & Wrightson P. (1974) Adult recovery of intellectual function after minor head injury. *Lancet* **ii**, 605–9.

Gronwall D. & Wrightson P. (1975) Cumulative effect of concussion. *Lancet* **i**, 981.

Kaste M., Vilkk J., Sainis K., Cumme T., Katevuo K. & Meuralao H. (1982) Is chronic brain damage in boxing a hazard of the past? *Lancet* **ii**, 1186–8.

Lindsay K. W., McLatchie G. R. & Jennett B. (1980) Serious head injury in sport. *British Medical Journal* **281**, 789–91.

McLatchie G. R. (1976) Analysis of karate injuries sustained in 295 contests. *Injury* **8**, 132–4.

McLatchie G. R. (1979) Recommendations for medical officers attending karate competitions. *British Journal of Sports Medicine* **13**, 36–7.

229

*Chapter 17
Combat sports:
common injuries
and their
treatment*

McLatchie G. R. (1981) Injuries in combat sports. In *Sports Injuries*, ed. T. Riley, pp. 168–74, London: Faber and Faber.

McLatchie G. R. (1982) *Injuries in Combat Sports*. Oxford: Offox Press.

McLatchie G. R. (1986a) Prevention of injuries in combat sports — a 10-year study of competition karate. World Congress of Sports Medicine, Brisbane, Australia.

McLatchie G. R. (1986b) Team doctor. In *Essentials of Sports Medicine*, ed. G. R. McLatchie, pp. 25–9. Edinburgh: Churchill Livingstone.

McLatchie G. R., Davies J. E. & Caulley J. H. (1980) Injuries in karate — a case for medical control. *Journal of Trauma* **20** (11), 956–8.

McLatchie G. R., Brookes N., Galbraith S., Hutchison J. S. F., Wilson L., Melville I. & Teasdale E. (1987) Clinical neurological examination, neuropsychological electroencephalography and computed tomographic head scanning in active amateur boxers. *Journal of Neurology, Neurosurgery and Psychiatry* **50**, 96–9.

Mantland H. S. (1928) Punch drunk. *Journal of the American Medical Association* **91**, 1103–7.

Montanoro M. & Francone A. (1966) Roentgencinematographic study of the hand in boxers. Proceedings of the 6th Major International Boxing Association Medical Congress, Rome.

Roberts A. H. (1928) *Brain Damage in Boxers*. Tunbridge Wells: Pitman Medical.

Tysvaer A. T. & Storli O. V. Association football injuries to the brain — a neurological and electroencephalographic study of active football players. Unpublished observation.

Tysvaer A. T. & Storli O. V. Association football injuries to the brain — a neurological, electroencephalographic and echoencephalographic study of former football players. Unpublished observation.

18 The doctor at the boxing ring: amateur boxing

L. M. ADAMS AND P. J. WREN

'Under the bludgeonings of chance my head is blooded but
unbowed'
William Ernest Henley

Background

The nature of the sport

Amateur boxing is a unique sport which has as its objective the
landing of legal blows with force upon the opponent. A boxing
match therefore tests both offence and defence in this form of
individual combat, and the sport caters for boys and young men
with a particular combination of physique, physical skills and
psychological make-up. As with many sports, amateur boxing
demands an extremely high standard of physical and mental fitness;
the few minutes spent in the ring in a competitive bout are the
climax of many hours and weeks of hard physical and technical
training. Those who participate find in amateur boxing a healthy
and enjoyable form of training for life, developing self-confidence,
discipline and true sportsmanship. Amateur boxing clubs have a
friendly yet competitive atmosphere and, as well as the techniques
of the sport, teach their boxers respect for themselves and each other
and a sense of social responsibility.

After joining a club, a boxer must train in the gymnasium for
many months before he is ready to box competitively. During this
period, he will learn the basic skills and discipline of the sport, and
develop his physical fitness. A competitive bout consists of three
rounds, each lasting from one and a half minutes in a junior under-
15 contest to three minutes at senior level. During this time the
boxer must demonstrate his ability to deliver blows to the front
and side of his opponent's head, chest and abdomen above the
umbilicus. To score points, these blows must be delivered 'with
force' with the knuckle part of the gloved hand in the absence of foul
play such as holding. The only direct contact should be that which
occurs when a punch lands. Three judges independently score each
bout and award points to each boxer for the number of legal blows
landed. The great majority of bouts are decided 'on points'. Each
judge must nominate a winner — if points are equal, the bout is
awarded to the boxer who has done most of the leading off, who has

shown the better style or who has shown the better defence (in that order).

A boxer is considered 'down' if he touches the floor with any part of his body other than his feet, or if he falls outside or hangs helplessly on the ropes, or if, following a hard punch, he is in a distressed condition and cannot, in the opinion of the referee, continue the bout. In this situation, the referee will start to count; if the boxer is not recovered and ready to box after ten seconds, this is a knock-out. A good referee will stop the boxing and start a count if he considers that a boxer has received a particularly hard blow which requires a recovery period. The minimum count is eight seconds. If a boxer receives three such counts in one round or four in the entire contest then the bout is stopped in favour of his opponent. Contests may also be decided by disqualification, by voluntary retirement or if one boxer sustains an injury which, in the referee's opinion, renders him unfit to continue.

The referee remains inside the ring throughout the bout and is in sole charge of the contest, he does not normally judge the result. His functions are to protect the boxers and to ensure that the rules are kept. Standards of refereeing and judging are monitored by adjudicators — themselves senior referees — who report on the performance of these officials from time to time and at major tournaments. Other officials present at a tournament include the time-keeper, who regulates the number and duration of rounds and the intervals between them, and the official-in-charge, who has ultimate responsibility for all aspects of the tournament and has powers commensurate with this.

In non-championship tournaments, contestants are matched by the competition secretary, usually an experienced official or coach of the organising club or body. His objective is to select two boxers who are evenly matched by age, weight and ability. There are three age divisions within the junior category (12–15 years, 15–16 years and 16–17 years) and one category of senior (over 17 years). Only a certain amount of weight may be given away and boxers may not compete outside their age category. Senior boxers are classed by experience as novice, intermediate or open, but for juniors the competition secretary must take account of the number of contests, the standard of opponents and the calibre of the boxer himself. Matching is a most important task, as confidence and skill can only be developed when boxers are evenly matched. Good matchmaking is also crucial to maintaining the safety of the sport.

Administration

The Amateur Boxing Association of England (ABA) is the body which governs amateur boxing in this country. Similar but independent bodies control the sport in Wales, Scotland and other countries. Regulations governing the administration and technical aspects of the sport are only made or amended at the Annual Meeting of the National Committee, which carries representation from all geographic areas and affiliated bodies. An elected council is responsible for the implementation of policy and rules determined at the annual meeting. The council also has the important reciprocal role of guiding the annual meeting in its decisions, and recommending new regulations to it.

The sport is organised on a geographical basis. The country is divided into a number of areas, each of which is independently administered. These are the London and several provincial amateur boxing associations, each of which is governed by its own council. Each association is further split into a number of divisions, which often represent single geographical counties. The sport is run at divisional level, the governing body again being a council, elected annually by those clubs and organisations affiliated to it.

Tournaments are promoted by the amateur boxing clubs themselves or, for championships and representative matches, by divisions, associations or the ABA. The arrangements for each tournament must be authorised by the division/association, which allocates the officials for these tournaments. The London association and the provincial divisions each has a duty to train and keep a register of their officials-in-charge, referees, judges and timekeepers. They also have the authority to discipline their boxers and officials and to disaffiliate any club or organisation which fails to abide by the rules.

Boxing activities are provided by the amateur boxing clubs, each of which has its own training facilities and registered members and normally promotes a number of tournaments in a season. A club is affiliated to the division in which it is situated. Other bodies which represent a sectional interest are also authorised to promote amateur boxing. The more familiar of these are the Schools Amateur Boxing Association, the Combined Services Boxing Association and the National Association of Boys' Clubs. When tournaments are promoted by these organisations, they are obliged to apply the regulations of the ABA.

Medical involvement in Amateur boxing

Is is important to realise that doctors contribute far more to amateur boxing than simply attending at ringside in a 'first-aider' capacity. Doctors have had an increasingly close association with amateur boxing throughout this century and this relationship was formalised in 1970 when the 'medical' rules were drawn together to constitute a 'medical scheme' within the regulations of the sport. This was the achievement of Drs J. L. Blonstein and R. W. Barr–Brown, who summarised the regulations of the medical scheme in the first edition of *Medical Aspects of Boxing* in 1972. Since then, the scheme and its regulations have continued to evolve, and the second edition of this book is now published. The medical regulations, which are now part of the rules of boxing, are strict and precise, and are accepted by all as an intrinsic component of the sport, implemented for the protection and benefit of the boxers. These rules are rigorously enforced — from local club tournaments to international contests — and breaches of them have lead to disciplinary proceedings against the officials and clubs concerned.

Some aspects of the medical scheme will be discussed in detail later in this chapter. However, it might be helpful at this point to summarise the general principles and main provisions of the scheme:

1 The medical scheme is national, and all associations are required to take part in it.

2 The scheme is organised at association (London) or divisional (provinces) levels, where it is under the supervision of a local registrar. A central registrar (a salaried official of the ABA) receives copies of all documentation relating to all registered boxers and tournaments.

3 The medical scheme provides for:

(a) an initial medical examination of every entrant before he is allowed to box competitively;

(b) the medical re-examination of every boxer at intervals not exceeding five years up to the age of 30 years. It is recommended that the eyes of every boxer be examined by an ophthalmic practitioner every three years;

(c) the medical re-examination of every boxer at yearly intervals after the age of 30 years;

(d) the compulsory retirement of every boxer who reaches the age of 35 years;

(e) the medical inspection of every boxer immediately before he boxes;

(f) the full documentation of every boxer's career, to include a record of every competitive bout entered, all injuries and compulsory rest periods and every medical examination;

(g) the administration of the scheme by local and central registrars;

(h) the appointment of a medical officer's assistant to be in attendance and administer the medical scheme at every tournament.

There are three main ways in which doctors contribute to amateur boxing. First, they carry out the full medical examinations required initially and at intervals by the medical scheme. These examinations take a prescribed form, and are broadly similar in scope to the medical examinations performed for insurance purposes. Secondly, a doctor is required to be in attendance at every boxing tournament; this is to perform the medical inspections of the boxers to determine their fitness to box at that tournament, and subsequently to deal with any injuries which may occur. Thirdly, doctors contribute in a major way to the sport by their appointments as club doctor or as honorary medical officers of the divisions and associations and of the ABA.

There are five honorary medical officers of the ABA, who together comprise its Medical Commission. They are ex-officio members of the National Committee and of the Council of the ABA and shall 'advise the Association on all matters which come within their province'. The commission is responsible for the administration of the medical scheme, and is the final arbiter in decisions regarding an individual's fitness to box. In this, the commission works closely with the central registrar. The Medical Commission also has the duty to review the statistics generated by the central registrar and discuss ways in which the safety of the sport may be improved. Recommendations for changes in the regulations are considered from both medical and boxing aspects before they are sponsored by the Medical Commission for adoption by the Annual Meeting of the National Committee.

The Medical Commission also undertakes to organise an annual symposium which is open to all doctors with an interest in boxing, to learn of difficulties experienced and advise accordingly, and to develop a consensus of opinion on medical matters which are to the fore. By means of invited talks from specialists in their own field, the symposium also serves an educational role. Members of the commission also perform a very important educational role within amateur boxing circles, lecturing in the training courses for coaches and referees, and giving guidelines to other doctors who might assist them in this. For the 1988 Olympic Games in Seoul, an 'Olympic Squad Support Group' was also set up under the supervision of the Medical Commission, consisting of a physiotherapist, nutritionist, psychologist and physiologist. The objective of this group was to advise on the preparation of the British squad for the Olympic Games. In this, the group worked closely with the national coach. The work of the group continues in the anticipation that the lessons learned at élite level may be incorporated into the training regimens operated in the boxing clubs. The Medical Commission also normally provides the medical officers for major tournaments.

Honorary medical officers of the provincial associations and their divisions are also expected to officiate at representative tournaments and stages of the national championships which take place within their areas. However, a more important role is the advice they give their local registrar — particularly regarding the fitness to box of individual boxers. In this they may wish to examine a boxer themselves, or discuss the medical history with the boxer's general practitioner or seek a specialist opinion before deciding whether to pass an individual 'fit for boxing'. Association and divisional medical officers should maintain contact with other doctors who give their services to clubs in their area to discuss matters of mutual interest and concern, and should contribute to the training of club and ABA officials.

Many amateur boxing clubs have a relationship with a local doctor who will carry out medical examinations on the club's boxers and act as tournament medical officer for the club's shows. Whether this is a formal appointment or an informal attachment, the conditions of the relationship and any remuneration for these services are entirely matters for the club and doctor concerned. The club doctor is encouraged to take an interest in the welfare of the officials and boxers of the club (in some cases, he may be their general practitioner). He is in an excellent position to recognise medical problems in boxers at an early stage, and to recommend appropriate action. By knowing the coaches and gaining their confidence, the club doctor can help to educate them and their boxers on the reasoning behind the medical regulations, and on the safety value of good defensive technique and physical fitness. He may also be able to give advice on hygiene, diet, first-aid and the likelihood of medication affecting the results of a drug test.

Medical risks

It is inevitable in a combative contact sport that there is a risk of injury. Injuries and other medical problems may derive either from the specific nature of the sport — the landing of blows — or, as in other sports, from the physical activity which is part of both training and competition. The injuries which give rise to most concern are those which do not heal completely and thus may leave some permanent functional deficit, whether or not this is apparent at the time. This includes acute and chronic brain injury and some eye injuries. The major purpose of the medical scheme is to minimise the risk of these injuries. The most common injuries experienced in boxing are minor — bruising, lacerations and abrasions (mostly around the eyes, mouth and nose) and epistaxis. An intermediate category of injury, including fractures, dislocations and strains, is rare.

Acute head injury

In the ring, unconsciousness following a knock-down rarely lasts more than a few seconds and recovery is very rapid. One in every 24 bouts ends by a knock-out (KO) and one in every 51 as referee-stopped contest — head (RSCH) (Tables 18.1 and 18.2). For a boxer competing in the maximum permissible number of contests (18 per year plus championship matches for seniors), these would together average about once a year. For an averagely active boxer such minor

Table 18.1 Numbers of bouts of amateur boxing in England in the last five completed seasons (excluding bouts governed by the Combined Services Amateur Boxing Association; figures provided by the Central Registrar of the Amateur Boxing Association of England)

Boxers	1983–4	1984–5	1985–6	1986–7	1987–8
Junior — under 15	8 529	6 593	5 591	5 280	5 182
Junior — 15–17	2 611	2 552	2 359	2 332	2 224
Senior	8 238	6 828	7 752	6 145	6 258
Senior internationals	166	119	143	157	192
Total	19 544	16 092	15 845	13 914	13 856

head injury would be expected to occur once every two to four years — perhaps two or three times over a ten-year career of forty to sixty bouts (which represents a longer and more active career than many). Repeated KO or RSCH in the same boxer is unusual — one in 27 KO/RSCH occurred within three months of the previous one, and only one in 149 was the third such result within a calendar year (Tables 18.1 and 18.2).

In an attempt to obtain information about the severity of concussion following knock-out, since 1986 this has been graded by the delay until full recovery is attained. Grade 1 knock-out is defined as immediate recovery; grade 2, full recovery delayed for up to two minutes; grade 3, full recovery delayed for more than two minutes. Of necessity, this is a crude quantitation, but it should give some idea of the severity of the knock-out. It is to be regretted that, so far, this grading has not been recorded by officials with sufficient frequency or consistency to have yielded useful figures, despite the circulation of a detailed information sheet from the Medical Commission. When considering the severity of concussion resulting from amateur boxing, the definition of 'down' should also be remembered — in most cases, a count is started not because the boxer has been rendered prostrate and unresponsive, but because he is distressed and unable to protect himself fully. In many (perhaps the majority) of the contests ended by knock-out, there has been no 'loss of consciousness' at all. When compared to the 'minor' head injuries seen in hospital accident and emergency departments, these are very minor indeed.

Table 18.2 Numbers of bouts of amateur boxing in England which ended by knock-out (KO) and 'referee-stopped contest — head' (RSCH) for the last five completed seasons (excluding bouts governed by the Combined Services Amateur Boxing Assocation: figures provided by the Central Registrar of the Amateur Boxing Association of England)

	1983–4	1984–5	1985–6	1986–7	1987–8
KO	691	685	654	662	586
RSCH	350	400	290	299	208
KO/RSCH twice within 3 months	26	30	20	29	16
KO/RSCH three times within 1 year	4	3	6	7	2

KO includes all knock-outs from both head and body blows.

Serious acute head injury is extremely rare in amateur boxing. Since 1940 four fatalities and two cases of non-fatal intracranial haemorrhage have been recorded in English amateur boxers. Two deaths occurred in the armed forces, and unfortunately no medical records have been made available to the ABA. A third fatality was due to rupture of a berry aneurysm. Sadly, the others have occurred recently. In 1987, a youth of 16 years died 72 hours after his contest. Post-mortem examination reported rupture of a major blood vessel within the skull due to a blow to the head. It is not known whether a congenital vascular abnormality underlay this, nor was it known whether such a defect was specifically sought or could have been detected. In early 1989 two boxers suffered intracranial haemorrhage immediately after a bout. One had been knocked out in the ring and recovered consciousness after half a minute or so; when seen at this stage by the medical officer, he was fully conscious with no neurological signs. The other had not been down during his contest, losing on points. In both cases, conscious level suddenly and rapidly deteriorated 15–20 minutes after the bout finished, with localising signs appearing equally suddenly a few minutes later. In each case, the doctor was a highly experienced tournament medical officer, a resuscitation ambulance was called immediately, and the haematoma was evacuated without delay. Both boxers are improving postoperatively at the time of writing, a few weeks after surgery.

So far as is known, the mechanism of acute brain injury in boxing is the same as that in other instances of head trauma, except that skull fracture has not been recorded in the modern sport. Most of the intracranial haematomata associated with boxing and reported in the literature have been subdural.

Chronic brain injury

The main discussion in boxing is whether or not repeated and minor disturbances of brain function are associated with physical damage and, if so, whether such small pathological changes are cumulative and ultimately lead to permanent functional deficit. The term 'punch-drunk' has been in use for 60 years and describes a person with slurred speech, unsteady and uncoordinated limb movements and gait and slowed thought processes. Over the years, a number of studies have correlated this clinical picture with an unusual pattern of pathological change — cortical atrophy, enlarged cerebral ventricles, cavum septum pellucidum and abnormalities in the adjacent periventricular grey matter, degeneration of the substantia nigra, neurofibrillary change (especially in the limbic pathways and medial temporal grey matter), and scarring of the inferior cerebellar cortex (in particular the cerebellar tonsils) associated with marked loss of nerve cells. Individually, these changes are not remarkable but, when occurring together and in the absence of other pathology, it is reasonable to conclude that the 'punch-drunk syndrome' is a clinical entity caused by repeated minor trauma to the head.

The clinical and pathological studies which lead to this conclusion have largely related to professional boxers who boxed long before there were medical controls in the sport (the 'booth boxer' is, thankfully, seen no more). Studies which purport to investigate the modern sport are contradictory in their assessment of the risk of chronic brain injury, although the majority do suggest or conclude that clinical and/or pathological changes occur as a result of boxing today, and that their severity is more closely correlated with the number of bouts than any other factor. However, critical review of many of these reports shows that most are flawed. Many still examined boxers who were active before the modern medical regulations were instituted, controls are usually absent, statistical analysis is often defective or not used at all, the reporting of investigations (such as computerised tomography (CT) scans) is biased and not blind. Many studies are anecdotal or report very small series. Added to this, a degree of prejudice and a lack of objectivity in both reporting and discussion of observations which is not seen in other areas of medical research and journalism, make it very difficult indeed to derive an accurate assessment of the risk of chronic brain injury in modern amateur boxing. The most recent investigations have been more thorough and better controlled, and have used such methods as formal psychometry, creatinine kinase isoenzyme assay, auditory and visual brainstem evoked responses, CT and electroencephalography (EEG) with excitation procedures to study active boxers — both professional and amateur. Their results remain contradictory. The time-lag for the development of the clinical and pathological features of chronic brain injury may be measured in decades, and the effectiveness of current medical controls can only be accurately assessed in the light of experience over future years, by properly controlled, objectively performed and properly analysed prospective clinical research using the most sensitive methods of measuring brain function and structure.

Eye injury

Theoretically, the eyes are at risk of any of the injuries which might result from blunt trauma, which are legion. Reports of eye injuries in all forms of boxing are mostly anecdotal, and objective surveys of boxers' eyes, examined with fully dilated pupils by an experienced ophthalmologist, are few. Eye injuries reported to have been caused by boxing include lid lacerations, squint due to damaged extraocular muscles, corneal abrasions, contusion of the angle of the anterior chamber (but not glaucoma secondary to this), traumatic cataract, vitreous haemorrhage, choroidal and macular damage and retinal tears and detachment. Of these, retinal detachment has received most attention as the most commonly reported serious eye injury. The gloved fist is unable to enter the orbit, and it is widely believed in boxing circles that eye injuries such as these are the direct result of illegal use of the thumb. In this respect, it is interesting to note that there was a sudden reduction in serious eye injuries in New York State following the introduction there of thumbless gloves in 1982. The risk of many of these injuries, and particularly of retinal tears and detachments and cataract, which are the most common ocular injuries, gives cause for concern because any loss of vision is permanent.

Thumbless gloves are not used by the Amateur Boxing Association of England, although the Medical Commission would prefer that they were. Despite this, no serious eye injuries have been recorded at tournaments under the control of the English ABA. The only eye injuries reported have been periorbital lacerations and bruising (Table 18.3). However, it is recognised that this is not proof that significant eye injuries have not occurred in recent years. It is well known that retinal tears (and other vision-threatening trauma) may initally be asymptomatic, and not easily diagnosed without dilatation of the pupils and examination by an expert ophthalmologist. Such injuries will almost certainly be missed by the tournament medical officer and possibly also by the doctor carrying out the initial medical examination and subsequent re-examinations — although there is a requirement here for thorough ophthalmoscopic examination of the fundi and a formal test of visual acuity using Snellen charts. Unfortunately, a systematic record giving the reason for failure of a medical examination is not kept by the ABA, so that it is possible that serious eye injuries have been detected, but

Table 18.3 Injuries requiring seven or more days' rest recorded for the last four completed seasons of amateur boxing in England (excludes bouts governed by the Combined Services Amateur Boxing Association; figures provided by the Medical Registrar of the Amateur Boxing Association of England)

	1984−5	1985−6	1986−7	1987−8
Periorbital lacerations	146	147	159	134
Other lacerations	20	18	28	19
Periorbital bruising	18	26	24	17
Wrist, hand and digital injuries	17	16	36	20
Dislocated shoulder	3	6	3	2
Other pectoral girdle/upper limb injury	4	9	14	8
Other soft-tissue injury	2	12	0	5
Fractured mandible	1	2	2	1
Rib injury	0	0	0	2
Fractured fibula	0	0	1	0
Fractured nose	0	0	1	0
Perforated ear-drum	0	1	0	1
Back strain	3	2	0	0
Total	214	239	268	209

because they result in the boxers not being passed fit have been subsequently lost to the records of the ABA. It is also possible that boxers have noticed visual symptoms after leaving the tournament, so that their examination and treatment have been under the supervision of their general practitioner or optician and never reported to the ABA.

Other injuries

Other injuries recorded at ABA tournaments during the last four years are detailed in Table 18.3; there are few suprises. It is not possible to give an accurate breakdown of the wrist, hand and digital injuries as radiology is required to confirm bony injury, and the results of such investigation would be learned after the tournament records have been returned. Within these four years, it has been possible to confirm the following fractures: finger (14), wrist (1), thumb (13) and hand (1). Personal experience would suggest that the single record of a fractured hand over two years is a significant underestimate; a number of the unspecified hand injuries must be fractures of a metacarpal neck. Experience would also suggest that nasal fractures occur more commonly than once in two years — perhaps in the sparring ring, thus avoiding being recorded on the tournament record sheet or boxer's medical card. Nosebleeds are common, but are rarely difficult to control. Dental and alveolar injuries have been virtually eliminated since wearing a well-fitting gum-shield has been compulsory, although occasional mandibular fractures are recorded. Haematuria as a result of an (illegal) blow to the loin is a theoretical possibility, but has not been reported. Blows to the groin are also illegal and occasionally require a brief suspension of the bout for recovery. Again, there has been no record of testicular injury.

The prevention of injury

There is hardly a single rule or regulation in amateur boxing which does not have some bearing on the safety of the sport. As these rules have evolved over the years, they have come to identify a number of basic principles which limit the risk of injury. Supporting objective evidence is often lacking, and they are mostly based on personal experience and prudent medical practice. Many of the regulations, and particularly those of the medical scheme, are designed to minimise the risk of acute the chronic brain injury in particular.

An underlying principle is that for some individuals the risks are simply too great to allow them to take part. These are boys or men who have a particular medical condition or previous injury which may itself be seriously aggravated by taking part in the sport. This may be because there would be an unacceptable degree of morbidity or risk of mortality should a blow land on the diseased or injured part, or because there is a reduction in the functional reserve of the organ or part which it would be unreasonable to risk reducing further. Others are excluded from boxing because a disease process or previous injury has a general effect on mobility or exercise tolerance, so that they would be physically unable to develop the technical skills required to defend themselves safely, or would be unable to maintain these skills for the full duration of a bout. Less commonly, a boxer will be rendered unfit because of the risk he would impart to his opponent, officials or others in the sport; this would generally be due to a risk of transmission of infection. It is the function of the full initial medical examination and of the subsequent regular re-examinations to detect such conditions as will always present an unacceptable risk to boxers. Other conditions may be transient and the pre-bout medical inspection is designed to detect these — normally intercurrent infection or minor injury. The scope of examinations and inspection is discussed fully below, but specific mention could be made here of the rationale for the tests of visual acuity. The main reason for insisting that visual acuity be better than 6/12 in the better eye and 6/24 in the worse eye has little to do with a lesser ability to see the opponent clearly or to detect an oncoming blow early: the vision would have to be very bad indeed for this to be the case within the confines of the boxing ring. What is deemed unacceptable here is the much greater risk of retinal detachment in the abnormally shaped myopic eye.

A second principle is that both the frequency of competition and the total length of activity in the sport should be limited. It is assumed that, by so doing, injury which is either 'physiological' or otherwise minor and perhaps unnoticed will be given time to recover or heal, and not be compounded by further injury. A hard contest is very tiring, both psychologically and physically, and it is recognised that a recovery period is necessary to allow a boxer to return to full physical fitness and mental sharpness before stepping into the ring again. There is also an underlying fear that chronic brain injury might still occur in modern amateur boxing, and that this might be related to the frequency and total number of bouts. Regulations which come under this heading include the 'three-day rule', which prohibits boxing within three days of the previous contest (except in a few defined situations), the limitation to 14 bouts (junior) or 18 bouts (senior) plus championship matches in any one calendar year, and the compulsory retirement of all boxers when they reach the age of 35 years.

A third theme is the application of a compulsory rest period to a boxer who receives an injury during a bout, in order that it may heal completely before he next boxes. This again is to prevent the unnecessary compounding of physical damage which has already been detected, and the rest period applies to sparring as well as competitive bouts. In some cases, minimum compulsory rest periods are defined by the regulations, as in the case of knock-out and RSCH. The minimum rest period here is 28 days clear, increased to 84 days if it is the second instance within 84 days and to 12 months if it is the third instance within a year. The length of lay-off following other injury is at the discretion of the tournament medical officer. If he is not available to give his opinion at the time, the boxer's medical record card is withheld until he has been examined by a medical practitioner and passed fit to box again. Many of the regulations which determine the detailed administration of the medical scheme are directed to this end, particularly to ensure that the boxer and all officials who need to know are informed of the length of rest period or requirement for further examination.

Once in the ring, many regulations aim to reduce the incidence of injury during a bout. The matching of contestants is very closely controlled. In a senior contest, a novice may not compete against an open boxer, and a junior boxer may not compete against a senior. In a junior contest, there may not be a difference of more than 12 months in age or more than 2.25 kg in weight; it is recommended that a junior boxer should not concede both age and weight. In seniors the weight bands cover 3–10 kg intervals, ranging from light-flyweight (up to 48 kg) to super-heavyweight (over 91 kg). Other regulations prevent the extremes of tiredness, such as those which determine the lengths of each round for the different ages, and which prevent boxing after 10.30 p.m. for juniors under 15 years, after 11 p.m. for juniors 15–17 years old and after 11.30 p.m. for seniors. The construction, materials and condition of equipment (ring, gloves, boxers' dress including gum-shield and abdominal protector) are all tightly defined, and the referee will stop the contest if the conditions are not completely satisfactory (e.g. the lace of a glove becoming undone, or a rope becoming slack, or a dangerous object being on the ring apron).

The definition of 'down' was given on p. 231, and the requirement of the referee to stop the boxing when a boxer is down and start to count was one of the earliest safeguards introduced into the sport. The minimum count is now eight seconds before boxing may be resumed, so that the injured boxer is given the greatest opportunity to recover without gaining undue advantage. If a boxer receives three counts in one round, or four during one contest, the bout must be terminated in favour of his opponent. The referee is also required to halt a contest if one boxer is clearly outclassed or if one of the boxers receives an injury on account of which he should not continue. Perhaps most importantly, he is required to prevent a weak boxer from receiving undue and unnecessary punishment. If a boxer loses by knock-out to the head and has not fully recovered within two minutes, the regulations require that he is immediately transferred to hospital. Finally, only water may be used by the boxer immediately before a bout or during the intervals between rounds; grease, Vaseline and other embrocations are prohibited in amateur boxing.

Regulations are only as effective as those who implement them, and the standards of those who officiate in the sport, particularly referees and officials-in-charge (who have the ultimate responsibility for the conduct of the tournament and are the only officials at many tournaments with an authority superior to that of the referee), are always under review. Judges, referees and timekeepers are required to undergo a training course and pass an examination before being admitted to the register of officials maintained by the London association, provincial divisions or the ABA itself. A referee may not start his training until he has officiated as judge for at least two years, and, once qualified, referees and judges are periodically assessed by adjudicators, who are the most senior and experienced referees in the country. Any referee who fails to give adequate protection to the boxers during a tournament may be withdrawn from that tournament by the official-in-charge or the adjudicators, and, if his standards are repeatedly inadequate, he will be removed from the referees' panel. The training courses for referees have a medical component, normally given by one of the medical officers of the division, association or ABA. Improving the standards of the referees and other officials across the country is a slow and difficult process, but over the years a steady progress has been maintained. A fact which may surprise those outside the sport, and is a source of concern for the medical officers within it, is that it is not a requirement for these officials to maintain a valid first-aid certificate. The fact that many other sports are in a similar situation does not make this any more acceptable.

Perhaps the greatest improvement in standards over the last decade has been seen amongst the coaches. This is the result of the hierarchical system of courses and examinations instituted by the national coach, initially training a selected group of coaches to regional posts, who in turn help him train club coaches to three grades — assistant coach, coach and senior coach. The training courses for coaches also have a medical input, and a senior coach is required to maintain a valid first-aid certificate. This is particularly important as coaches routinely direct training in the gymnasium where medical help is not immediately available. The first objective of the national coach, that every amateur boxing club in England should have at least one trained coach on its staff, is now virtually achieved. The improved standards of coaching are particularly encouraging, as a responsible attitude to training programmes and preparation of boxers and good training in technical aspects — particularly defensive skills — will probably be the most important factor in the next decade for improving the safety of the sport.

Administration of the medical scheme

Records

The general principles of the medical scheme have been stated above, but it might be helpful to enlarge on them here. The following records are used in the scheme:

ME1 — medical officer's medical examination card (completed by the practitioner who performs the initial medical examination or re-examination, and contains the findings of his examination).

ME1a — medical officer's medical examination notification form (which provides a record for the local registrar that the examination has taken place).

ME2 — master medical record card (retained by the central registrar, and updated as necessary with details of medical examinations, injuries and compulsory rest periods for the boxer).

ME3 — boxer's medical record card (issued by the division or association and kept by the boxer or his coach, it carries a record of every bout boxed by the holder, every injury and compulsory rest period and the dates of medical examinations — this is the boxer's 'passport').

ME4 — medical officer's assistant's report form (completed by the medical officer's assistant at each tournament, to record all injuries, including head injuries, and compulsory rest periods for that tournament).

Enrolment

It is the responsibility of the honorary secretary of the club and/or the prospective boxer himself to arrange for the initial medical examination by a medical practitioner. This will normally be the boxer's general practitioner or club doctor. Forms ME1, ME1a and ME2 are required; the initial sections of these three forms should have been completed in advance by the club secretary and given to the boxer to take to the examining doctor. Where the boxer is under 18 years of age, his parents should have completed the sections for personal and family medical history. Consent for the entrant to box is also required from his parents; this is indicated by their signature on the master medical record card (ME2). When he has performed his examination, the doctor should complete the three forms and send them directly to the local registrar (a stamped addressed envelope should have been provided for this purpose), or return them to the boxer or his coach.

When he receives these forms the local registrar retains the examination notification form (ME1a) for his own records, and sends the other two forms to the central registrar. He scrutinises them and seeks advice from the Medical Commission if necessary, and a decision is made regarding fitness to box. Forms ME1 and ME2 are retained by the central registrar. The local registrar is told of the decision and, if this is 'fit', only then may he issue the boxer's medical record card (ME3) to the club secretary. The entrant may then box under ABA jurisdiction.

The local registrar

A local registrar is appointed by each division or its parent association to administrate the medical scheme within that division or association. He has an important role to play in enrolling new boxers, as outlined above. If further information is required before the boxer can be passed fit — from his general practitioner, from an association medical officer or from a specialist — then the local registrar will arrange this, usually with the help of one of the medical officers of the division or association.

The local registrar is also responsible for monitoring the careers of the boxers registered with him. After each tournament in his area, he will receive a copy of both the medical officer's assistant's report form (ME4) and the tournament record sheet (ME5), which gives full details of every contest. He may also receive instructions from the central registrar which require a boxer registered with him to be medically examined following injury or compulsory rest period, and he must arrange this and ensure that the club secretary is fully informed of what is required in this respect. He has to be alert to boxers whose records give cause for concern, such as repeated stoppages, repeated injuries or reports of concern from tournament officials-in-charge. In such cases, he will take advice from his association medical officers and council, and advise accordingly. He is also responsible for issuing replacement or duplicate medical record cards to boxers, for registering changes of club and for advising club secretaries when their boxers are due for medical re-examination or retirement.

The central registrar

The central registrar is a salaried employee of the ABA, and it is his duty to keep records regarding all boxers and all tournaments which take place under its authority. In this, he has duties which complement those of the local registrar in the enrolment and routine medical re-examination of boxers and in the continuing documentation of their careers. The central registrar receives and retains the medical examination card (ME1) and the master medical record card

(ME2) when a new boxer enrols (only form ME1 is completed when a boxer is re-examined). He must ensure that they are properly completed and discuss with the Medical Commission of the ABA any cases of doubt regarding fitness to box. He also receives the tournament record sheets, the medical officer's assistant's report form and the new injury forms for every tournament; he may also receive other reports of injury, illness and rest period or other information relating to individual boxers.

The central registrar is pivotal in passing information between local registrars, the Medical Commission and the Council of the ABA, particularly when a boxer competes outside his home association and receives an injury and compulsory rest period. It is the central registrar who must communicate this to the local registrar of the boxer's own association. The central registrar has overall responsibility to ensure that the medical scheme is operated correctly in all divisions and associations. If he detects a breach of regulations, he must instruct the local registrar accordingly, or refer the case to the Medical Commission or the Council of the ABA as necessary.

The principal records for every registered boxer in the country are held by the central registrar and he must amend these as he receives information about injuries, rest periods, medical examinations and retirement. An increasingly important duty is to prepare an annual statistical report to show the number of contests, the numbers of stoppages under the various categories, the numbers of injuries recorded and any other information requested of him by the Medical Commission or by the Council of the ABA.

The medical officer's assistant

Each division or association must train and keep a register of medical officer's assistants, one of whom must be appointed for each and every tournament. If the medical officer's assistant is unable to act at a particular tournament, then the official-in-charge at that tournament must appoint a suitable replacement or act in this capacity himself. It is possible, if the tournament medical officer is experienced and willing, for him to assume the duties of the medical officer's assistant. The function of this official is to administrate the medical scheme at the tournament. In this, he must work closely with both the tournament medical officer and the official-in-charge, and must provide a pathway for communication between them. In practice, there is often a sharing of duties between these three officials, but it remains the particular responsibility of the assistant to ensure that the requirements of the medical scheme are met and that the tournament medical officer receives the advice and guidance about the regulations that he requires.

The official-in-charge

The official-in-charge at a tournament has overall responsibility for its administration and safe conduct. Most of his responsibilities have some impact on the safety of the sport. This includes ensuring that the correct equipment is available and in a satisfactory condition, that boxers wear the necessary protective items of dress and that all tournament officials carry out their duties to a satisfactory standard. The latter is particularly important with respect to the standard of refereeing, in which the official-in-charge has the authority (and the responsibility) to advise or report to the divisional or association secretary any referee who is not adequately protecting the boxer.

The official-in-charge has overall responsibility to see that the medical scheme is properly administered at the tournament, and the duty to bring to the attention of the tournament medical officer any boxer who receives an injury. If the doctor is no longer present at the tournament, then the official-in-charge must take the ultimate responsibility for the health and safety of the boxers, and must make the decisions regarding the need for treatment and compulsory rest periods for boxers receiving injury.

The club secretary

The honorary secretary of an amateur boxing club is the point of contact within the club for the local registrar. He will often share his duties with the club's senior coach. The club secretary arranges the medical examination of his boxers, has to ensure that the instructions of the local and central registrar are enacted, and is responsible for the safe and confidential keeping of his boxers' medical record cards. When his club is promoting a tournament, it is his duty to arrange for the attendance of a tournament medical officer. If the doctor is new to the sport, the club secretary must explain his duties to him. He must also arrange the attendance of first-aiders and other facilities required for the tournament, such as a suitable medical examination room, an official delegated to supervise the transport and escort of injured boxers (should this be necessary) and a working telephone.

The boxer's medical record card (ME3)

The ME3 is the critical document in the operation of the medical scheme. It is not issued to a boxer who is under 11 years of age, and is only issued through the club of which the boxer is a member. No boxer is able to compete in a tournament unless he presents his own ME3 at that tournament. To be valid, a boxer's medical record card must:

1 be complete (all pages are now numbered);
2 have all the personal details of the holder correctly entered;

3 bear a photograph of the holder;
4 bear the medical stamp of the association.

When a boxer is medically examined, the date and result of the examination are indicated on the card, as will be the date on which the boxer eventually retires from amateur boxing.

Full details of every contest are recorded on the ME3:

1 date of contest;
2 opponent's name;
3 opponent's registration number;
4 opponent's club;
5 result (in detail: won/lost; if stopped the reason and round);
6 nature of any injury and resulting compulsory rest period;
7 doctor's signature.

The initial medical examination and re-examinations

These examinations are similar in scope to the routine examinations carried out for insurance purposes. The objective is to decide upon the fitness to box, remembering that boxing demands a high standard of physical fitness to be maintained over a period of time, with short periods of extreme activity. The presence of a condition preventing the attainment of full physical fitness and not detected at the examination will cause underachievement at best and a risk of serious injury at worst. The examination includes all body systems and the aim is to identify those individuals with a significantly higher-than-average risk of suffering injury or illness from congenital defect, previous injury or disease process (or who place others in the sport at unacceptable risk of infection) and select them out of boxing (see also Chapter 5).

The boxer attending for examination will bring the necessary forms with him, and it is a requirement that all abnormal findings of the examination are entered on the medical examination card (ME1). Guidelines for these examinations are issued by the ABA and are reproduced in full as Appendix 18.1. These illustrate the extent of the examination, and list a number of specific conditions which will prevent the boxer being passed fit or indicate the need for further specialist advice.

The examining doctor is required to give his opinion regarding fitness to box. His examination findings will form the basis of this opinion; no guidelines can be comprehensive. If the doctor is unable to form a definite opinion from his examination, he has to make this clear on the form and state his reasons. This will then be taken up by the local and/or central registrar when he receives the form, and further information or advice will be sought as necessary.

If the doctor is unable to declare that the boxer is definitely fit to box, this has to be disclosed to the boxer and, if he is under 18 years of age,[*] also to his parents. Consideration should also be given to the disclosure of the information to his general practitioner. If further information is required from the boxer's general practitioner, or special investigation or specialist opinion is advised, this too should be discussed with the boxer and/or his parents so that they are fully informed of his health, do not suffer undue anxiety and are encouraged to co-operate with the referral and any advice and treatment which may result from it.

Medical re-examinations are required every five years to the age of 30, and annually thereafter to compulsory retirement at 35 years. They take the same form as the initial examination, and should be carried out with the same degree of diligence. It is always possible that an important condition or injury was missed at an earlier examination, or that the boxer might previously have been unaware of his own or his family's medical history. It is particularly important to look for conditions which might have arisen since the previous examination, as well as for significant injury. Visual acuity must be examined critically as myopia may continue to worsen through adolescence and into adulthood. 'Degenerative' conditions are unusual in the age range of boxers, but towards the end of a long career, especially if the family history is suggestive, such conditions as ischaemic heart disease and spinal degeneration should be borne in mind.

The importance of these regular and full medical examinations cannot be overemphasised. The officials in the sport, the boxer and the tournament medical officers all rely on the fact that a thorough medical examination has been performed and any underlying abnormality likely to expose the boxer to unacceptable risk of injury has been excluded. In the past year, a number of instances have come to light in which the initial examination appears to have been scantily performed, particularly with respect to visual acuity and ophthalmoscopic examination. This is deplorable and potentially negligent: the boxers often pay a substantial fee to be examined and are entitled to expect as competent and thorough attention as that given to any other patient; they will be exposed to unknown risk if the examination is not performed as directed and with care.

The tournament medical officer

A medical practitioner is required to be present at every amateur boxing tournament to carry out a medical inspection of all boxers before they can box. The regulations do not require that he be present throughout the tournament, but the strongest possible recommendation is given that he stays until the last bout has been completed. (If the tournament medical officer is unable to stay for the duration of the tournament, the organiser is required to arrange trained first-aid cover.) The tournament medical officer need not be

[*] Section 8 of the Family Law Reform Act 1969 provides that any person of sound mind who has attained the age of 16 years may give a legally valid consent to medical or dental treatment or procedures. It follows therefore that for a person above this age a duty of confidentiality is owed. Therefore, for a boxer between the age of 16 and 18, in law the boxer's consent is required before information is disclosed to a third party. This includes his parents.

totally familiar with the medical regulations of amateur boxing, as an assistant will have been appointed specifically to advise him/her on his duties and to assist him in their execution. However, it will have been helpful if the tournament secretary has informed the doctor of his duties and responsibilities, particularly the guidelines for the pre-bout medical inspection. Payment for acting as tournament medical officer is between the tournament secretary and the doctor. Agreement on this beforehand will avoid later embarrassment.

When he arrives at the venue, the tournament medical officer should be met by the medical officer's assistant and introduced to the other officials for the tournament. It is recommended that the medical officer accompanies the official-in-charge when he inspects the ring to ensure that there is adequate and effective underfelt, and that the ropes are taut and tied together and the corner-post padding properly fixed.

The pre-bout medical inspection

Inspecting the boxers immediately prior to a contest is the only duty specifically required of the tournament medical officer. If he is unavailable for this, the boxing tournament simply cannot take place. Any doctor undertaking the role of tournament medical officer should remember this, as failure to attend will cause cancellation of the tournament. This would waste an enormous amount of work on the part of the organisers, who will also lose a substantial sum of money, and the results could be disastrous if the boxing tournament is part of a major charity occasion or championship.

In some specific championships, boxers are permitted to compete twice in the same tournament. Although it is not a regulation, the strongest possible recommendation is given that the boxer receive a further medical inspection prior to his second bout.

The medical inspection is of necessity brief and cannot attempt a full clinical examination of each boxer. The purpose of the inspection is to assess the risk of recent illness and injury for the boxer and his opponent. Although the boxer will have been thoroughly examined within the previous five years, the tournament medical officer should be alert to the possibility that significant disease or injury might have developed since then or might have been missed at this examination. It is not the purpose of the pre-bout inspection to detect such conditions, but if observed the boxer must be prevented from competing. The boxer and his coach should be informed of the problem, as well as the official-in-charge through the assistant, so that the local registrar may take the necessary action. The usual guiding principle prevails: any condition affecting the boxer's general fitness renders him open to receiving excessive blows; if in doubt, the boxer must be protected by refusing to pass him fit.

Guidelines for the medical inspection are given as Appendix 18.2. The description 'medical inspection' is well chosen. Apart from auriscopic examination of the ears and auscultation of the heart and lungs, the process is one of taking a brief history and then observing the boxer in an orderly fashion. Time is often short and it is best if a fixed routine is developed for this inspection.

It is the duty of the assistant to gather the boxers together at the examination room in an orderly manner (preferably in the order in which they expect to box), each boxer having his gum-shield in place and carrying his medical record card (ME3). If, after the inspection, a boxer has been declared unfit, the reason for this and recommendations regarding a compulsory rest period or follow-up should be entered on the boxer's medical record card by the doctor. This information should also be entered on the medical officer's assistant's report form (ME4) by the assistant.

During the tournament

The doctor is required to sit at a neutral corner of the ring, and should be accompanied here by his assistant. The official-in-charge and referees should be aware of his position in case he is needed urgently. It is recommended that the doctor has immediately available (i.e. in his pocket) a disposable plastic glove and packet of sterile gauze swabs, and perhaps an oral (e.g. Guedel) airway.

The medical officer may only enter the ring on the instruction of the referee, and must do nothing to attract his or the judges' attention once the bout is under way. The doctor has no authority to stop or interfere with the conduct of the bout.

In all things medical, the tournament medical officer is the highest authority, and other officials are obliged to follow his advice and recommendations. In some situations, the rules of boxing define minimum rest periods, e.g. following a knock-out; the doctor may increase these if he thinks this is indicated. In other cases he will have to make up his own mind about advice to give to the referee or official-in-charge (for example, if he is asked to give an opinion regarding a cut during a bout, treating an injury, deciding on a compulsory rest period after injury or referral to hospital). The doctor must use his own experience and judgement, and if in doubt he must 'play safe'.

The medical officer has a general responsibility for the health and safety of the boxers. He should watch each contest so that he is aware of the mechanism should an injury occur, and he should also form an opinion regarding the performance of the referee and the closeness of matching of contestants. If the medical officer thinks that the standard of refereeing is such that a boxer does not receive proper protection, he should inform the adjudicator (if present) or the official-in-charge of his opinion. Only the official-in-charge of a tournament has authority over and above that of the referee, and he may withdraw the referee if he is not up to standard. However, doctors who are inexperienced as tournament medical officers should take care not to form an opinion regarding dangerous refereeing too hastily. The effects of many apparently hard blows are nullified by good defensive technique, and a boxer who is apparently under attack may be quite in control of his situation and deflecting or avoiding the blows. The assistant is very familiar with the sport and discussion of these aspects with him is invaluable.

Knock-out and 'referee stopped contest — head'

If a boxer is knocked unconscious, the medical officer should immediately prepare to enter the ring. He must remember, however, that even in this situation he can only enter the ring on the instruction of the referee. The immediate requirement is to maintain the boxer's airway by removing his gum-shield and any other obstruction. Holding his jaw forwards will lift the tongue out of the airway. The level of response must be assessed quickly and, if indicated, the boxer should be placed in the recovery position. Consideration should be given to inserting an oral (e.g. Guedel) airway, but if a gag reflex is elicited this should not be persisted with because of the risk of inducing vomiting. The level of response should be monitored continuously until he recovers, and the time taken for the boxer to recover his faculties completely must also be noted.

The boxer must not be moved simply in order to continue the contest, and smelling-salts must not be used. After recovery, the boxer should be thoroughly examined in the examination room, and his further management decided upon. In this, the doctor will be guided by the severity of the blow(s), the period and degree of reduced responsiveness, the rapidity of recovery, residual symptoms and signs of concussion, where the boxer lives and who is at home with him. In minor cases, the boxer may be given a head injury card (form D) and escorted home by a responsible adult. In more serious cases, he will need to be escorted to the local accident and emergency department for further assessment and perhaps observation; a letter giving the relevant details (form C) should be sent with him. (These forms should be carried by the official-in-charge.) Rarely, an ambulance will need to be called. It is the responsibility of the tournament organiser to provide transport and escort, and the medical officer's assistant should help in organising this.

Even though a boxer may not be knocked out, the referee may decide that he has received sufficient blows to the head for the decision to be RSCH. The doctor should examine any boxer who has lost RSCH before he leaves and, if necessary, refer him to hospital as above.

The regulations regarding knock-out and RSCH are given as Appendix 18.3.

Lacerations

The referee should stop any bout as soon as a sizeable laceration occurs. This is to minimise the extent of damage to the wound, which in turn reduces the risk of infection and promotes rapid and strong healing with the least likelihood of recurrence in the future.

The referee may ask the doctor's opinion as to whether a boxer with a cut should be allowed to continue. He may be unsure in his own mind about the severity of a laceration, or he may wish for the support of the medical officer if stopping the bout might be contentious. If the medical officer is requested to advise the referee in this way, he must first of all thoroughly examine the wound by removing blood with sterile, dry swabs. It is recommended that he first don a disposable glove. He must then consider the position, depth and size of the cut and the extent to which it is bleeding (particularly if it is above the eye and obscuring vision). The importance of the contest and the length of time remaining in it are also factors which may reasonably be taken into account in deciding whether or not to allow the bout to continue.

Whether or not the tournament medical officer sutures a laceration is for him to decide. This will depend upon his expertise in minor surgery, the position and severity of the laceration, the equipment he carries with him, the suitability of the facilities at the tournament (minimum requirements are a couch or table for the boxer to lie on, a hard, clean surface which can be used as a sterile area, good light, privacy and a nearby sink with running water, soap and towel) and the proximity of a hospital accident and emergency department.

When suturing lacerations, particularly on the face, it should be remembered that this injury will be a potential site of weakness throughout the rest of the boxer's career, and if not sutured correctly might cost him a national title or national or area representation. All wounds should be sutured with great care and under sterile conditions, preferably using a fine monofilament (such as 6/0 Ethilon) ready-fixed to a cutting needle. If the laceration is small, the boxer will usually tolerate such fine suturing without the use of local anaesthetic. This has the advantage that the tissues are not distorted by the injection and more accurate apposition of the skin edges is attained. If the laceration is larger, then the advantages and disadvantages of suturing the wound immediately but under non-ideal conditions must be weighed against those of the delay for transfer to hospital and the availability of a proper minor surgery theatre.

Arrangements must be made for the sutures of be removed at the correct time, by instructing the boxer to attend his own general practitioner or the local accident and emergency department. It is courteous to give him a letter requesting the removal of sutures by the general practitioner or casualty officer.

Other injuries and compulsory rest periods

The action to be taken regarding other injuries must depend upon the particular circumstances. If there is any doubt about the presence of a fracture (most commonly of the hand or nose) or of serious joint injury, then the boxer must be referred to the local accident and emergency department for X-ray, with a suitable letter. In any injuries in which there is bruising and/or swelling, an ice-pack should be applied immediately and the injured part elevated if possible. Heat in any form must not be applied in the first two days, as this will only increase the bleeding.

The tournament medical officer has to determine the length of the compulsory rest period during which the boxer may neither compete nor spar, to allow the injury to heal. The boxer or his coach may encourage the doctor to advise a shorter rest period if an important championship or representative match is planned for the near furture. In general, the doctor should not allow himself to be swayed by such arguments, but it may not be altogether unreasonable for the doctor to consider making some compromise to accommodate this, *provided* that he discusses the situation fully with the boxer and his coach, particularly the risks of exacerbating the injury by boxing before it is completely healed. If a boxer is nearing the final stages of a championship, it may be acceptable that he risks reopening a laceration for the chance of gaining a national title.

It is very difficult to give examples of compulsory rest periods for injuries, as each individual case is different. The regulations lay down minimum rest periods for knock-out and RSCH (see Appendix 18.3); the tournament medical officer may extend these at his discretion. In Table 18.4 the authors offer suggestions for lay-off periods which are derived from their own experience, but wish to emphasise that they can only be regarded as a broad indication for any individual case.

Where the boxer is treated by his general practitioner or a hospital specialist for his injury, it is reasonable to require that either he be discharged from their care or the doctor treating him be asked to confirm that the injury has healed and he is fit to box before returning to the ring. This would certainly be the case for more unusual injuries such as perforation of the ear-drum.

Documentation and communication

Reasons for failing the pre-bout inspection and details of injuries sustained and lay-off periods advised must be entered on the boxer's medical record card. The doctor should also complete the injury form, which provides more detailed information about the nature, site and severity of the injury. These forms have been introduced recently in the hope that they will provide a valuable source of

Superficial laceration (through skin only)	3−6 weeks
Deep laceration (involving facial muscles or other deep structures)	6−12 weeks
Fractured nose	12 weeks
Fractured mandible	6 months
Dislocated shoulder	12 weeks
Fractured metacarpal	3−4 months
Fractured finger	8−12 weeks
Fractured thumb	3−4 months
Muscle strains	2−6 weeks
Joint strains	2−8 weeks
Periorbital haematoma	7 days−3 weeks

Table 18.4 Authors' suggestions for lay-off periods

information to help quantify the injury risks in boxing. This documentation should be completed by the medical officer and countersigned by him; he will be aided in this by his assistant if necessary. It is only courteous to write a short letter to go with the boxer when referring him to hospital or his general practitioner for further examination or treatment.

Communication between the medical officer, tournament officials, coaches and the boxers themselves is very important if the rules, regulations and recommendations regarding rest periods and follow-up after injury are to be understood and accepted by those concerned. Explaining the doctor's decision and requirement for a rest period do much to educate the boxer and his trainer in the medical aspects of the sport and to foster a co-operative spirit between all officials.

The doctor's bag

The items carried by the doctor to a boxing tournament will depend on factors such as his own experience and personal preference, the geographic location of the venue in relation to hospital services and the facilities provided at the venue. He must at least have sufficient to examine the boxers, maintain an airway, clean and dress skin wounds, support an injured hand and write a letter. He should bear in mind that he may also be called upon to assist members of the public who have collapsed, fallen or otherwise injured themselves.

The following probably represents a minimum:

1   stethoscope, auriscope (which can also serve as a nasal speculum and pen torch), ophthalmoscope, thermometer, sphygmomanometer and tongue depressor;

2   oral airway (e.g. Guedel; it is advisable to have small and large sizes to cover the younger juniors as well as seniors);

3   sterile gauze swabs (5 cm square suggested), cotton wool, Steristrip or butterfly sutures, assorted self-adhesive dressings (such as Elastoplast), antiseptic (such as cetrimide), sachets of sterile saline (for eyewash), antiseptic swabs (e.g. Sterets), non-adhesive plastic

dressings (e.g. Melolin), adhesive tape, bandages (crêpe or cling), triangular sling;

4 disposable gloves;

5 correspondence paper and envelopes.

If he intends to suture minor lacerations, the medical officer should come prepared to provide all items: soap and sterile towels to wash hands, sterile surgical gloves, local anaesthetic, sterile syringe and needle, sutures (preferably a fine monofilament (e.g. 6/0 Ethilon) ready-mounted on a needle), sterile stitch pack or instruments for suturing (needle-holder, toothed forceps, small scissors, gallipot, gauze swabs, cotton wool balls) and sterile towels or cloths to provide a clean area.

The medical officer may also wish to include such items as assorted crêpe bandages, surgical tapes (Micropore is particularly useful), tubular stockingette and elastic adhesive tape for strapping sprains, sterile eye pads, fluorescein to stain for corneal abrasions, Bactigras tulle, etc. The application of plastic spray-on dressings to the face is not recommended, and a nasal pack should not be introduced unless the doctor is experienced in the technique, he has the correct materials and other methods of controlling the haemorrhage have been unsuccessful.

There is little advantage in carrying full resuscitation equipment (laryngoscope, endotracheal tubes, hand inflation bag, mask and portable oxygen-giving set) unless the doctor is experienced in its use and has ready access to it. Simple first-aid measures should always be enough to maintain the airway until arrival at hospital. Consideration may be given to carrying hand-operated suction equipment.

It is recommended that the carriage of drugs and medication to a boxing tournament is kept to a minimum. No such treatment should be instituted which will need medical supervision; this should be left to the boxer's general practitioner or the accident and emergency department. Care must be taken to ensure any medication given will not compromise the result of a drug test, should the boxer be selected for this in the near future. The risk of theft must also be considered. The doctor may wish to carry minor analgesics (such as paracetamol), tetanus toxoid, sterile syringes and needles and chloromycetin eye ointment. If the medical officer is likely to be the boxers' general practitioner, then he may wish to carry a wider selection of drugs so that he can initiate and continue treatment with, for example, stronger analgesics, non-steroidal anti-inflammatory drugs or oral antibiotics.

Alcohol and drugs

Boxers are strongly discouraged from taking alcohol whilst in training during the competition season (approximately September to May), and are advised to consume none in the 36 hours before a contest. Abstention is particularly important in boxing because even low levels of alcohol slow the reflexes and impair balance and co-ordination, having a significant effect on defensive ability. Body-weight also needs to be very tightly controlled, and the high calorific values of beers make them doubly inappropriate for a boxer in training.

The taking of (or the encouragement to take) illegal substances is absolutely forbidden by the regulations of the sport, and is not con-doned under any pretext. Drugs taken to enhance performance or the effects of training or to obscure the detection of those which are (steroids, beta-blockers, stimulants, depressants or diuretics) have their own medical risks and represent a cheating ethic which has no place in amateur boxing. In fact, it is little advantage to a boxer to take many of these drugs — he gains no benefit from increased muscle bulk and stimulants and depressants have a potentially disastrous effect on such a technical sport as boxing. One English amateur boxer was found to have low levels of an illegal substance in his urine when tested after a performance. It later transpired that he had taken a proprietary cold cure, which was compatible with the findings, and disciplinary action was discontinued. Another admit-ted to taking Pro-plus (a mild stimulant containing caffeine) when selected for testing, but the caffeine in his urine was within per-mitted levels. There has never been word 'along the grapevine' that drug-taking for enhanced performance occurs in amateur boxing.

The Amateur Boxing Association of England has followed the advice and requests of the Sports Council in determining its drug-testing scheme at tournaments and the list of banned substances. This started in 1984, when the national squad had to be tested during its preparation for the Olympic Games. Thereafter the ABA organised its own drug tests at major tournaments without prob-lems until 1987, when this duty was taken over directly for all sports by the Sports Council. At the same time, the Sports Council proposed to institute random drug testing at all grades of tourna-ment (from club shows to internationals) and also to test boxers during training. The ABA fully suports these moves, and co-operates fully with the Sports Council in its drug-testing programme.

Drug testing in boxing is no different from that in any other sport. The only problem is a practical one — that many boxers are dehydrated at the time of the contest. Despite intensive rehydration following the bout, there may be a delay of up to two hours before sufficient urine can be voided for the test. This can cause transport problems for those supervising the test (and boxers and coaches) if the tournament extends into the later part of the evening.

Current issues

The scope of the pre-bout inspection

The existing form of the pre-bout medical inspection probably represents the most that can be achieved with the time and facilities normally available. For major tournaments held in large sports arenas, there is often a fully equipped medical room which provides privacy, space, light and quiet in which to carry out the inspection quite thoroughly. In these situations, there is normally more than one medical officer at the tournament, so that more time is available as well. These advantages do not obtain at most club shows, where a single tournament medical officer will have to inspect 20 or more boxers in an hour or so, in more cramped and less private surroundings. Having said that, when experienced in the role of tournament medical officer, it is quite possible to carry out an effective inspection in these circumstances following the guidelines given in Appendix 18.2 and the doctor should never be pressured into doing anything that is less than adequate. Ultimately the tournament medical officers will set the standards for the facilities they require to carry out their inspections and possible treatments in the case of injury.

The scope of the medical examinations

Whether the initial medical examination and re-examinations should be extended is a more vexed question. The Association Internationale de Boxe Amateur (AIBA) has recently recommended that all boxers who are to participate in international tournaments should have an exhaustive medical examination before their first international bout, including full blood count, Wassermann test, electrocardiogram (ECG), urinalysis (for glucose and ketones), EEG, skull X-ray and CT scan of the head. AIBA also recommends that international boxers should have further examinations before each international tournament, annually and before each bout — but does not specify the nature of these examinations. It is possible that such investigations might detect the very occasional abnormality which would render a boxer medically unfit, but the cost of extending this battery of investigations to every registered amateur boxer in the country would be utterly prohibitive. Amateur boxing is not a rich sport, its participants and officials being drawn from the less advantaged sections of society, and the money is simply not there to pay privately for investigations of this sort. Many boxers and clubs struggle to find the fee to pay for the basic medical examinations, and many rely on the benevolence of their club doctors or a kindly general practitioner to carry out these examinations for a nominal fee or for no fee at all.

The EEG has traditionally been used as the investigation carried out on (professional) boxers who have suffered repeated knock-outs. The main reason for this was that, until the advent of CT, the EEG was almost the only non-invasive investigation of the brain, and was relatively simple and cheap to perform on selected boxers. However, the information gained is minimal. Normal variation is enormous and, in the absence of neurological symptoms or signs, an abnormal EEG is rarely of diagnostic value. It is of no value in determining the seriousness or otherwise of a closed head injury, and is of no value in predicting those boxers who have a high risk of acute brain injury from a blow which produces shearing or concussional forces on the brain. The likelihood of recording a frankly epileptic EEG in a boxer who has not suffered fits or other disturbances of consciousness is remote. (Only 20% of those with epilepsy actually have an 'epileptic' standard EEG; epilepsy has a prevalence of about 0.5% and the proportion who have 'epileptic' EEGs without clinical epilepsy must be small indeed.)

The only preventative advantage of skull X-ray would be the detection of an abnormally thin skull. However, the skull would have to be very thin indeed to be at real risk of fracture from boxing — whether by the force of the blows landing on the head or by hitting the head on the floor when falling. Only the temporal and frontal regions of the vault are in the target area, and the thinner parts of the vault would only be at significant risk from an accidental clash of heads. The force of a blow is spread over a large area by the padding of the glove, so that point loading of the skull is relatively low; likewise the ring floor is composed of canvas on a layer of felt supported by a sprung wooden floor. A skull X-ray would show a fracture, but the normal practices of medical care for a person suffering concussion following head injury provide adequate indication for X-ray in the acute situation.

The main advantage of CT would be to show cortical atrophy, ventricular dilatation and cavum septum pellucidum if these were to occur as a result of chronic head injury. It would also detect hydrocephalus or a porencephalic cyst which would make a person unfit for boxing — but these must be exceedingly rare in the absence of neurological symptoms and signs. It is possible that CT would detect a large berry aneurysm or vascular malformation, but these are also very rare in the general population.

The Medical Commission of the ABA has taken advice on these three recommended investigations and, from the arguments above (which are taken from this advice), has concluded that the possible benefits cannot justify the enormous cost. It is also doubtful if the facilities currently exist in the National Health Service or the private sector to carry out regular CT on all registered amateur boxers. For the present, EEG with excitation procedures, skull X-ray and CT must remain research tools in amateur boxing, to help quantitate the risks to its participants, or for diagnosis of the individual case where this is indicated by the clinical situation.

The one form of investigation which does appear to give an earlier indication of chronic brain injury than simple clinical examination or CT is expert psychometric assessment by a clinical psychologist. This form of investigation certainly merits closer attention, and a number of studies utilising this technique have recently been published or are currently under way. We await further developments in this field with interest.

The other major concern for 'boxing doctors' is the risk of eye injury. There can be little doubt that full ophthalmological examination with fully dilated pupils is the only way to be sure of detecting retinal and choroidal damage. Routine ophthalmoscopic examination of the fundus by a non-specialist will miss at least small lesions and those in the periphery, if not more. The Medical Commission of the ABA recognises this, and as a compromise measure currently recommends (but cannot insist) that every boxer should have his eyes examined by an ophthalmic practitioner at intervals not exceeding three years. The recent imposition by the Government of charges for this routine examination must undermine this recommendation and raise the question of routine expert eye examination in the future. Ophthalmological out-patient clinics are notoriously busy, and it is unlikely that they could cope with the regular examination of many thousands more 'patients' nationwide. On a private basis, costs would again be prohibitive for most boxers and clubs. This makes it all the more important that the doctor carrying out the full medical examinations performs the test of visual acuity and fundoscopy to the best of his ability.

In an ideal world, it would be advantageous to include, as part of the initial medical examination for enrolment, full ophthalmological examination of the eyes, psychometric testing and, perhaps, high-resolution CT of the brain. These would pick up some (but not all) retinal and congenital neurological disorders which would put the boxer at increased risk. For boxers competing regularly and frequently, it would also be to their advantage to have annual ophthalmological examinations and psychometric testing, perhaps followed by CT if indicated by an abnormality in the latter. This would give the best chance of detection of the first signs of chronic brain injury, given the techniques available at the moment.

Contact lenses

The regulations prohibit a boxer from wearing spectacles or any form of contact lenses during sparring or competitive boxing. The reasons for prohibiting spectacles and hard contact lenses are obvious — there is a real risk of laceration of the cornea or sclera. The situation regarding soft (hydrophilic) contact lenses is less clear-cut, and this subject has been given some consideration by the Medical Commission in the last year.

Soft contact lenses are larger, covering the whole cornea, are not sharp and do not fracture; there is no risk of laceration from them. Indeed, it might be argued that soft contact lenses would give some protection against corneal abrasion. The visual acuity of the boxer would be rendered normal, improving the judgement of distance and movement. However, in the confines of the boxing ring (maximum size 6 m²), the benefit of this improvement in vision can only be marginal given that visual acuity must be at least 6/12 in the better eye and 6/24 in the worse eye to be boxing in the first place.

The reasons that soft contact lenses are banned in amateur boxing are threefold. First, if a lens were to fall out during a contest, there would be no way of replacing it hygienically, without causing such a delay as to render the bout void. The boxer would, of course, be gloved and there are not normally washing facilities in the immediate vicinity of the ring. (The alternative — a sudden change in vision during a bout — would be disconcerting and potentially dangerous.) Secondly, the nature of the sport means that there are always dust and small particles in the air, with the risk that they may be carried into the eye by the opponent's glove. Such particles resting on the surface of an exposed cornea are rarely irritating but, when trapped between a contact lens and cornea, pain, irritation and watering start suddenly and unexpectedly and may be debilitating. Thirdly, in the often less-than-ideal situation in which the pre-bout inspection is carried out, it may be difficult for the tournament medical officer to be sure that contact lenses were of the soft variety and not of the hard. The reasons against the wearing of soft contact lenses, in the opinion of the Medical Commission, outweigh the marginal advantage of improved visual acuity.

Head-guards

Head-guards are mandatory in all other countries, but are optional in domestic tournaments under ABA rules. They must be worn, however, by English boxers who compete in international tournaments, whether home or away, as these are boxed under AIBA regulations. To our knowledge, no studies have been performed to investigate the balance between risk and advantage in the wearing of head-guards for boxing and, in the absence of such objective evidence, the theoretical advantages and disadvantages have to be considered.

A well-fitting head-guard in good condition should reduce soft tissue bruising and cuts about the eyes and face, although when it has become saturated and hardened with sweat the converse is true (members of the Medical Commission have witnessed quite severe periorbital laceration when head-guards have been worn, apparently caused by lines of stitching and such hardening of the fabric). By increasing the contact area of a blow, a head-guard should reduce the point force of the impact and therefore reduce more serious injuries to the facial skeleton. Against this, the field of vision is reduced, the balance of the head is disturbed, and boxers report feeling uncomfortable and claustrophobic, making concentration difficult.

The value of head-guards in reducing the risk of brain injury is equally unclear. If made of high energy-absorbing material, the force transmitted to the head should be reduced, but their physical bulk increases the target area (and therefore the chance of a blow landing) and, perhaps more importantly, the turning moment which a blow might impart to the head. Senior coaches, reporting observations on their boxers who have worn head-guards in tournaments abroad, report that the style of their boxers often changes, so that they pay less attention to defensive technique, making less effort to parry or slip a punch. The result is that they receive more and harder punches than when boxing without head-guards. Coaches and many doctors fear the sense of false security which boxers seem to feel when wearing head-guards, and have expressed concern that the compulsory wearing of head-guards may encourage boxing to become more of a static, slugging sport rather than an exhibition of fleetness of foot and defensive technical skill.

The wearing of head-guards has been introduced in other countries without proper assessment of their risks and benefits. It is possible that, if the compulsory wearing of head-guards is introduced as an expedient response to external opinion, boxers may be exposed to greater risk of brain, eye and facial injury, and the development of the higher skills, which are the essence of good boxing, would be neglected. The great problem is that, once introduced, it would be impossible to withdraw their use without this being seen as a retrograde step by the general public, even if their use should ultimately prove to increase the danger to the boxer. The recent occurrence of two serious acute brain injuries in English boxers who were not wearing head-guards has brought this issue to prominence, and makes it unlikely that the compulsory wearing of head-guards will be resisted for much longer.

Infection with HIV and hepatitis

Currently, blood-borne hepatitis is much the more serious risk, but it has been the publicity about AIDS which has brought both of these topics of the fore. Bleeding occurs quite commonly in boxing — bloody noses are frequent, and lacerations occur in more than 1% of bouts. At particular risk of infection would be those who will examine and treat the bleeding wound between rounds and after the bout — the referee, coach and doctor — as well as the opponent and ringside officials, who are occasionally spattered with blood. For these reasons, boxers who are known to be hepatitis B- or HIV-positive are prohibited from amateur boxing in England. At present, there is only provision to determine this from the personal medical history of the boxer, although it would be reasonable for any boxer who declares a history of jaundice to be required to be tested for hepatitis B before being given his medical card. A personal medical history of a coagulation disorder also renders a boxer unfit, as does major surgery. These should incidently eliminate most instances of infection via transfusion of blood or blood products. Current regulations do not prevent a person who has previously taken drugs intravenously from boxing (perhaps they should?), but the examining doctor is required to record any suspicion of this on the examination form. Again, non-infection with hepatitis B or HIV would need to be proved by testing. In all these situations, these tests would have to be fully discussed with the boxer (and his parents if he were under 18). There is no suggestion that they would be carried out in the absence of fully informed consent.

Apart from these specific regulations, the approach is to educate boxers and officials about the nature and transmission of these diseases in their training courses and through advice published by the ABA. Specific advice is simply that good basic hygiene be demanded in the gym as well as at tournaments. A new recommendation is that referees and coaches (and doctors) put on a disposable glove whenever they examine or treat a bleeding wound.

The situation is being watched carefully by the Medical Commission, particularly in respect of the increasing prevalence of these diseases, and of the practices adopted by other contact sports. It is not the intention to require positive vetting of every entrant, although this would have to be considered if AIDS continues to spread rapidly through the population and tests for HIV become socially accepted and even expected in situations where there will be contact with fresh blood.

The boxing debate

History

In 1962, the Committee on Medical Aspects of Sports of the American Medical Association recommended 'that boxing be banned at all times and places where optimum protection for the participants cannot be provided', in addition to many specific measures to improve the safety of the sport. In the early 1980s, a concerted attack on boxing was led by the medical establishment in the United States. It became a major issue of debate in 1983–4 with the publication of leading articles in the *Journal of the American Medical Association*, in which the editor delivered a prejudiced and personal attack on the sport. The lack of objectivity in such a prestigious journal was disturbing, but nevertheless the journal and the American Medical Association provided a rallying point for those of similar persuasion. They drew support from confused medical arguments and articles of such a scientific standard as would probably not have been accepted for publication were they on any other medical topic.

At the same time, the American Academy of Paediatrics adopted the principle that 'boxing, with its potential for head trauma and the primary goal of producing injury, is not an appropriate sport for any young person'. Its proposal to eliminate boxing from any sports programme for children and young adults was endorsed by the US Committee on Sports Medicine in 1984. The World Medical Association advocated a ban on boxing and strict reforms until that could be obtained, and the Canadian Medical Association also recommended to their Government that all boxing in Canada be banned.

In Europe, moves against boxing by the medical profession had started earlier, but had received less publicity. Professional boxing was banned in Sweden in 1969 and in Norway in 1982. In that year, Britain joined the fray when the British Medical Association (BMA) adopted the resolution 'that in view of the proven ocular and brain damage resulting from professional boxing, the Association should campaign for its abolition'. Having accepted in this resolution that ocular and brain damage from professional boxing was 'proven', the Board of Science and Education of the British Medical Association was instructed 'to consider the medical effects of boxing and to make recommendations in relation to the Annual Representatives Meeting resolution of June 1982'. Its report was published in February 1984, following which the BMA adopted a policy of promoting a campaign to ban all forms of boxing.

Prejudice, ignorance and confusion

In fairness, medical reports of injuries sustained in boxing, both acute and chronic, have continued to be published, and there is a genuine desire in the medical profession to reduce unnecessary injury to a minimum — especially brain and eye injury because of the failure of these organs to repair without leaving a deficit. To those who share the desire to restrict unnecessary injury but are also familiar with amateur boxing, it is clear that the proponents of 'ban boxing' are often confused about the difference between amateur and professional boxing, and are ignorant of the nature of the amateur sport and the benefits it brings to the community which supports it. The conclusion emerges that theirs is a personal, prejudiced and emotional reaction to a sport with which they are unfamiliar and unsympathetic. The style of language used does discredit to a prestigious journal which purports to lead medical opinion: 'This editor believes personally that boxing is wrong at its base. In contrast to boxing, in all other recognised sport, injury is an undesired by-product of the activity. Boxing seems to me to be less sport than is cock-fighting; boxing is an obscenity. Uncivilised man may have been bloodthirsty. Boxing, as a throwback to un-civilised man, should not be sanctioned by any civilised society.' (*JAMA*, Editorial, 1983).

How true!

A large culture gap exists between many doctors and the boxing community, whether it be amateur or professional. Boxing and its people are outside their experience. Too many doctors are all too ready to assume a position of moral superiority, and with a con-fidence born of ignorance condemn out of hand a sport in which the only "benefit" they can see is inevitable brain injury for each and every participant.

Those with a foot in each camp, the medical and the amateur boxing, see a rather different picture — a gymnasium full of young people, often a truly integrated mixture of many races and religions, coming together to enjoy their sport. Many are disadvantaged, non-achievers at school, with manual jobs or unemployed. Many boxing clubs are associated with social clubs, and they provide a real service in helping to unite the local community and give their members stability and purpose. For many, boxing is their only sphere of achievement, the only environment where they may perform in front of their peers and others to display their skills. The club gives them a stimulating environment where they are given a goal, where their energies are channelled into physical fitness. They encounter firm but fair discipline, which they learn to respect and accept, and in turn they develop respect for other individuals and their property. They learn self-discipline and, perhaps for the first time, are able to develop a pride in one aspect of their own performance. They become part of a close-knit and mutually supportive community, with a true spirit of camaraderie and fair play. They receive instruc-tion in hygiene and diet, develop physical fitness and are dis-couraged from smoking, drinking, drug-taking, vandalism and other antisocial behaviour.

Every sport is unique, providing for individuals with a particular combination of physique, physical skill and psychological make-up. Boys and young men participate in a particular sport simply because they enjoy the particular nature of its activities; in boxing, they have the basic attributes the sport requires, and they wish to test themselves in this form of individual combat and self-defence. Facile comments such as, 'Why do we need boxing — can't they play football?' are counter-productive. Boxers are good at boxing and they enjoy it. If boxing ceased to exist, then they would not only have lost their sport but with it, for many, the chance for personal achievement, self-development and social education.

Doctors who have given their time to amateur boxing and who have seen all of these benefits make a more balanced judgement. They are well aware that there must be some danger of injury in a contact sport which has as its objective the landing of blows with force on the opponent (the objective is not to injure the opponent, as this is often paraphrased). Because the benefits are seen as well, they support the sport and try to bring their medical expertise to bear to educate and guide its participants in its safety aspects as well as the general aspects of health, hygiene, diet, training routines and so on. In one way, the medical attacks over the last few years have been to the benefit of the sport. They made 'boxing doctors' examine the evidence which has been cited in support of their arguments, and their own philosophical and moral standpoint. The sport is healthier and better informed as a result. If boxing is to be criticised because the risk of injury is deemed too great, then it behoves the critic to apply the same high degree of objectivity in the interpretation of his 'facts' as he would in advancing any other medical argument, and he has a duty to direct his argument against an equally objective assessment of the benefits derived from the sport — of which he has a duty to inform himself.

There is one area of confusion which does much to muddy the water of the boxing debate. The media largely promote the professional sport. Amateur boxing is normally broadcast in England only on such occasions as the National Championship Finals and the Commonwealth, European and Olympic Games, where it still receives only a small proportion of the overall sports coverage. Much of the case against boxing has been based on the common perception of the professional sport as seen through the media. This has been to the disadvantage of amateur boxing, which, whilst sharing some technical aspects with the professional sport, has its own ethos, principles and traditions, has its own standards of medical care and refereeing, and is administered by bodies and individuals who are entirely independent of and divorced from those of professional boxing. The Amateur Boxing Association of Engand has no links — at individual or corporate level — with its professional counterpart, the British Boxing Board of Control. Officials, coaches and boxers gain no financial advantage from amateur boxing — in fact, they are usually out of pocket (expenses often do not cover expenditure and are not covert payment). There is no factor to compromise the basic tenet of the sport, that the boxers' safety always comes first. In many sports which have both amateur and professional wings, there is little difference in the way the sport is promoted and played. In others which are now 'open' the amateur principles of sportsmanship and fair play are subjugated or lost altogether. This is not the case in boxing, where the amateur and professional sports are far removed from each other.

267
Chapter 18
The doctor at the
boxing ring:
amateur boxing

The medical question

That brain function is sometimes temporarily disturbed is undeniable: knock-out and concussion occur as a result of blows received whilst boxing. What is not known is the extent to which small degrees of structural damage occur at the same time (or as a result of even less forceful blows which do not disturb brain function), and which over a period of time may add up to a significant and irreversible degree of brain damage. It is likely that chronic brain injury (the 'punch-drunk' syndrome) occurred in the past as a result of boxing. The great majority of studies which have reported this examined boxers who were active long before medical controls were instituted, who had taken part in an enormous number of contests, and in whom other causes of chronic brain damage could often not be ruled out with certainty. Similar conditions have also arisen in people who have never boxed. However, the weight of evidence does suggest that repeated brain trauma — even though each individual injury may be minimal — can cause brain damage which is permanent. The essential medical question is, does amateur boxing in England today with its improving standards of refereeing, coaching and medical supervision expose the participants to significant risk of chronic brain injury? Many of the investigations which have attempted to prove such a risk in the modern sport have been scientifically flawed, as mentioned above. The time-lag for the development of chronic brain injury is so long that it is only now becoming possible to study modern amateur boxers for evidence of this. The results of such studies are contradictory and inconclusive. That said, the potential for this type of injury in boxing is fully acknowledged by those in the sport, and its prevention is their prime concern.

The moral question

Whether or not the benefits of amateur boxing justify the medical risks is a question which must be clearly separated from the philosophical question of whether or not modern society should accept a sport in which the objective is to land blows with force on the opponent. We respect those who hold the opinion that a sport with these aims has no place in the society in which they would wish to live; equally, we expect others to respect our own opinion that amateur boxing in its current form does have a place in the sporting community, especially as this opinion results from our intimate knowledge of the sport and its participants and officials as well as its medical aspects. Desirable individual qualities (sportsmanship, mutual respect, mutual help and support) are more often exhibited in amateur boxing than in many sports which have a more prominent and accepted place in society.

The philosophical question of the acceptability of the sport is for each individual to decide. It is a particular example of a general question: to what extent should an individual's activity be curtailed by state legislation? Should the state adopt a libertarian or restrictive attitude? The authors' stance is basically libertarian, which, of course, implies a corresponding degree of responsibility and respect for others' wishes. In the case of amateur boxing, the participants are willing and there is no intrusion into the lives of those who do not wish to take part, and no harm done to 'defenceless animals' or personal property. A society should give all of its members the maximum opportunity for achievement and self-development, which means allowing the widest range of activities and experiences compatible with a social responsibility. The more avenues open to an individual to develop skills, expertise and self-respect, the richer and happier society is. The small cost of providing health care for the few injured in any sport is more than repaid by the fulfilment of the individual's who participate and the pleasure they give to those who spectate. Many do not care to live in a protective and restrictive society in which the recognition of natural aggression and a sporting form of individual combat is taboo and becomes channelled into disruptive antisocial behaviour. But it is appreciated that others may disagree with this view. The role of the medical profession should be to research and publish, to inform and educate, objectively within the sphere of its expertise — in this case, the actual and potential risks to those who take part in all sports, and the costs to individuals and society of providing the health care needed as a result. Individuals would then be fully equipped to make their own informed decisions about risks versus benefit and the nature of the society they wish to create.

In the context of sport in general

The medical risk versus individual and community benefit equation should be applied to all sports, and not just boxing. As far as can be determined on present evidence, boxing is probably at least as safe a sport as many others which gain ready acceptance in society. Few other sports can have such close medical involvement and supervision, or be as informed about *every* contest which takes place and the injury rates which result. If the argument is to be sustained that the medical risks are too great to allow boxing to continue, then a similar detailed analysis of risk and benefit should be applied to every other sport and the same criteria of judgement applied to each, without the intrusion of personal prejudice. The acute death-rate in boxing is much lower than in many other sports, and there is evidence of chronic brain injury in other sports as well (rugby, horse-riding, soccer, American football).

Appendix 18.1: Requirements for the initial medical examination and re-examinations

General points

1   These are similar to the routine examinations carried out for insurance purposes. It must be remembered that the objective of these examinations is to decide upon fitness to box, which demands an extremely high standard of physical fitness to be maintained over a period of time, with short periods of extreme activity. The presence of a condition preventing the attainment of full physical fitness and not detected at the examination will cause underachievement at best and the risk of potentially serious injury at worst. The examination must include all systems and the aim is to identify those individuals with a significantly higher-than-average risk of suffering injury or illness from congenital defect, previous injury or disease process, and select them *out* of boxing.

2   *All* abnormal findings of the examination must be entered on the medical examination card (ME1).

3   The examining doctor is required to give his opinion regarding fitness to box. The medical examination forms the basis of this opinion and no guidelines can be comprehensive. If the examining doctor is unable to form a definite opinion from his examination, he should make this clear on the form, stating his reasons. This will then be taken up by the local registrar when he receives the form, and further information or advice will be sought as necessary.

4   If the examining doctor is unable to declare that the boxer is definitely fit to box, this should be disclosed to the boxer and, if he is under 18 years of age, to his parents. Consideration should also be given to the disclosure of the information to his general practitioner. If further information is required from the boxer's general practitioner, or special investigation or specialist opinion is advised, this also should be discussed with the boxer and/or his parents so that they are fully informed of his health, do not suffer undue anxiety, and are encouraged to co-operate with the referral and any advice and treatment which may result from it.

5   The importance of these full medical examinations cannot be overemphasised. The officials in the sport, the boxer and the tournament medical officers all rely on the fact that a thorough medical examination has been performed and any abnormality likely to expose the boxer to unacceptable risk of injury has been detected.

Medical re-examination

1 This must be carried out with the same degree of thoroughness as the initial examination. It is always possible that an important condition or injury was missed at an earlier examination, or the boxer might previously have been unaware of his own or his family's medical history. The guidelines and procedures outlined above for the initial examination apply equally for medical re-examinations.

2 It is particularly important to look for conditions which might have newly arisen since the previous examination, as well as for significant injury. Visual acuity *must* be re-examined critically as myopia may continue to worsen through adolescence and into adulthood. 'Degenerative' conditions are unusual in the age range of boxers but towards the end of a long career, especially if the family history is suggestive, such conditions as ischaemic heart disease and spinal degeneration may appear.

Guidelines

1 Height, weight and general physique. Obesity does not debar unless suggestive of hormonal imbalance, in which case further investigation is required. Departure beyond the 20th or 80th centile for height and weight requires special consideration.

2 Family history.

(a) A family history of tuberculosis requires a chest X-ray and information from the general practitioner regarding its current activity in the family.

(b) Conditions with a known genetic inheritance (e.g. Huntington's chorea) must be recorded; most will debar from boxing.

(c) A family history of epilepsy, insulin-dependent diabetes, asthma, sickle-cell anaemia or trait or coagulation disorder will all require further investigation in the boxer to determine the extent to which he is affected.

3 Personal medical history. A previous history in the boxer of the following conditions renders him unfit:

(a) epilepsy, infantile or other convulsions or fits, blackouts or any history of faints of unknown cause; skull fracture or other severe head injury; severe migraine, meningitis, encephalitis or other major disease of the central nervous system or any form of brain surgery;

(b) insulin-dependent diabetes;

(c) congenital heart disease, rheumatic heart disease;

(d) severe asthma, spontaneous pneumothorax;

(e) sickle-cell anaemia (not the trait), coagulation disorders;

(f) bilateral deafness requiring regular use of hearing-aids;

(g) significant congenital abnormality of the genito-urinary system, renal calculus, nephritis;

(h) proven infection with hepatitis B or HIV;

(i) peptic ulceration, pancreatitis, gallstones, severe inflammatory bowel disease;

(j) malignancy of any sort;

(k) tropical infectious diseases or infestations;

(l) porphyria;

(m) nephrectomy, orchidectomy, transplant or other major surgery.

4 Eyes and eyesight.

(a) Visual acuity must be assessed separately for each eye by the Snellen method, *without* contact lenses or spectacles being worn. Visual acuity which is worse than 6/12 in the better eye and/or worse than 6/24 in the worse eye automatically renders a boxer unfit to box.

(b) Squint or visual field defect requires referral for a specialist ophthalmological opinion.

(c) The eyes must be ophthalmoscopically examined for evidence of corneal scarring, cataract and retinal tears, detachment or haemorrhage.

5 Ears and hearing.

(a) Significant bilateral deafness debars from boxing, whatever the cause.

(b) Unilateral deafness in itself does not prohibit boxing, providing hearing is adequate in the other ear.

(c) Otitis externa, otitis media, mastoiditis, a moist or discharging perforation of the pars tensa and the presence of a grommet all prevent a boy from boxing until the infection has fully resolved and any grommets are removed. An attic perforation and/or cholesteatoma permanently debar, but a simple, dry perforation in itself does not.

6 Nose. Gross nasal deformity, including the septum, leading to severe nasal obstruction debars from boxing. Hay fever, if severe, might debar, as might a large polypus. Submucosal resection (SMR) or other nasal surgery requires special consideration.

7 Mouth and throat. The following debar from boxing:

(a) Excessively protruding front teeth, or malocclusion such that the lower incisors cannot gain location on and support from a gum-shield.

(b) Active dental sepsis, excessive caries of the incisors and/or canines.

(c) Fixed braces or any other form of orthodontic treatment.

(d) Tonsillitis (until resolved).

(e) Repair of cleft palate may need referral for specialist opinion if a defect still remains.

8 Chest.

(a) Expansion should be at least 3.7 cm; deformity of the chest wall which compromises ventilation would debar.

(b) If there is evidence of obstructive airways disease, full details including peak expiratory flow and medication must be recorded.

(c) Evidence of parenchymal lung disease will require referral for specialist opinion.

9 Cardiovascular system.

(a) Cyanosis, evidence of cardiac failure, cardiomegaly, dysrhythmia and valvular disease all debar from boxing.

(b) In cases of doubt, exercise testing may be necessary as part of a specialist cardiological opinion.

(c) Blood-pressure should be average for age; in senior boxers, a systolic pressure higher than 140 mmHg and/or a diastolic higher than 90 mmHg requires further investigation. Examination of the fundi may be helpful in deciding whether marginally raised blood-pressure is due to anxiety or organic disease.

10 Abdomen.

(a) Full examination of the abdomen must be performed (rectal examination is not required). Hepatomegaly, splenomegaly, absence of or undescended testis and hernia (inguinal, femoral or incisional) all debar from boxing.

(b) A soundly healed surgical scar does not in itself debar from boxing, but the examining doctor should satisfy himself of the nature of the operation.

(c) Abnormally delayed puberty should be referred for investigation.

(d) If there is doubt, all details should be recorded and further information sought from the general practitioner.

11 Central nervous system.

(a) Full examination of the CNS is required — pupils, cranial nerves, power, tone, reflexes and co-ordination; speech and higher functions will be appreciated during the course of the examination.

(b) If any abnormality is found it must be recorded and the boxer referred for neurological opinion.

(c) Formal psychological examination is not required, but the examining doctor should be alert to and record grossly subnormal intelligence, obvious personality disorder or any suggestion of the abuse of drugs or solvents.

12 Spine and limbs.

(a) Significant spinal deformity (scoliosis, kyphosis) or stiffness debar from boxing. Spinal surgery or previous fracture/dislocation also debar.

(b) Any deformity in the limbs (congenital or acquired) must be recorded. Abnormally reduced or excessive mobility of the joints may debar from boxing.

13 Skin. Problems with the skin rarely lead to long-term unfitness to box. Severe pustular acne, impetigo, infected eczema with marked excoriation, fungal dermatosis, herpes and unhealed inoculation scars all debar until the condition is adequately controlled or healed.

14 Urine. The urine must be passed at the time of examination and tested by dip-stick. A trace of albumin can be ignored, but sugar, blood, significant albumin or ketones all require further investigation.

Appendix 18.2: Guidelines for the pre-bout medical inspection

The following represents the recommended procedure for the medical inspection, and gives some indication of findings which should prevent a boxer being passed fit to box.

1 Medical record card (ME3). The boxer's medical record card must be inspected to confirm the following:

(a) that it is valid;

(b) that it relates to the boxer being examined;

(c) that the boxer has been medically examined within the stipulated period (five years up to 30 years of age; one year between 30 and 35 years of age);

(d) that the boxer is not in a period of compulsory rest from previous injury or illness;

(e) that the minimum prescribed time has elapsed since the previous contest, whatever the result.

Specific injury or illness will be documented and, if recent, should direct the tournament medical officer to pay particular attention to that region.

2 History.

(a) In practice, the history is perhaps the most valuable part of the inspection. It will direct the doctor's attention to recent specific problems, and alert him to more generalised illness, such as a viral illness.

(b) Boxers are always very keen to box, and may deny any recent injury or illness. For this reason, it is stongly recommended that the coach accompanies his boxer(s) to the inspection and reports his boxer's recent performance in the gym. It is useful to ask if there has been recent illness or injury, recent loss of time from work or school, absence from regular training sessions or recent visits to the general practitioner or hospital.

3 General condition.

(a) A few seconds should be taken to stand back and look at the boxer. He should appear well and be mentally alert and desiring to box. Pallor, lethargy or mouth-breathing in association with a runny nose or cough should alert the medical officer to recent or continuing illness.

(b) Colds and sore throats, whilst having little specific effect on a boxer's skills, will take the edge off his alertness, concentration and performance, and will generally lead to the decision 'unfit'.

(c) More significant viral illness (cervical and axillary lymphadenitis, pyrexia and rash are pointers, in addition to any specific effects) definitely prohibit boxing, and a minimum rest period of two weeks is suggested. In these conditions, performance is well below par, and the risk of extreme exercise in the possible presence of viral infection of the myocardium, pericardium or lungs is not justified.

4 Skin. Severe pustular acne, impetigo, open cold sores and un-healed inoculation scars all prevent boxing, because of the risk of spread of infection (to the eye or opponent).

5 Face.

(a) The periorbital regions are common sites for laceration and should be closely inspected. The scar of any recent laceration should be well healed — two weeks is probably the absolute minimum time required before boxing, and then only in the course of a major competition, after explaining the potential risk of chronic problems for the boxer and trainer, and after alerting the referee to the potential for the cut to reopen.

(b) Minor recent bruising and older bruising in the absence of swelling do not necessarily debar from boxing.

(c) The hair must not be so long as to be drawn into the eyes by a punch.

6 Eyes.

(a) The boxer should be specifically asked if he has suffered a recent change in vision. If he has, this demands testing of visual fields and full ophthalmoscopic examination, as well as a test of visual acuity. Whatever the outcome, it would be difficult to allow a boxer to box with such a history, and he should be referred to an optician or ophthalmologist.

(b) Otherwise, a superficial inspection of the eyes is required, specifically looking for conjunctivitis, large subconjunctival haemorrhage (as indication of more serious injury to eyeball or orbit), evidence of injury to the cornea, iris or sclera, or hyphaema.

(c) No boxer may spar or box in a competitive bout wearing spectacles or contact lenses (this applies to all types of contact lenses).

7 Nose.

(a) A discharge or obstruction should be assessed.

(b) A recent fracture of the nose should be healed, with no swelling, bruising or tenderness, and the nasal airways should be clear.

8 Gum-shield.

(a) The gum-shield must be closely examined in position in every boxer. It must extend beyond the premolars on each side and fit well; it should not fall out when the facial muscles are relaxed and the mouth opened.

(b) Many gum-shields are moulded from plastic blanks after warming in hot water; if one of this type does not fit well at the inspection, it may be reheated and the fit improved by further moulding.

9 Mouth and pharynx. Dental caries of a degree that will weaken the anterior teeth prevents boxing, as does tonsilitis and marked pharyngitis. Fixed orthodontic braces and bridgework debar. Pharyngeal erythema alerts the attention to a viral illness.

10 Ears.

(a) Both ears must be examined with the auriscope.

(b) Otitis media (purulent or serous), severe otitis externa, attic perforation or a grommet *in situ* all render the boxer unfit and require referral to the GP if not currently under review by him.

(c) A boxer may box with a dry inferior perforation, provided that he can hear the referee's instructions.

11   Heart.

(a) The rhythm, rate, and force of the pulse should be felt, and the heart sounds auscultated. If indicated, the blood-pressure should be measured.

(b) Any suggestion of organic disease automatically renders the boxer unfit, and necessitates referral for further advice.

(c) It must be remembered, though, that boxers are highly trained athletes, and at rest often have a low pulse rate with relatively high pulse pressure. They are also anxious at the pre-bout inspection, as competition is imminent — in some, therefore, there may be a tachycardia. There should be no disturbance of rhythm, except for sinus dysrrhythmia, which is sometimes quite marked. Gross bradycardia or tachycardia render unfit and require investigation.

12   Lungs.

(a) The breath sounds should be auscultated, particularly at the lung bases.

(b) Noticeable loss of air entry or persistent adventitial sounds render a boxer unfit; if in doubt, pyrexia is a useful indicator for significant infection.

13   Abdomen.

(a) The anterior abdominal wall should be inspected for hernia, particularly in boxers employed in heavy manual labour.

(b) Beware the boxer who has recently been discharged following abdominal surgery. This may not be regarded as an 'illness', and he may truthfully answer 'no' to the question, 'have you seen your doctor recently?'

14   Central nervous system. Examination of the central nervous system is not indicated, but lethargy, confusion, disorientation, incoordination and difficulties with balance should be recognised during the rest of the inspection. It must be remembered that minor head injury can occur in training and normal daily activities and might not be indicated on the boxer's medical record card. Any indication of a continuing state of concussion renders the boxer unfit, and requires referral for full examination.

15   Hands. A recent injury, particularly to the metacarpophalangeal joints (evident from swelling, bruising and tenderness) must be assessed. Loss of range of movement and pain on clenching the fist are significant in this respect.

16   Limbs.

(a) Specific examination of the lower limbs is only indicated if abnormal posture or gait is observed during the course of the inspection, or is suggested by the declaration of recent injury in the history.

(b) A crude examination of pectoral girdle, shoulder and elbow joints and associated muscles is provided by asking the boxer to place both hands behind his head and then his back. Any pain or loss of mobility in these actions requires closer examination, and probably the decision 'unfit'.

Appendix 18.3: Regulations for knock-outs

1   If a boxer is rendered unconscious then only the referee and the doctor summoned should remain in the ring, unless the doctor needs extra help.

2   A boxer who has been knocked out during a contest or wherein the referee has stopped the contest due to a boxer having received hard blows to the head, making him defenceless or incapable of continuing, shall be examined by a doctor immediately afterwards and accompanied to his home or suitable accommodation by one of the officials on duty at the event.

3   A boxer who has been knocked out during a contest or wherein the referee has stopped the contest due to a boxer having received hard blows to the head, making him defenceless or incapable of continuing, shall not be permitted to take part in competitive boxing or sparring for a period of at least 28 days after he has been knocked out.

4   A boxer who has been knocked out during a contest or wherein the referee has stopped the contest due to a boxer having received hard blows to the head, making him defenceless or incapable of continuing twice in a period of 84 days shall not be permitted to take part in competitive boxing or sparring during a period of 84 days from the second knock-out or RSCH.

5   A boxer who has been knocked out during a contest or wherein the referee has stopped the contest due to a boxer having received hard blows to the head, making him defenceless or incapable of continuing, three times in a period of 12 months shall not be allowed to take part in competitive boxing or sparring for a period of one year from the third knock-out or RSCH.

6   The referee will indicate to the OIC and judges to annotate the score card 'RSCH' when he has stopped the contest as a result of a boxer being unable to continue as a result of blows to the head.

7   The KO to be divided into three classes.

(a) Immediate recovery.

(b) Recovery within two minutes.

(c) Recovery over two minutes.

In the case of (c) the boxer concerned should be referred to hospital immediately.

Further reading

Adams L. M. (1989) *Medical Aspects of Amateur Boxing*, 2nd edn. London: Amateur Boxing Association of England.

Amateur Boxing Association of England (1984) *Memorandum, Articles of Association and Rules*. London: ABA.

American Medical Association Council on Scientific Affairs (1983) Brain injury in boxing. *Journal of the American Medical Association* **249**, 254–7.

Atha J., Yeadon M. R., Sandover J. & Parsons K. C. (1985) The damaging punch. *British Medical Journal* **291**, 1756–7.

Barns R. J. (1986) Boxing and the brain. *Australian and New Zealand Journal of Medicine* **16**, 439–40.

British Medical Association (1984) *Report of the Board of Science and Education Working Party on Boxing*. British Medical Association, London.

Corsellis J. A. N., Bruton C. J. & Freeman-Browne D. (1973) The aftermath of boxing. *Psychological Medicine* **3**, 270–303.

Cruickshank J. K., Higgens C. S. & Gray J. R. (1980) Two cases of acute intracranial haemorrhage in young amateur boxers. *Lancet* **i**, 626–7.

Editorial (1976) Brain damage in sport. *Lancet* **i**, 401–2.

Giovinazzo V. J., Yannuzzi L. A., Sorenson J. A., Delrowe D. J. & Cambell E. A. (1987) The ocular complications of boxing. *Ophthalmology* **94**, 587–96.

Gunby P. (1986) Epidemiologic study to examine amateur boxers' potential risks. *Journal of the American Medical Association* **255**, 2397–9.

Jordan B. D. (1987) Neurologic aspects of boxing. *Archives of Neurology* **44**, 453–9.

Jordan B. D. (1988) Medical and safety reforms in boxing. *Journal of the National Medical Association* **80**, 407–12.

Kaste M., Vilkki J., Sainis K., Kuume T., Katevuo K. & Meurala H. (1982) Is chronic brain damage in boxing a hazard of the past? *Lancet* **ii**, 1186–8.

Lampert P. W. (1984) Morphological changes in brains of boxers. *Journal of the American Medical Association* **251**, 2676–9.

Ludwig R. (1986) Making boxing safer: the Swedish model. *Journal of the American Medical Association* **255**, 2482.

Lundberg G. D. (1983, 1984, 1986) Boxing should be banned in civilised countries; Round 2; Round 3. *Journal of the American Medical Association* **249**, 250; **251**, 2696–8; **255**, 2483–5.

McLatchie G., Brooks N., Galbraith S., Hutchison J. S. F., Wilson L., Melville I. & Teasdale E. (1987) Clinical neurological examination, neuropsychology, electroencephalography and computed tomographic head scanning in active amateur boxers. *Journal of Neurology, Neurosurgery and Psychiatry* **50**, 96–99.

Maguire J. I. & Benson W. E. (1986) Retinal injury and detachment in boxers. *Journal of the American Medical Association* **255**, 2451–3.

Martland H. S. (1928) Punch drunk. *Journal of the American Medical Association* **91**, 1103–7.

Morrison R. G. (1986) Medical and public health aspects of boxing. *Journal of the American Medical Association* **255**, 2475–80.

Palmer E., Lieberman T. W. & Burns S. (1976) Contusion angle deformity in prize fighters. *Archives of Ophthalmology* **94**, 255–8.

Patterson R. H. Jr (1986) On boxing and liberty. *Journal of the American Medical Association* **255**, 2481–2.

Ross R. J., Cole M., Thompson J. S. & Kim K. H. (1983) Boxers — computed tomography, EEG, and neurological evaluation. *Journal of the American Medical Association* **249**, 211–3.

Ross R. J., Casson I. R., Siegel O. & Cole M. (1987) Boxing injuries: neurologic, radiologic and neuropsychologic evaluation. *Clinics in Sports Medicine* **6**, 41–51.

Royal College of Physicians (1969) Report on the medical aspects of boxing.

Ryan A. J. (1987) Intracranial injuries resulting from boxing: a review. *Clinics in Sports Medicine* **6**, 31–40.

Smith D. J. (1988) Ocular injuries in boxing. *International Ophthalmology Clinics* **28**, 242–5.

Thomassen A., Juul-Jensen P., de Fine Olivarius B., Braemer J. & Christensen A. L. (1979) Neurological, electrocephalographic and neuropsychological examination of 53 former amateur boxers. *Acta Neurologica Scandinavica* **60**, 352–62.

World Medical Association (1984) Statements on terminal illness and boxing adopted by the 35th World Medical Assembly, Venice, Italy, October 1983. *Medical Journal of Australia* **140**, 431.

19 The doctor at the boxing ring: professional boxing

A. L. WHITESON

'The bigger they come the harder they fall'
Robert Fitzsimmons

The first control of professional boxing was instituted in this country in the nineteenth century with the introduction of certain rules and regulations that were used to govern the sport by the Marquess of Queensberry and the National Sporting Club, which at that time, was the controlling body as far as the sport was concerned.

In 1929 the Boxing Board of Control took over as the acknowledged ruling body for professional boxing and has governed the sport ever since. The Boxing Board of Control has always been an independent organisation with none of its members having any financial interest in the sport whatsoever. This body is responsible for the introduction of the rules and regulations, and, from the inception of the National Sporting Club, a doctor has always been in attendance at contests. With the passage of time, the doctor's role has become more demanding as the dangers of the sport have become more clearly recognised. The prevention of medical hazards has become a major concern, both of the lay members of the boxing board and its medical panel.

In the early 1960s the board resolved that two medical officers should be in attendance at all contests and that no contest would be allowed to commence or continue without at least one doctor sitting at the ringside.*

The British Boxing Board of Control is responsible for governing professional boxing throughout the UK, which for administrative purposes is divided into eight areas, each of which is controlled by an area council. Each council has its own medical officer and

---

*The moral arguments against boxing are well known and rely on the notion that it is abhorrent for a sport to allow within its rules the deliberate infliction of injury between participants. The doctor attending such a sport is therefore faced with the dilemma of deciding whether it is morally acceptable to offer tacit support for such a system by providing medical cover, both in the pre-contest assessment of fitness to box and in the treatment of injuries as they arise during the contest. The doctor in attendance should remember, however, that, provided the participants are adequately aware of the dangers which they face in taking part in the sport, the final decision whether or not to compete as fit and mentally competent individuals rests with the boxers themselves. The doctor does, however, have a role in identifying and reporting individuals whose physical condition makes them unsuitable for competition.

278

279

*Chapter 19
The doctor at the
boxing ring:
professional
boxing*

medical panel, who are responsible to the board's chief medical officer and which report to him on a regular basis if any untoward problems occur. There is an annual meeting of the medical panel at which the medical rules and regulations are updated and amended from time to time, to improve safety for the boxer. Close contact is maintained throughout the year between the area medical officers and the chief officer. Each area medical officer is responsible for the appointment of his deputy and other doctors who will be in medical control of the tournaments. It is his duty to satisfy himself as to the competence of the doctor working at the ringside. All must have a working knowledge of sports medicine and trauma management. In particular they must be able to recognise and treat injuries that are peculiar to the sport itself. No tournament is allowed to take place without two doctors in attendance and they must ensure that all the safety regulations of the board are upheld. They must be prepared to give advice not only on the medical aspects of the sport, but also on training methods and diet, and on tournament days are expected to attend the lunch-time medical examination and to arrive at the tournament well before the start. They will probably be the last to leave.

All promoters, managers, boxers, trainers and seconds must be licensed by the Board and the tournament venue must also have official approval. No tournament can take place without an adequately equipped medical room being available. This must have hot and cold running water, an examination couch, adequate lighting, and facilities for minor operative procedures such as suturing, should it be required. There must be resuscitation equipment available at the ringside and it is the doctor's duty to ensure that it is working properly, and that he and his colleague can use it efficiently. An ambulance should be on site or readily available and the local hospital, in particular the casualty and neurosurgical unit, should be pre-advised that a tournament is taking place.

Every professional boxer must be licensed by the Boxing Board of Control and must have an annual physical examination. This includes an in-depth questionnaire, including present and past medical history, family history and social habits. A general physical examination is required with particular attention to the skeletal system, the eyes, including visual acuity, and an in-depth neurological and neuropsychological assessment. Skull X-rays are mandatory as is a urinalysis. CT scanning and/or nuclear magnetic resonance imaging of the skull is now a prerequisite for most boxers. Should any problem arise then the boxer is referred for specialist investigation, and all the reports are sent to the chief medical officer for consideration by the medical panel, whose recommendations are then placed before the Boxing Board of Control. Detailed physical examination of boxers occurs annually, and also whenever a boxer loses a contest

280

Chapter 19
The doctor at the
boxing ring:
professional
boxing

or at any other time the medical panel deem it to be necessary. The boxer also undergoes medical examination at the 'weigh-in', which takes place normally at lunch-time on the day of the tournament. He is again seen prior to going into the ring and then after he has finished his contest, regardless of whether he has won or lost. Any untoward features, either in his performance during the contest or subsequently, must be reported to the area medical officer who will pass these reports to the board in order that a complete medical dossier is kept, on each registered boxer.

Each doctor wanting to join the medical panel must satisfy the area medical officer or his deputies of his competence and his interest in the sport and of his awareness of the problems that may arise. In order to do this he is invited to sit at the ringside on several occasions with an experienced doctor so that he can be assessed, and only then will he be invited to join the medical panel. All doctors must be fully trained in the management of the unconscious patient and also be able to make competent decisions on other medical matters pertaining to boxing, including the assessment of a cut. At the cessation of each contest one of the two doctors must examine the boxers and must satisfy himself that they are in good health and be prepared to institute treatment should it be required prior to returning to the ringside. In the case of an unconscious boxer the senior of the two doctors should take immediate emergency action, removing the boxer's gum-shield, maintaining an airway, placing him in the recovery position and assessing his general condition. Should recovery not occur immediately, then the boxer must be transferred by ambulance to hospital and it is the task of the second doctor to ensure that this is effectively carried out.

In all tournaments run by the British Boxing Board of Control the referee is in sole charge of the contest and it is the duty of the area medical officer to instruct referees as to the medical hazards of boxing and as to how he should be able to recognise and prevent these problems. At European and World level the doctor may be invited by the referee to assess an injury, but it is important to realise that the doctor can only offer advice, and it is the referee's ultimate responsibility to decide whether or not a contest can continue. When the injury is a laceration, it is the doctor's role to be able to assess rapidly whether the cut is serious enough to warrant the stoppage of a contest and to advise the referee accordingly.* It has been argued that the doctor should have the power to stop a contest but this may be fraught with dangers. A doctor sitting at the ringside may not have a good view of the two contestants and will not be able to assess from any distance whether the boxer is or is not

---

* The doctor is the agent of the Boxing Board of Control and his professional responsibility is to provide sound advice. The responsibility for the safe running of the competition rests with the Board of Control or its delegated area council.

distressed, whereas the referee is in an ideal position to decide whether the boxer is fit to continue or not. If the doctor were able to stop the contest, the referee might have a tendency to allow it to continue rather than exercise his own judgement, and this might result in more serious damage than would otherwise occur. Providing the medical education of all referees is adequate and constantly being updated, as it is in this country, then the referee, in the opinion of the author, should continue to be in sole charge of the contest.

Medical problems arising from boxing, can be divided into acute and chronic.

Sudden death in the ring, or soon after a fight, is fortunately very rare in the UK. There have been just 12 deaths in the British ring in the past 43 years: 11 were subdural haematomas (the commonest cause of death in the boxing ring) and the other was probably a sensitivity to aspirin, which a boxer had taken for a headache prior to going into the ring. (Incidentally, nowadays no boxer is allowed to box when taking any form of medication and must be totally free of all symptoms and complaints both at the weigh-in and prior to the contest. It is the responsibility of the examining doctor to ensure that this is the case.)

The commonest injury in the boxing ring is a 'cut eye'. This in fact is a laceration of the eyelid or eyebrow, not of the eye itself. The majority of these are of no significance to a boxer's future health, for even if they are severe, competent suturing and a two- to three-month exclusion from the ring will allow any cut to heal satisfactorily and soundly. The importance of a cut is not only its severity but also its location. Should it occur on the eyebrow or upper eyelid then blood running downward into the eye will impair vision, causing the boxer to alter his stance, and may seriously impair his ability to defend himself. Lacerations away from the eye do not have the same significance. Lacerations of the scalp and cheeks bleed profusely but do not cause any problems, and can normally be controlled by the trainer or second. Prior to being licensed, these personnel are taught how to treat a cut by using 1/1000 aqueous solution of adrenaline, which is applied into the wound on a sterile swab stick. This treatment is harmless, and causes local vasoconstriction and thus cessation of bleeding. Following this the cut is covered with a thin layer of Vaseline. In the past various other substances have been used to achieve haemostasis, including Monsel's solution and ferric chloride, both of which are now illegal. Various other haemostatic agents have also been used such as thromboplastin, but they are not readily available throughout the world and should only be used under the direct supervision of medical personnel. These are therefore not recommended for use in the boxing ring. It is the doctor's duty to ensure that the correct haemostatic agents only are used. In title bouts, it is his responsibility to provide

282
Chapter 19
The doctor at the
boxing ring:
professional
boxing

the two bottles of 1/1000 aqueous solution of adrenaline to each contestant's corner.

The cauliflower ear, once a characteristic feature of a boxer, is now very rarely seen. Damage of the small joints of the hand does occur quite regularly, but rarely progresses to arthritis or joint deformity, and can be prevented by use of correct punching technique, adequate bandaging, and taping of the hands beneath the boxing gloves. Friction burns around the neck and chest are not uncommon as a result of rubbing against the ropes during a contest. These injuries are of minor significance and are self-limiting.

Intraocular damage is very rare in professional boxing. Detachment of the retina has received a great deal of publicity but is far less common than has been suggested in the recent BMA report on boxing. This injury was thought to be due to accidental use of the thumb in a punch. This mechanism is now prevented by the use of gloves in which the thumb is tethered. The injury is also probably prevented by the rule which excludes severely myopic people from holding a professional boxing licence. Traumatic cataracts can occur, but are not common. Their presence, however, would preclude a boxer from continuing to hold a licence. Penetrating wounds of the orbit do not occur in boxing. Whether a boxer should be allowed to resume his career after retinal detachment is a controversial matter, but usually when this occurs the boxer's licence to box would not be renewed. Fractures around the orbit do occur, as do blow-out fractures of the maxillary sinus; both are correctable surgically but would usually herald the retirement of the boxer. Occasionally, bruising into the intrinsic muscles of the eye will cause double vision, but this is transient and settles with adequate rest, and, providing recovery is complete, then a boxer's career would not be in jeopardy.

As far as the skeletal system is concerned the commonest injury apart from bruising of the joints is a fracture of the metacarpals and carpals of the hand and thumb, normally due to bad punching technique and/or poor strapping support to the hand under the gloves. Operative treatment is sometimes required but would not preclude the boxer from continuing boxing subsequently, although several months of recovery may be required. Fractures of the ribs are rare, and recovery is rapid with rest. Dislocation of the shoulder, patella and the ankle have been recorded on several occasions in the past 20 years. There have been four documented cases of fracture of the mandible in professional boxing, all of which required surgical treatment. In each case the boxer was able to resume his career. On all four occasions this occurred in association with carious teeth and a boxer is always advised therefore to maintain regular dental check-ups. Fractures of the vault of the skull are unknown in boxing.

283

Chapter 19
The doctor at the
boxing ring:
professional
boxing

The most important complication that has been associated with boxing, and one which fortunately is rare, is the punch-drunk syndrome, or accumulated brain damage. This was well documented by Professor Corsellis in the 1970s. He carried out post-mortem examinations on deceased boxers of yesteryear and described mid-brain and cerebellar changes which were common to all. It is generally held that the reduction that has occurred in the number of rounds in boxing contests and also the reduction in the number of contests taking place have brought about a lower incidence of brain damage in boxers. Clearly, the institution of stricter medical examinations and the use of sophisticated scanning equipment and neuropsychological tests have played a significant part in this. Constant scrutiny of the boxer's performance in the ring and reports from officials and medical officers have led to medical dossiers being compiled on all registered boxers. Both have helped to bring about a reduction in the frequency and severity of punch-drunk boxers, and hopefully will eliminate this very distressing condition in the not-too-distant future.

The use of stimulants of all types is strictly forbidden by the Boxing Board of Control and boxers are randomly tested for drug abuse after contests. Should illegal substances be found, the boxer would risk permanent disqualification from the sport. During a contest, no boxer is allowed to use any form of stimulant. Even the use of smelling-salts is illegal and, should the use be suspected or confirmed, disciplinary action would be taken with the possible disqualification of the boxer.

The moral aspects of boxing are controversial but it is the view of the board and the medical panel that, providing a boxer and his family are fully aware of the dangers of the sport and providing he is prepared to keep himself in good physical condition, then he must make a conscious decision as to whether he does or does not wish to box. He must at the same time realise that when he becomes a professional he joins a very select club, whose rules and regulations, medical and otherwise, are very strict. In the event that medical advice is given to the boxer regarding retirement from a bout, or rest after injury, this should be heeded to safeguard not only his own health but also the reputation of the sport. The boxer should be as fit when he returns from the ring as when he started. Medical advice should not be given lightly but only after full examinations with due consideration for the boxer and his future health.

There are few differences between the medical problems facing amateur and professional boxing. Although an amateur boxer will only box three, or occasionally four, three-minute rounds, and a professional may box anything up to 10–12 rounds, an amateur will box far more frequently than a professional and at the end of a season the number of rounds boxed may not be very different. The

284
Chapter 19
The doctor at the
boxing ring:
professional
boxing

brain does not recognise any difference between a blow delivered by an amateur or a professional boxers, any more than a blow resulting from a football or a clash of heads in a rugby scrum.

In conclusion, it is not denied by those governing sport that boxing has attendant risks, some of which are minor and some of which are major, but, providing that the control, both medically and through the rules governing the sport, is good and that the boxer is prepared to make the necessary sacrifice to keep himself at peak fitness, then the individuals involved can only benefit physically, emotionally and of course, in the professional sport, financially. To ban the sport, as some advocate, would be counter-productive. The sport would be driven underground where unlicensed shows would occur, as some do already, with no control of any type (let alone medical) and that can surely do no good whatsoever. The administrators of the sport and its medical advisers are not complacent, and are always looking for better investigative procedures in order to ensure that a boxer is as fit when he leaves the sport as he was when he started.

Medical problems in competitive and recreational swimming 20

J. M. CAMERON

'In the world, who knows not to swim goes to the bottom'
Outlandish proverb by G. Herbert

The Amateur Swimming Association (ASA), the governing body for the sport in England, was founded on 7 January 1869, although in fact was not known by this name until 17 years later.

Also founded on 7 January 1869, following a Swimming Congress held at the German Gymnasium in King's Cross, London, was the Metropolitan Swimming Association, or, as it was known originally, the Associated Metropolitan Swimming Clubs and then the London Swimming Association. This amalgamation of London clubs received much approval but no active support (Besford 1971). Its influence was purely local and its development hampered by lack of funds. Early in February 1874 the title of the association was again changed to the Swimming Association of Great Britain (SAGB), in order to include all the clubs in the country. In 1884, following a breakaway led by the Otter Swimming Club of London, a rival body, the Amateur Swimming Union (ASU) was set up. A desperate struggle for supremacy went on, with continual rows concerning amateur and professional status, until 1886 when these two bodies agreed to dissolve and agreed on a set of 135 rules, based on those of the Amateur Athletics Association and the National Cyclists Union, which have been the basis of the ASA administration ever since and have been copied by bodies throughout the world.

Though primarily concerned with England, the ASA by virtue of its greater size and number of clubs (by 1987, approximately 17 500 clubs were affiliated), has dictated the policy of British swimming, in which Scotland and Wales also participate.

In March 1970, an era probably unparalleled in sports administration ended when, after 49 years as honorary secretary, Harold E. Fern retired. His successor was Norman Sansfield, who was appointed by the ASA to be its first professional secretary, after almost 100 years of amateur administration.

The ASA is divided into five districts — Midlands, North, Northeast, South and West — together with a number of affiliated bodies such as the Services, English Schools and British Universities.

286
Chapter 20
Medical problems
in competitive
and recreational
swimming

Competitive swimming: types of injury

Shoulder injuries are some of the most common types of injury among competitive swimmers. The great freedom of movement at the shoulder is due to the anatomical construction of the joint. The capsule is loose with little ligamentous restraint to movement, joint stabilisation with activity being maintained primarily by the muscles of the shoulder. The commonest shoulder injuries among swimmers are muscle strains and tendinitis. The aetiology of the strains is simply through overstress either in or out of the water; improper or poor technique; inadequate and/or inappropriate rehabilitation of initial symptoms with return to activity too early. All injuries to the shoulder either directly or indirectly involve the muscles of the shoulder. The aetiology of shoulder tendinitis is often difficult to identify but the majority would appear to be secondary to an initial injury such as strain that has been inadequately or inappropriately rehabilitated, resulting in a residual weakness and thus affecting the muscular stabilisation of the shoulder. The tendon(s) can as a consequence become inflamed by impingement (contact) with ligaments and/or bones which normally do not impinge on the tendon(s) when adequate stabilisation exists. Swimmers with such secondary tendinitis experience a gradual onset of deep pain, noted mostly with overhead subluxation of the tendon from the groove, and this can eventually lead to tendon rupture (Aronen 1985; Blatz 1985).

Butterfly back syndrome

One of the most frequent complaints seen in swimmers, of all levels of achievement, in the last 10–15 years, is low back pain, particularly in butterfliers and more recently in breaststrokers.

To remind you, the 'fly', with its dolphin-like leg action in its modern form, originated as a 'mutant' of the breaststroke. Swimmers who were dissatisfied with the maximum speed they could develop with this style sought to make greater use of the potentially powerful arm action than was possible in the traditional breaststroke. It has developed as a competitive event following the 1952 Olympic Games (Helsinki). The use of the breaststroke kick has virtually disappeared and now is performed using the dolphin undulation. In the fly stroke the buttocks remain fairly well fixed in relation to the surface of water and act as basal fulcrum around which the top and bottom halves of the body work. The range and power of the kick depend greatly on the degree of lumbosacral mobility as well as the flexibility of the feet and ankles. The movement of the lumbar spine is essentially repeated flexion/extension, the latter being necessary

Table 20.1 Results of X-rays

Minimal change	25%
Old Scheuermann's disease	
Possible narrowing facet joints	
Scoliosis	
Radiologically normal	75%

to elevate shoulder and forearms to clear the surface of the water in recovery.

Repeated powerful flexion/extension movement of the lumbar spine has been implicated previously in gymnasts in the mechanism of the production of the stress fracture of the pars interarticularis of the zygoapophyseal arch (Jackson *et al.* 1976).

In research carried out at the London Hospital in an investigation of some 50 swimmers with low back pain and who regularly compete in butterfly events, the findings were as follows:

1 The common complaint was non-specific low back pain with no specific localising.

2 On examination all had vague tenderness in lumbosacral region.

3 Assessment of mobility of the lumbosacral spine revealed that 40% had full range, 35% some limitation of flexion and 25% limited lateral flexion rotation.

4 All swimmers underwent radiological examination of the lumbosacral spine. This was found to be abnormal in a quarter of the athletes examined, although the abnormalities were of a minor nature (Table 20.1).

The investigation concluded that the majority of symptomatic swimmers were associated with a proven spondylolysis — occasionally spondylolisthesis, an impending stress fracture in pars interarticularis, may be inferred by a 'hot' bone scan, preceding radiological change. Using a cadaveric spine in flexion and forced hyperextension, clear impingement of the apex of the facet joints L4–5 is seen and is exactly the point at which spondylolysis occurs. This point provides the fulcrum across which 'bending movement' occurs in the dolphin leg kick.

By fixing the shoulders in the water (which is the effect produced by use of a hand-held float), a 'whiplash' originating from the fixed point of the shoulders and imposed upon and increasing in the lumbosacral junction occurs in butterfly stroke. It may be postulated that by shoulder fixation there is a much greater degree of energy expenditure in the region of the lumbosacral joint than when the shoulders are free to move. When a 'dolphin' undulation method and a kick practice are used one returns to the dolphin movement or rolling 'S' and the lumbar spine is not fixed for long periods of hyperextension but relieved periodically, following the dipping of the head into the 'dive' part of the stroke.

288

*Chapter 20
Medical problems
in competitive
and recreational
swimming*

Table 20.2 Review of injuries occurring amongst swimmers (after Hunt 1987)

Head
  Concussion
  Laceration of forehead
  Laceration of chin
  Epistaxis × 2
  Supraorbital haematoma
  Fractured skull

Neck
  Fracture dislocation lower cervical spine
  Fracture cervical spine C3–4
  Strained sternocleidomastoid
  Strained trapezius muscle

Shoulder
  Bruise
  Dislocation
  Strained trapezius
  Old fractured clavicle: acromioclavicular pain
  Joint
  Supraspinatus tendinitis
  Strained ligaments of shoulder
  Biceps strain
  Strained deltoid bursitis
  Strained deltoid
  Biceps tendinitis

Forearm
  Tenosynovitis
  Bruising

Elbow
  Chronic 'tennis elbow'
  Acute 'tennis elbow'
  Strained ligaments of elbow from indirect blow on hand

Hand
  Laceration to ring finger
  Injury to metacarpophalangeal joint
  Bruising
  Dislocation of thumb
  Ruptured ligaments of two fingers
  Extensor tendinitis of wrist

Back
  Strained back muscle
  Sacroiliac strain
  Non-specific low back strain

Legs
  Torn hamstrings
  Patellofemoral pain
  Patellofemoral pain with crepitus
  Strained medial ligament of knee
  Dislocation of patella
  Strained vastus medialis

Ankle and feet
  Strained lateral ligament of ankle
  Bruising of tendo Achilles
  Extensor tendinitis of foot
  Laceration of feet
  Torn medial ligaments of ankle
  Bruising of perineum
  Dislocation of hip

Neck injury C3–4 distribution	1
Acute supraspinatus tendinitis	3
Acute biceps tendinitis	2
Acute deltoid strain	1
Chronic biceps tendinitis	1
Chronic supraspinatus tendinitis	2
Chronic tendonitis of shoulder	2
Osteoarthritis of shoulder	1
Strained trapezius muscle	2
Strained pectoralis major	2
Acute tendinitis of flexor and rotator muscles of forearm	1
Strained rectus abdominis	2
Chronic sacroiliac strain	1 (butterfly)
Adductor strain	1
Injury 2–3 fingers (collision with ropes)	1
Flexor injury both wrists (collision with finish)	1
Blistering of toes (start-practising on rough-surface starting-blocks)	2
Abrasion of fingers on starting-block	1
Laceration of foot (broken tile)	1
Laceration of finger on starting-block	1
Injury to toe	1

Table 20.3 Injuries occurring amongst international swimmers 1985–7

References and further reading

Aronen J. (1985) Swimmer's shoulder. *Swimming World* April, 43–7.

Besford P. (1971) *Encyclopaedia of Swimming*. London: Robert Hale & Co.

Blatz D. (1985) Swimmer's shoulder. *Swimming World* Jan., 41–2.

Cameron J. M. (1986) The Butterfly Back Syndrome. *Swimming Times, technical supplement*, Jan., 4–7.

Hunt D. J. (1987) Personal communication.

Jackson D. W. *et al.* (1976) Spondylolysis in female gymnasts. *Clinical Orthopaedics* **117**, 68–73.

21 Scuba-diving and its medical problems: the role of the doctor

J. C. BETTS

'If their lungs receive air that moment they are free'
William Cowper

While scuba-diving, of all amateur sports, is probably the sport most dominated by medical and physiological factors, litigation involving medical issues has fortunately been rare.

Diving takes place in a hostile environment where extremes of pressure, cold and poor visibility combine to make diver selection, training and self-discipline essential for safe enjoyment of this rewarding sport. Before discussing the medico-legal problems, it will be necessary to outline, albeit briefly, the techniques and hazards of diving.

Equipment

Nearly all amateur diving is carried out using a supply of compressed air (not the oxygen of popular myth) carried in cylinders on the diver's back and fed via a demand valve which supplies compressed air at the pressure of the water surrounding the diver to a mouthpiece. The equipment has only a limited duration which decreases with depth. The use of a mouthpiece implies that, if unconsciousness occurs underwater, death from drowning results inevitably.

This system is in marked contrast to that of professional divers, who are supplied from compressors or large capacity compressed gas supplies, via pressure hoses, and use masks or helmets which completely cover the face and ensure that an unconscious diver, provided that he or she continues to breathe, may survive. For reasons of cost and also because of the need to retain mobility, this type of equipment is almost never used by amateur divers.

The amateur diver protects his or her face and ensures adequate vision by using a face-mask covering the eyes and nose. In all but tropical water, thermal protection in the form of a diving-suit is used. Until recently this was a so-called 'wet suit', which consisted of a close-fitting garment made of foam neoprene. The 'dry suit', which is a watertight suit made of foam neoprene or of rubberised fabric, with a waterproof entry zip and watertight seals at the wrists and neck, is now coming into use. Under this, thermal undergarments are worn and compression of these at depth is avoided by a manually regulated supply of air into the suit.*

Safety equipment carried usually includes a *weightbelt* (whose primary purpose is to balance out the additional buoyancy of the suit but which can also be dropped in emergency), a *life-jacket* capable of being inflated at depth and which frequently can provide a supply of air in emergency, and a *knife*.

*With increasing depth the compressive effect of water pressure increases at 1 atmosphere per 33 ft (10 m)

Medical hazards

For obvious reasons, most divers who die in the water ultimately die of drowning, whatever the primary cause. This has often led to misleading post-mortem results and erroneous coroner's verdicts, where important preceding pathology such as air embolism or acute pulmonary oedema has been overlooked.

Decompression sickness

Decompression sickness, 'the bends', is a problem peculiar to diving, compressed air work and aviation. At depth, because of the increased partial pressure of nitrogen in the compressed air breathed, nitrogen dissolves in the blood as it passes through the lungs and is diffused throughout the body, but tends to end up in fatty tissues, such as the brain and spinal cord, in which it is more soluble. On return to the surface, the reverse process takes place. However, if any individual tissue has too great a nitrogen level for a particular depth, the excess nitrogen will bubble out of solution, producing a wide variety of clinical pictures depending on the site involved. To avoid decompression sickness, divers make 'stops' in the water, in which they remain at prescribed depths for periods of time to allow the surplus nitrogen to be safely eliminated. For this purpose, diving tables are employed which specify the depth and duration of stops according to the length and depth of the dive.

When bubbles appear near a joint, usually one of the larger limb joints, pain will result. If occurring in the bloodstream, they usually appear in the systemic venous return and are filtered off in the pulmonary vascular bed of the lungs, leading to symptoms of chest pain, acute shortness of breath, cyanosis, haemoptysis and eventually unconsciousness if sufficiently severe. When occurring in the spinal cord, a wide variety of symptoms may result. Depending on the exact location of the bubble the resulting symptoms may include: paraplegia, monoplegia, paralysis of any muscle group or loss of any type of sensory function with paraesthesia, numbness, loss of light touch, pinprick, thermal or postural sensation. When affecting the brain, hemiplegia, vertigo or unconsciousness may represent the more severe type of presentations but often far more subtle changes may occur.

292
Chapter 21
Scuba-diving and
its medical
problems: the role
of the doctor

With such protean manifestations of this condition, which can present at any time from surfacing to 36 hours later, the potential for mistaken diagnoses by both diver and doctor is large. This is particularly unfortunate since prompt recompression treatment in a hyperbaric chamber not only is diagnostic but can be curative. However, the beneficial effects of recompression diminish hour by hour as treatment is delayed.

Barotrauma

Because the body has many air-containing spaces, these have to be filled with compressed air during descent or be squeezed. Similarly, during ascent these have to be vented or the compressed air will find an alternative escape route, sometimes with disastrous consequences. This type of injury is collectively termed 'barotrauma'.

Amongst the cavities of concern are the ears, the paranasal air sinuses and the lungs. Failure to inflate the middle ear via the Eustachian tube during descent may result in rupture of the tympanic membrane or haemorrhage into the middle ear or sometimes in rupture of the round window.

Air embolism

The compressed air breathed by the diver will expand as he or she approaches the surface. The diver is taught to breathe normally during an ordinary slow ascent and to breathe out continuously in an emergency ascent. If the breath is held, expanding compressed air in the pulmonary alveoli will enter the pulmonary venous circulation and thence via the left heart pass into the systemic circulation where, because of the upright posture of the diver in ascent, it ends up in the brain, giving rise to similar symptoms to those of cerebral decompression sickness. However, in the case of air embolism, the onset of symptoms is usually within the first minute of surfacing, although it may be delayed in minor cases for up to half an hour. Typically a diver will surface and give the OK signal before becoming unconscious.

As well as failure of breath control during ascent, air-trapping lesions of the lung such as lung cysts or stenosed bronchi from old pulmonary tuberculosis may not vent quickly enough during ascent and result in air embolism. For this reason, although positive findings are exceptionally unusual, both the British Sub Aqua Club (BSAC) members and professional divers are required to have chest X-rays at first medical examination. A preventable accident arising from this cause would be impossible to defend in court without a normal X-ray. Unfortunately, many cases of air embolism seem to arise from undetectable or transient lesions in the lung and, apart from banning further diving by the individual concerned, there is little that can be done in the way of prevention.

One misleading clinical feature of air embolism that has caused problems in the past is that spontaneous recovery frequently occurs. This is thought to be due to the air bubbles eventually passing on through the cerebral circulation into the systemic veins, but it may be followed by relapse, thought to be caused by cerebral oedema developing in the damaged areas of the brain, which can be difficult to treat by recompression.

293

Chapter 21
Scuba-diving and
its medical
problems: the role
of the doctor

Hypothermia

The wet suit provides barely adequate thermal protection in the cold UK waters and most dives involve moderate loss of body heat. This is principally because the wet suit is compressed at depth and its insulation value considerably reduced. Subclinical degrees of hypothermia reduce physical and mental efficiency and are often a silent factor leading to diving accidents. For this reason there is now a revival of interest in dry suits, which do not lose their protective value against heat loss at depth.

Nitrogen narcosis

The increased volume of nitrogen circulating in the blood during a dive acts as an anaesthetic, the effects increasing with depth and first becoming noticeable from depths of 30 m onwards. From 45 m onwards disorientation of the diver becomes increasingly severe and this is a major reason why the British Sub Aqua Club discourages amateur divers from going deeper than 50 m. The Health and Safety Executive ban professional divers from working beyond this depth using compressed air.

Natural hazards

Except in tropical waters, the diver has little to fear from the natural underwater fauna and flora. Even in the tropics, shark attack is comparatively rare and is seldom without previous warning except in low visibility or in a feeding frenzy. Many fish and invertebrates have poisonous spines which can be exceedingly painful and lead to temporary disablement but are not usually fatal. Fire coral also has the capacity to inflict painful burns.

Incidence of diving accidents

In spite of its reputation as a risk sport, diving does not figure in the list of the ten most dangerous sports. In the UK in 1987, which was a fairly representative year, there were 162 incidents, of which about

294

*Chapter 21
Scuba-diving and
its medical
problems: the role
of the doctor*

115 were medical in nature. These included eight deaths, six cases of air embolism, 69 of decompression sickness, five of injury, four of ear damage, four of hypothermia, five of unconsciousness, five resuscitations, six cases of breathlessness and four of narcosis. (Some cases appear under more than one category.)

This is against a background of some 600 000 dives carried out by members in the year, an incidence of about one in 5000 dives for medical incidents and an average fatality rate of one in 100 000 dives. (Only six of the fatalities were BSAC members.)

Diving-related illnesses

Probably the most dramatic problem to present as a medical emergency is decompression sickness or air embolism. When this occurs during or immediately after diving operations and there are severe symptoms, the diagnosis is not likely to be in much doubt. For England and Wales the Royal Navy provides an emergency telephone line for diving emergencies, when the duty diving medical officer on HMS *Nelson* will be contacted for advice. When the victim is still at sea, the coastguard is usually contacted by radio-telephone and will pass on details to HMS *Nelson*. Depending on the location of the incident, arrangements will be made for transport and treatment in the nearest available recompression chamber.

Scotland and Ireland have similar centres from which advice may be obtained.

Fortunately, with the increasing popularity of diving as a sport, NHS hospitals near the sea in areas of diving activity are recognising the risks that may occur, and are alerting their casualty officers to the possibility of receiving diving casualties and advising them as to where they may seek advice.

When the diver returns home, help may be sought from the local GP in the event of delayed-onset symptoms, who may not possess the relevant specialised knowledge and may possibly put off a decision in the hope that spontaneous improvement will occur. The BSAC maintains a list of medical referees, most of whom are also active divers, to whom the symptomatic diver or his GP may also turn for advice.

A recompression facility has recently been established at a diving centre in the south-west of England, which also acts as an advice and treatment centre for amateur divers.

To overcome the problem of widespread medical ignorance of diving illnesses, the BSAC has made available to divers a small card similar to those carried by epileptics, detailing the signs and symptoms of decompression sickness and air embolism and emphasising the urgency of prompt treatment by recompression.

Although in retrospect many errors of diagnosis and treatment may have been made in the past, surprisingly little litigation has resulted. There are probably several factors involved. First, diving is perceived as a 'risk sport', although in truth it is probably less dangerous than the drive to the coast. Secondly, it is emphasised in training that decompression sickness and air embolism are avoidable conditions and when a diver develops either he is often presumed to have been guilty of poor diving practice. Many divers have imperfect knowledge of recompression procedures or lack any standards by which to judge the quality of their treatment, which is mainly carried out by a relatively small group of doctors, well known to one another, who are well aware of the difficulties of both diagnosis and therapy.

Nevertheless, when casualty officers or other doctors are told by a diver that his symptoms are likely to be due to a recent dive, they run the risk of failing to diagnose a potentially serious and eminently treatable disease if they fail to seek expert advice.

295

Chapter 21
Scuba-diving and
its medical
problems: the role
of the doctor

Litigation

While the BSAC has been the subject of litigation on several occasions, these have usually involved indefensible diving procedures, usually novice divers taken into conditions totally unsuitable for them. There has only been one case of note involving the BSAC in which the medical aspects predominated. In many ways, this exemplifies the problems which may befall the unprepared casualty officer.

An insulin-dependent diabetic business executive joined the BSAC at a time when, subject to certain safeguards, diabetics were still accepted as divers. While still an inexperienced diver, he went on a boat to dive to a depth of 30 m. Before diving he explained to his companions that he was a diabetic and that, if he became unconscious, he should be given sugar. He was accompanied on his dive by two very experienced members, who said that his maximum bottom time was not exceeded. On surfacing his legs became weak as he swam back to the boat and he had to be assisted on board where, shortly afterwards, he became unconscious. As instructed, he was given sugar and partly regained consciousness. It took some time to get him ashore, where he was taken to the local casualty department.

Unfortunately his apparent response to sugar was misinterpreted as evidence of hypoglycaemia and he was given further quantities of glucose. It was not until several hours later that a blood glucose was taken and was found to be above 30 mmol/l. He was sent to the local recompression chamber, where he was found to be paraplegic. Unfortunately, management of a hyperglycaemic diabetic in recompression proved extremely difficult and there was no response to treatment. He emerged after three days almost tetraplegic, with only a little power in one hand. Eventually he committed suicide

296

Chapter 21
Scuba-diving and
its medical
problems: the role
of the doctor

and his widow sued the BSAC, its officers, the diving officer and the buddy diver, the casualty officer and the area health authority.

The history of rapid onset of symptoms after a normally safe dive would suggest that he sustained an air embolism and the case was fought on this basis, although the subsequent post-mortem showed the changes of decompression sickness in the spinal cord. It is conceivable that this resulted later from his recompression treatment, compromised as it was by his gross hyperglycaemia.

Interestingly enough, no criticism was made in court of the original decision to accept him as a diabetic diver. Very substantial damages were awarded against the area health authority and casualty officer while the BSAC and its members were exonerated.

Subsequently the Medical Committee of the BSAC, when reviewing the case, felt that it had identified a hitherto unforeseen problem, namely the extreme difficulty of making a diagnosis in an unconscious diabetic diver at sea and advised the club that in the light of this case it would be indefensible to allow diabetics to continue as diving members of the club.

Medical administration of the BSAC

The BSAC was founded at the time of the first flowering of the National Health Service, when it was felt to be almost immoral to make a charge for any medical service and consequently it was impossible to persuade members to pay for medical examinations. However, continued pressure from the medical officer and from diving officers of the branches, who were unhappy about taking out divers whose fitness was an unknown quantity, eventually resulted in medical examinations decided on by the local branch committee. Later on, compulsory medical examination and chest X-ray on entry were made a club rule, although repeat medical examination remains at the discretion of the branch committee. In practice, most do insist on them because of their possible legal liability in the event of an accident occurring due to some preventable medical cause. The chest X-ray is carried out almost entirely for medico-legal reasons.

Diving, in common with most risk sports, has a high turnover with an annual entry of over 6000 would-be divers. The comparatively small number of active diving medical members would find it impossible to carry out all these examinations and so a very successful and innovative medical reference system has been set up. In this system, the prospective diver is given a medical examination form on which he or she fills in basic details and medical history. The diver then takes it to his or her GP, who is able to carry out the examination aided by a reference chart included on the form containing the basic medical standards required by the club. For certain conditions and in any case of doubt, he is encouraged to contact by

297
Chapter 21
Scuba-diving and
its medical
problems: the role
of the doctor

telephone or letter any of the medical referees, also listed on the form, for advice and a decision as to the diver's fitness. This system works extremely well and has never yet resulted in litigation, although often advice is given by telephone. It is something of a grey area as to where the responsibility for such a decision would lie were it ever to be in question, given that the GP from whom the primary advice is being sought is himself/herself seeking expert guidance from one of a panel of experts on the subject. Each case will inevitably depend upon its individual merits, and perhaps the only concrete advice that can be offered is for all practitioners to keep good notes of the consultation and advice given in order that their position may subsequently be defended.

Where written advice is given by the medical referee in response to a letter from a medical colleague, responsibility for the advice given must lie with the medical referee, provided that the information on which it is based is correct.

Because of their knowledge of diving medicine and the average GP's reluctance to treat diving conditions, the medical referees are often called upon to treat divers, usually with diving-related ENT conditions. Here the medical referee may choose to treat the patient in the first instance, although referral to the relevant specialist opinion would perhaps be wise in cases of doubt.

Administering the medical referee system is the Medical Committee with a chairman who is its spokesman on the National Diving Committee, the chief technical committee of the BSAC. In addition to this the Medical Committee is responsible for setting and maintaining the necessary medical standards to permit safe diving. The Medical Examination Board is the ultimate court of appeal in deciding on a diver's fitness, and gives advice on medical and physiological matters to the club. It also liaises with the Diving Incidents Panel, carries out research projects and organises regular symposia on matters relating to sports diving medicine.

The Medical Committee of the BSAC has traditionally adopted a liberal stance in respect of medical standards and, unless there are firm medical grounds on which a condition should be considered a disqualification for diving, the applicant has been accepted pending further evidence. This is in contrast to the attitude of many authorities who take the view that in any case of doubt one should impose a ban on diving. Thus divers with some types of asthma, old poliomyelitis and carcinoma in remission have been accepted by the BSAC and, provided that a member has been accepted as fit to dive in accordance with the standards set by the Medical Committee, the club insurers will continue to give cover.

Although the British Sub Aqua Club is recognised as the governing body for underwater sport, it has no legal powers to enforce rules or decisions on its members and the most severe sanction that can be visited on a member is to be expelled from the club, a procedure

298
Chapter 21
Scuba-diving and
its medical
problems: the role
of the doctor

which is rarely invoked. This does not prevent the expelled member from continuing to dive, since there is no legal requirement for membership of a club or diving qualification for amateur divers. In spite of this inability to enforce decisions, the club enjoys a high reputation for the responsibility and standard of training of its members.

Medical hazards of water sports — and how to avoid them 22

F. NEWTON

'The sea will wash all man's ills away'
Eurypides

Water seems to have a fascination for man — sometimes a fatal fascination. It is, perhaps, not too strange that this should be so, since we spend the first nine months of life in a 'watery' environment, and it may be for this reason that, from time to time, we seek to return. Man has devised a number of ways of playing in this environment; some on the surface, some partly submerged and others deep below in the 'murky depths'.

Sailing in its various forms — either recreational or competitive — takes place in vessels varying in type from sailboards to transglobal racers. Whether racing or pursuing more leisurely activities in modest craft, the sport may none the less be hazardous. When craft are provided with engines which contrive to give greater speed, there is a correspondingly greater risk, not only to competitors, but perhaps to onlookers and officials involved in organisation of events.

Hazards

Annual statistics of water sports casualties provide a sad reminder that water is an inhospitable environment to man. The critical range of temperature that we must maintain and the fact that our respiratory apparatus is ill-equipped for aqueous survival remind us that we can only ever be visitors to this danger zone, and are always at the mercy of wind, tide and weather. Trauma, however minimal, occurring to sailors whilst afloat may present problems out of proportion to the degree of injury sustained.

The most effective way of bringing about a reduction in water sports-associated morbidity and mortality is through prevention. Education to prevent the taking of undue risks by the ill-prepared will undoubtedly reduce figures. However, if man wishes to try a dangerous sport because of the peculiar and particular thrill that can be derived from conquering the difficulties of that sport, risks will inevitably occur.

Drowning, or near drowning, would appear to be the greatest risk in water sports. It is not, however, necessary to travel out of sight of land for this risk to arise.

The Report of the Royal Life Saving Society for 1982 into drown-

300

Chapter 22
Medical hazards
of water sports —
and how to avoid
them

ings in the British Isles indicated that in that year there were a total of 516 drownings. These were predominantly males (389, that is, 75.4%) with 127 victims being female. The peak time of the year for drowning was found to be June and July, with monthly totals of 79 and 65 respectively.

Contributory factors were analysed and it was felt that, in 1982, drug abuse was not a significant factor in drownings, being reported in less than 1% of cases. However, alcohol was an important contributory factor, being found in 26% of cases. There appeared to be no apparent trend in the contribution of either mental or physical disability to drowning, apart from a sharp upturn in the 70+ age group, where disability through the enfeeblement of old age may become a contributory cause. As far as swimming ability is concerned, it is of interest that 94% of those who drowned playing near water and 66% of those who drowned *en route* by foot (where the swimming ability was known) could not swim. However, of those drowned whilst boating and where the victim's swimming ability was known, 81% *were* able to swim, which would tend to suggest that the old square-rigger sailors may have had a point in not bothering to learn to swim as it might not have significantly increased their chances of survival if they were to have fallen in.

Comparatively safe situations may become dangerous in relation to drowning if the would-be sailor has a pre-existing medical problem such as epilepsy. Water sports undertaken as a group activity can be quite safe for the epileptic; however *but*, sailing solo can prove fatal. It is important to remember that an important contributory factor in drowning is exposure to the cold. A fall in the body's core temperature can occur even when the sailor is not necessarily actually immersed in the water, for example, in a life-boat awaiting rescue following an accident. A sailor showing symptoms and signs of the onset of hypothermia may become initially talkative, perhaps slightly uncoordinated, and somewhat excitable. Judgement may become increasingly impaired and the victim may or may not complain of the cold, and be shivering. When the core temperature falls to 35°C, movements become slow, as does thought, and decision-making is impaired. When the core temperature reaches 32–30°C, the victim may become semiconscious and, at 28°C, unconscious. With further fall in core temperature, the heart begins to beat irregularly and cardiac arrest may occur. Sudden immersion in cold water can cause a marked increase in heart rate with characteristic electrocardiograph changes.

When protective clothing is worn, it is important to remember that as far as the body is concerned the climate to be considered is that between the skin of the wearer and the clothing worn, and *not* the climate outside the clothing. It is possible that, even on a cold day whilst sailing in a strong wind, when wearing an efficient neoprene wet suit or an all-enveloping dry suit, the sailor may actually suffer overheating and hyperthermia.

301
*Chapter 22
Medical hazards
of water sports —
and how to avoid
them*

Following capsize, a sailor may be thrown a short distance from his craft and may be unable to get back to it. The golden rule in sailing is that one should never desert one's craft, even a large cruiser, until it is about to sink. *Always*, when capsizing, the dinghy sailor or crew should hold on to the tiller or a rope that is part of the boat during the moment of capsize.

In yacht racing the racing rules state that the officer of the day may, if conditions dictate, hoist the appropriate flag to compel personal buoyancy equipment to be worn by all competitors. The racing rules also explicitly indicate that 'it is for the skipper of a given boat to decide whether to take part in a race, should he consider that he, or his crew, are either too inexperienced to cope with the conditions expected, or that his boat is not well enough equipped to cope with the inclement weather'. There are British Standards for buoyancy. Flotation aids are *not* the same as life-jackets. A couple of kilograms of extra personal buoyancy from a foam-filled orange jacket may be reassuring, but it is not as good as the many extra kilograms of buoyancy available from a properly constructed inflated jacket.

The personal safety equipment may extend beyond the need for flotation. A board sailor, sailing offshore, would be well advised to take a small personal type distress flare, some of which are not much larger that a bulky fountain-pen and are waterproof. They release either a red flare or coloured smoke. A Dayglo brightly coloured nylon flag, which is lightweight and can be wrapped into an extremely small package, may be carried on the person without inconvenience for display in an emergency. The wearing of a buoyancy jacket with harness attachment, which will, in any case, make long-distance board sailing more comfortable and not significantly less exciting, may become a necessity in strong wind and wild water.

Seasickness is not necessarily the province of the feeble and inexperienced. Many a well-known international sailor has been affected with this problem. The author has known an Olympic sailor who had no problem until his race was over, but immediately afterwards was affected with the most violent form of motion sickness. Tension perhaps has a part to play. Certainly, it is easier for those whose minds and bodies are occupied with coping with the difficult motion of a boat in rough seas, particularly if they are in a position of responsibility. Those who are merely sitting as passengers can concentrate fully upon their malady. It is not only competitors who are so affected. At a recent Olympic Regatta, the writer, on his Committee boat, found that over half of the race officials were seriously affected on a day in which the anchored boat

302

Chapter 22
Medical hazards
of water sports —
and how to avoid
them

was spiralling wildly on the waves whilst they tried to set a course for the competitors.

Medication helps. During the Olympic Games in 1972, the German Organising Committee had thought about 'doping' and doing the dope-testing, but no one thought that sailors might be affected by seasickness! Ciba-Geigy manufacture a patch, which may be applied behind the ear where there is an accessible piece of smooth skin, from which hyoscine is absorbed. This does prove effective if used sufficiently long before the voyage is commenced. The patch may be left in operation for three days. Care should be taken not to rub the eyes after touching the patch, since vision may be affected. Acupuncture has been tried, and a wrist band, working on the acupuncture principle, has been worn by some with good effect. Unfortunately, Ciba-Geigy patches are not on sale in the UK.

Trauma is a common occurrence owing to irregular motion through the water. One of the commonest injuries is that of the head being struck by the boom, which swings across when tacking the vessel, striking the unwary. Many logged instances of persons being knocked overboard unconscious and then drowning are due to having been hit on the head with the boom. Falls from a height, producing multiple injuries, including fractured skull, fractured cervical vertebrae and broken limbs, are surprisingly common injuries associated with sailing. In Nelson's time and even more recently in the time of the clipper ships, the man who fell overboard from the yard-arm stood no chance of survival. If a boat were not cast off immediately, and that was unlikely since they were frequently stacked in tiers on the deck and well lashed down, there was no possibility of the boat turning round and retracing its steps in anything like adequate time. Those who fell overboard were lost.

In modern sailing there are other mechanisms of injury which may occur in racing boats — ocean racers or cruiser racers in particular. The winch, which is a device for winding in ropes to adjust the trim of the sails, is a very powerful instrument. A hand or digit may become trapped in the winch by a rope coil which may have, perhaps, several thousand pounds of 'load' upon it. Sharp objects protruding from the deck or the hull, in the form of fittings, may cause lacerations or puncture wounds, and, indeed, in close-quarter manoeuvring in rough water and strong winds, collisions between boats are not uncommon. Damage in a collision may not be solely to the boats. Crew members have indeed been killed in such instances. The writer remembers an Admiral's Cup Race in Cowes week in which a sailor attempted to fend off another ocean racer. His arm was broken in the process. He was a non-swimmer and he was catapulted into the water 25 yards astern of his craft before his fellow crew members realised what had happened. In Olympic-class racing a crew member of a Soling-class three-man keel boat was struck in the back by another boat; he was paralysed from the waist

303

Chapter 22
Medical hazards
of water sports —
and how to avoid
them

down and subsequently died. The violence of a collision on the water is no less than that of a collision on the motorway. Our aim, therefore, should be to control the hazards by adequate design of boats themselves and of their rigging and fittings, and by enforcing the clear 'right of way' rules which are learned by competitors so that the risk of collision is reduced.[*]

In powerboating, precautionary checks are taken of the surface of the water before racing commences so that floating flotsam is removed. The nature of the course is surveyed to eliminate dangerous hazards before a race permit is granted. Considerable alterations were made to the course at Bristol docks for the powerboat racing during the 1987 season following a tragic accident to a competitor whose hydroplane had collided with the gas ferry jetty in 1986. It was subsequently decided that this structure should be removed. Other parts of the course considered dangerous from the spectators' point of view were provided with safety fencing, and full visibility of the course for race officers was provided by video camera surveillance.

The changes were recommended by a board of inquiry set up by the Royal Yachting Association, of which the honorary medical officer was a member. The board sat for two days investigating the 1986 fatality and all aspects of the Bristol Grand Prix. The costs of implementing changes were undertaken by Bristol City Council, who were most co-operative and also anxious to make the event safe and to preserve it in the racing calendar.

In the 1987 race, after these alterations had been made, there was, happily, no fatality,[†] but there was a competitor who had an accident in precisely the same spot where the dangerous jetty had stood 12 months earlier — happily, with no significant consequences. Clearly the RYA was correct in insisting on expensive course modifications. It is not, unfortunately, always possible to legislate for 'all risks', and in 1987, sadly, three offshore powerboat racers died when their craft capsized at speed, having crossed the wash of a large craft whilst racing close to the Isle of Wight.

Risks to those who are on the water for prolonged periods are not always physical. The solitary sailor may thrive in his personal one-to-one battle with the watery environment in his attempt to be the first man to sail around the world in one or other direction, or the first one to go around twice; or the one to do it in the smallest boat, or one of a number of particularly peculiar methods of gaining

---

[*] There is perhaps no more graphic and disastrous example of the hazards of collisions on water than the *Marchioness* Thames pleasure-boat sinking with the loss of 57 lives in August 1989.

[†] This is a further example of the way in which medical input into a governing body's responsible inquiry may help to identify and eliminate risks for sports men and women and spectators alike, to help promote safer enjoyment of the sport (see Chapter 3).

304

Chapter 22
Medical hazards
of water sports —
and how to avoid
them

entry to the *Guiness Book of Records* or the 'Hall of Fame' in sailing. A famous board sailor — a great breaker of records — disappeared and was never found whilst attempting to sail from mainland China to Taiwan. A competitor in the round-the-world single-handed race succumbed to mental stress and was reduced to sending false messages as he despairingly sailed around the Atlantic. His empty boat was found many months later.

The writer conducted a survey of members of the Royal Yachting Association to attempt to determine the commonest causes of sailing injuries. With a mailing of 40 000–50 000 copies of *RYA News* it was hoped that a significant response would be obtained to provide much valuable information. Unfortunately, a return of only 229 served to demonstrate that sailors may not be as deeply interested in sports medicine as are other athletes who in similar circumstances might have provided a more significant response. Amongst those who responded the most commonly found trauma was that to the back, followed by head injury and knee injury. Various lacerations and injuries to the neck, shoulder, elbow and ribs were also recorded in the survey. An interesting finding, however, was the age distribution of sailing injuries, which ranged from under 10 years to over 70 years. The commonest age group was in the range of 30–40 years.

Injuries to the head were all from direct trauma. Those from the back frequently related to either unreasonable demands on the body when hauling up anchors or pulling ropes, or, perhaps, to the singularly uncomfortable 'hiking' position adopted by sailors with knees and back bent when sailing dinghies, particularly when wearing the 'heavy' jacket, which is water-filled to increase the weight of the sailor so that he may better sail the boat upright in strong winds. Significant to sailing, however, may be the knee injury. The average competitive racing dinghy requires that the sailor hangs over the side in the so-called 'hiking' position. In order to see where he or she is going, it is necessary to flex the back and hips, and to maintain this position by what is almost a constant isometric exercise for the muscle groups concerned. Chrondroma-lacia patellae appears to be common in young dinghy sailors, producing anterior knee pain. Individuals suffering this condition may be treated by medial quadriceps isometric exercises with the knee held in extension. After about six weeks about half of those treated will be free of pain.

It is likely that this discomfort is occasioned by the fact that prolonged sailing with the knees bent in certain types of dinghy leads to a significant development of certain groups of muscles. Sports men and women often feel that when they are taking part in their particular sport they are exercising *all* the muscle groups that matter. This is not necessarily the case, and in many sports time has to be taken out of normal competitive routine in order to give a particular muscle group a chance to catch up with those other groups used during the sport itself. For better performance and top-level competition, the author advises sailors, be they dinghy sailors or board sailors, to do a brief warm-up routine shortly before the start of the race. Most, if not reminded, tend to remain physically inactive before the start, worrying about technique, wind and the tide direction, and sundry other problems, so that when the starting gun is fired their bodies are physically unprepared for the active part of the competition.

305
Chapter 22
Medical hazards
of water sports —
and how to avoid
them

Precautions

One might think that some of the hazards described above might deter all but the most hardy from taking part in water sports. This, however, is not the case, and water sports figure high on the nation's list of most popular recreational activities. What precautions can we take to minimise these hazards? Although competence in swimming would seem an obvious precaution to avoid drowning, it is worth remembering that the teaching of survival routines to maintain buoyancy can be of great assistance in saving life even for the non-swimmer.

Trapping air in clothing may help in the absence of all other precautions. Likewise the shipwrecked sailor may be saved by heeding advice to stay with the boat until it sinks, or by clutching floating wreckage. Life-jackets or buoyant neoprene suits should be standard equipment for all yachtsmen and yachtswomen. A sailing dinghy should always carry a paddle and bailer. A small plastic whistle costs a few pence, weights a few grams, can be easily worn around the neck and is very useful for calling for assistance, particularly in time of bad visibility, for example in the dark, in fog and in driving rain.

A wide range of sailing clothing is available nowadays to offer protection against the cold. The neoprene wet suit has recently been replaced to some extent by the dry suit. The original wet suits were made of neoprene foam of varying thickness. The thicker suits provided more protection against the cold, but were more expensive and perhaps slightly more restricting. These suits, worn by sub aqua divers and by dinghy sailors, absorb water which the body subsequently warms and which, having been warmed, provides a thermal barrier, thus reducing the rate of heat loss from the body. Inadequate clothing will lead to rapid heat loss in the event of capsize. When immersed in water, heat will be lost at a rate which may be up to 27 times greater than would be the case in air of the same temperature. This rate of loss may be further increased by movement — e.g. attempting to swim or to right the dinghy. Therefore, if the sailor is wearing an efficient life-jacket and is floating well with head above the water, it is better in cold condi-

306

Chapter 22
Medical hazards
of water sports —
and how to avoid
them

tions to avoid unnecessary movement in order to conserve heat whilst awaiting rescue.

The dry suit consists of a thin layer of waterproof material with elasticated collar and cuffs, sometimes having cuffs at the ankles and sometimes having integral feet. More recent suits are made in two parts which overlap a waterproof waistband. In the dry suit it is possible to wear thermal, garments underneath the suit which further retain the heat. So efficient are these suits that, when removed, the inner garments are often wringing wet from perspiration which has accumulated during physical activity.

Hands can become so cold that it is impossible to adequately carry out one's task of sailing the boat properly, and, for this reason, protective leather gloves made of the finest chromed chamois leather are often worn. These may have exposed fingertips to preserve a degree of fine touch/sensation whilst at the same time protecting the fingers and the hand. The gloves are manufactured with tough leather palms and tough surfaces on the flexor aspect of the fingers so that rigging and abrasive ropes may be handled without undue trauma to what would otherwise be waterlogged skin. The dorsum of the glove often has open mesh material to allow for ventilation, sometimes in winter, however, having a neoprene foam-type backing for warmth.

The RYA in the course of its programme of education for the sailing of dinghies, boards and sailing craft has, as part of the training programme, instruction on coping with emergencies that occur on the water. It is an essential part of such coaching that one learns how to right a sailing dinghy which has capsized, or to cope with problems on a sailing cruiser. It is a requirement for RYA-approved sailing schools that there be such instruction and that there be adequate rescue and training craft during periods of tuition. It is also necessary that the pupils are seen to be adequately clothed and are provided with appropriate life-jackets, and that there is an approved ratio of instructors/rescue craft to the particular number of pupils who may be coached at any one time. The premises of such schools are regularly inspected by the RYA to see that these standards are upheld. Indeed, if they are not adhered to, official recognition of a training school is withdrawn.

Part of the education process involves training in the understanding of the wind, weather and tides. Most sailors in distress are untrained and inexperienced. Money-saving 'progress' towards a reduction in the number of lighthouses and other hazard warnings which have been under the care of Trinity House presents a risk and may usher in an era in which a significant reduction in the numbers of warning lights will be seen around our coasts. This reduction in warning, together with the dependence on more modern navigational aids, such as satellite navigators, will place considerable numbers of sailors at greater risk. In past generations navigation entailed the use of the sextant and the compass, and the log. Although these may be less accurate methods of navigation than techniques which employ up-to-date technology, they are probably less likely to fail.

The general increase in leisure time that has occurred in recent years has produced a significant increase in the numbers of people afloat. An increased number of individuals therefore are putting themselves at risk. A more widespread knowledge of the wind, weather and tides will be required if a significant increase in the loss of these new sailors is to be avoided. The satellite navigator is a very useful invention, but the absence of sound knowledge of traditional methods of navigation leaves no fall-back position in the event of equipment failure.

The treatment of medical emergencies

The medical emergency afloat is in essence no different from the same medical emergency ashore. The problem with the medical emergency afloat arises through the logistical problems of either moving the casualty to the doctor or moving the doctor to the casualty. Two-way radios now being relatively inexpensive, the average cruising sailor or racing yachtsman who is in a boat larger than a dinghy will be able to call for professional advice in the case of significant illness or injury to crew members, and it would be advisable to include such equipment as standard.

The possession of an adequate first-aid kit on board is desirable. Various other accessories for use in an emergency should also be on board: a smaller foresail to use in a storm, a spare impeller for the engine's water pump, and a distress rocket to fire in an emergency. The first-aid box itself should be fitted with a secure handle so that it can be carried about the boat. An ideal type of box is that used by fishermen for their tackle, opening in layers with compartments. This item has the advantage of also being waterproof. An airway of the Guedel or Brooke type should be carried and crew should be instructed as to its use. A foil exposure blanket occupies little space and is available quite cheaply from most sports or camping shops. An unconscious person is at greater risk on a sailing boat. On the shore it is possible to place the patient in the recovery position and to position the head to protect the airway. On board a boat rolling over a stormy sea, sometimes on one tack, sometimes on another, the safe recovery position of one tack is the aspiration and asphyxiation position of the next. The patient should be directly in view and placed as close to the companionway steps as possible since this is the position of least motion on the boat. A constant watch should be kept by a spare member of the crew. Movement about the boat of those with limb or back injury should be kept to the minimum. Splinting should be done before movement, if possible, and transfer

308

*Chapter 22
Medical hazards
of water sports —
and how to avoid
them*

into a heaving motorboat alongside, or even into a helicopter, should only be undertaken if absolutely necessary.

In the case of resuscitation of those who have suffered exposure in the water, a rough rule of thumb is that, if they have lost heat very recently then rewarming may be carried out quickly. But if they have been hypothermic for a long time rewarming should be gradual and prolonged. If facilities at the clubhouse allow, then the sailor brought ashore suffering from hypothermia should be rewarmed in a bath whose optimal temperature would be 41°C. Immersion in the bath should include limbs. This treatment should not be carried out if rewarming is delayed for more than half an hour.

If at sea, the victim should be wrapped in warm towels below decks after the wet clothing has been removed, and it should be remembered that, in the absence of any form of heat, a warm colleague, by his or her own body warmth, will provide significant heat if lying adjacent to the hypothermic patient. Some warmth may be available from the engine if this is running and warming the surrounding air; towels may be warmed by the running of the engine and, only if the situation is safe enough, by lighting the galley stove. Alcohol and any other drugs which cause peripheral vasodilation should not be given, as these may lead to further loss of heat.

Medical certificates

For powerboat racing it is necessary that a medical certificate be presented to show that the competitor is fit to race. This should certify that the competitor is free from serious illness, such as diabetes or epilepsy, etc., that there is normal power of movement of the limbs and that vision is not defective.

It is recommended that a driver's medical certificate should be lodged with the medical officer at the start of an event, and that, in the event of an accident during the competition, the medical officer should *retain* this certificate and determine whether a later re-examination is necessary before a driver who had had an accident is allowed to return to competition.

Safety in high-speed powerboat racing may also be achieved by the granting of 'super licences' which can only be held by persons considered to have sufficient driving skill and experience to compete in such a regatta. Basic standards of construction of the boat are also scrutinised to ensure safety for participants. The design of the 'safety shell' and minimum weight requirement must exceed minimum standards to ensure safety at high speed and in heavy seas. The keeping of clinical records by the team medical officer is vital. Reference to these records may be required later. The fact that one carries out a consultation with head bent in the small cabin of an ocean racer whilst trying to examine an injured crew member may not make a very plausible excuse when later one is accused of having missed a fractured cervical spine or a significant head injury. It is the nature of most sports that a medical officer is probably an ex-competitor in that sport himself. The team doctor will probably also be made use of to perform other functions in assisting the coaches and competitors on the water and at the venue, and may be used largely for these duties with only a small time allowed in the day for the medical part of his or her briefing. It is unfortunately difficult in such circumstances to ensure that records are always adequate.

It should also be remembered that, when travelling abroad, the Medical Protection Society will provide legal advice and offers its members the opportunity to apply for medico-legal indemnity for incidents occurring in any country in the world other than the United States and Canada, and the territorial waters or airspace thereof.

The satisfaction derived from the sport comes from returning home with a successful team, being proud of their endeavours and feeling an essential part of that team. Essentially the profile of the team doctor is that of the old-fashioned family doctor. He or she has to be professionally correct and competent, and must be seen to be so in relations with professional colleagues. He or she must give due deference to senior team officials, yet not be afraid to make a point and to press that point if he or she feels it is being ignored to the detriment of a particular competitor (patient) or of the team as a whole. He or she must have the courage to carry out therapy which will assist the competitor to compete if ill or injured, but not to do so if he or she feels it is not in the competitor's interests to compete and thus harm himself/herself.

309

Chapter 22
Medical hazards
of water sports —
and how to avoid
them

23 Medical aspects of competitive rowing

P. L. THOMAS

'Row brothers, row, the stream runs fast
The rapids are near and the daylight's past'
Thomas Moore

International rowing races are held over a straight 2000 m six-lane course. Competitions are held both for men and for women; the men have eight separate events, ranging from single sculls to eight-oared boats. Some boats are steered by a cox and in others one of the rowers controls the rudder through lines attached to the shoes fixed in the boat.

In addition to the open or heavyweight events, there are light-weight events for both men and women. Lightweights, however, do not have their own events at the Olympic Games, but they do compete at the annual World Championships, which are held in a different country each year. The weight limit for lightweight men in 72.5 kg and the average weight for the crew must not exceed 70 kg. Lightweight women may weigh up to 59 kg and their average weight may not exceed 57 kg.

The sport of rowing involves considerable athleticism and re-serves of endurance. The men's eights will take approximately 5½ minutes to race over 2000 m. The same distance may take up to 8½ minutes for a woman in a single scull. Racing at the Olympic and World Championships takes place over a period of eight days with *repêchages* and semifinals in the middle of the week. No crew will race more than four times in any one event although a few oarsmen and oarswomen may double up in two different events.

In Great Britain there is now a well-established national squad system, and any rower wishing to compete internationally is re-quired to register his or her intention. As a result the vast majority of the athletes who eventually gain international selection will have trained with the squad for most of the year. The team eventually selected will probably consist of up to 80% of the previous year's national team.

Training

During the winter, training is done in the small boats such as single sculls and pair-oared boats, the training consisting mainly of long stretches of endurance work. However, perhaps 50% of the work will be done on dry land, during the dark mornings and evenings, on static rowing ergometers. Weight training is undertaken less and less these days and indeed some of our top oarsmen and oarswomen have not trained with weights for the past two years. It is not uncommon in international-standard rowing, particularly in an Olympic year, for rowers to commit themselves totally to training and to give up their jobs. They will train for up to 12 sessions a week in the winter, rising to three training sessions a day during the summer.

As a winter season closes the rowers will be combined into larger boats (fours and eights) and the provisional team selection will be made during a training camp, perhaps abroad, in warmer weather, over the middle of April. The racing season for 2000 m competition starts at the beginning of May. The team will compete at weekend international regattas approximately every two weeks up to the final selection regatta in the middle of July. The selected team will then train together at a training camp for two to three weeks before moving to the World or Olympic Regatta a week before the first race. The venue of the training camp will be dependent on the conditions likely to be met with at the championship; for example in 1988 the team had a three-week spell in South Korea before the Olympics in order to get over the time difference of nine hours from Great Britain and in order to acclimatise themselves to the heat.

Each crew will have their own coach who will travel with them to the championships. In addition a team manager and assistant team manager will work with the team for the whole year, organising boat transportation, flights and regatta entries. Although each coach is ultimately responsible for his or her own crew, the team manager may overrule the coach in the interests of the team as a whole.

Team doctors and physiotherapists

The medical support for the national squad consists of a doctor for the men's team, one for the women's team and another for the junior team. We have a team of six physiotherapists, who look after the squad in the winter and early summer, and one physiotherapist will be selected to act as the senior team physiotherapist and another as the junior team physiotherapist. In Olympic teams, when the lightweights have their own World Championship instead of the Olympics, a further physiotherapist will be assigned to look after them.

In 1988 the Olympic team trained all year long in and around London together with 80% of the lightweights. The rest of the lightweights trained in Nottingham but met up with the remainder of the team at regattas and at occasional training weekends. This polarisation of the squads makes it much easier to provide medical support, in contrast to other national teams such as athletics and swimming. Both doctors and physiotherapists will get to know the athletes very well throughout the whole year and will not be expected to treat athletes they have never met before. The author has been looking after the men's team for ten years but the newer members in the first year or two are initially reluctant to put their confidence in someone they have not met before. The newer members of the team are more reluctant to seek medical advice at an early stage of illness or injury. Perhaps they see the doctor and physiotherapist as people who may jeopardise their chances of selection by passing on unfavourable comments about their state of health. They need reassurance that the support team is there to assist them, and we try to emphasise to the younger athletes the importance of coming to us early so that conditions can be corrected or eased before the important races.

One way of making the rowers feel more at ease with the doctor and physiotherapist is for us to perform our screening examinations every year. Preventative medicine plays a major part in the team doctor's and physiotherapist's role. As with any other routine medical examination, the history will establish if an athlete has any ongoing problems or any significant previous illnesses or injuries which may recur. It is also important to determine whether or not they are taking any medication. It may be that a rower is using a drug prescribed by a doctor or bought over the counter. It is essential to know the complete medication of all the athletes, in order to avoid any preparation that may be banned by the sport's governing boards. The doping categories for rowing follow the classes laid down by the International Olympic Committee. It follows also, therefore, that the doctor must familiarise him or herself with the doping regulations and methods adopted for dope-testing. Only some of the drugs are banned during the training period, namely amphetamines, cocaine, anabolic steroids and other controlled drugs.

During racing, however, none of the International Olympic Committee's banned drugs are permitted even though they may have been prescribed by a doctor, perhaps the athlete's own GP or a consultant. The drugs liable to cause problems are beta-blockers, codeine, ephedrine and pseudoephedrine, together with oral and depot corticosteroids (sometimes prescribed for severe hayfever or asthma). It should be possible for a team doctor, if given enough notice, to advise the athlete to switch to another drug which is permitted by the sporting authorities. It may be necessary for the team doctor to communicate with the athlete's own GP.

The purpose of the medical examination is to detect any defects and note them for future reference, should something go wrong, and to measure the basic physiological parameters such as blood-pressure, peak expiratory flow, skinfold thickness, weight and resting pulse. The systolic pressure is often raised a little in rowers and their resting pulse is usually in the order of 40 to 46 beats per minute. The athletes are encouraged to check regularly their resting pulses as it is a good indication of prodromal illness, as is a sudden weight loss. The skinfold thicknesses when converted on a body fat conversion chart enable both the doctor and rower to monitor his or her progress if trying to make the lightweight category.

The heavyweight rowers are also trying to reduce their fat content in order to perform more effectively. The chances of anorexia, a problem in some runners, will be minimised by calibrating the skinfold thickness rather than merely relying on total body-weight. It is important to emphasise to the athletes that the medical examination is not a test to be passed or failed. The mere fact that they are able to perform at a high enough level to be considered for the national team is sufficient to indicate that their general well-being is satisfactory.

The team should be followed up as often as possible, usually about once per week and perhaps more often in the summer. Frequently no one presents with any problem but, by merely putting in an appearance, both the athletes and their team doctor can familiarise themselves with each other. It also gives the coaches an opportunity to talk over aspects of training. The doctor may be the best person to interpret new physiological ideas which have been put forward by the physiologists whom they meet and are tested by. We now have the benefit of regular physiological testing at the new British Olympic Medical Centre at Northwick Park Hospital in London.

Research and continued attention to techniques can result in some useful preventative measures to the benefit of the individual rower and the team. Together with the physiotherapists we have been able to reduce the number and severity of knee injuries in the national team by recommending modifications to land training and the correction of techniques within the boats. The coaches may well pay more attention to the advice given by a doctor who has regularly been attached to the team than to one who appears only infrequently at major championships. They will also usually accept our advice when we advise an athlete to stop training for a specified time when an injury or illness occurs. Likewise the medical team become more competent in treating the injuries which arise. Regular follow-up also gives the doctor and physiotherapist an opportunity to get to know each other and to work as a team when dealing with a crisis, should it arise.

The medical support team receives no remuneration for the work that is involved but recently the Amateur Rowing Association have been able to pay some of the locum expenses incurred whilst we have been away with the team when it has been necessary to employ someone to do our normal work at home. They will also pay reasonable travel costs and will not expect us to pay for the flights and accommodation when accompanying the team at training weekends, training camps or championships. Needless to say, at the end of the season we are out of pocket but the rewards are greater than any financial return and rowing still remains an amateur sport.

The team doctor in Rugby Union football 24

K. W. KENNEDY

'A ruffians sport played by gentlemen'
Anon

Doctors who are considering providing services in the context of rugby football ideally should have a sound knowledge of traumatology and the kinesiology of the sport. Most importantly the doctor should have an affinity for the game and the people in it. It is helpful also if the doctor has good contacts within the profession in order to facilitate referral in cases where this is appropriate. Experience in rehabilitatory medicine or orthopaedics is invaluable and the ability to liaise concisely with physiotherapists is nowadays most important, so as to ensure the safe return of the player to his sport as quickly as possible. In rugby football the duties of a team doctor are mixed. On match days prior to the game the doctor will have liaised with the coach and manager to ensure that players are aware of, and ideally should have taken, an optimal pre-match diet. In the dressing-room the doctor will be expected to assist with strapping of joints where necessary. Often players will ask for a pain-killing injection prior to playing. This practice is to be avoided. Moreover, the request should not arise if the selectors and coach have agreed beforehand that an injured player should be rested until he is fully recovered. During the game, the doctor, although metaphorically 'in the background', should actually be in the forefront of availability, ready to help with any injury that occurs. The doctor should actually therefore be available somewhere near the touch-line, and not in the back of the grandstand or, worse still, in the committee bar!

The responsibility of the team doctor

The principles of preventive medicine should be high on the list of priorities when a team doctor is considering the list of his duties.

At the start of a season both the coach and the doctor must advise the players on many topics.

Training

Training involves consideration of the total musculoskeletal system and includes:
1 Mobility and flexibility training.
2 Breathing controls.

315

3   Muscle training and building.
4   Co-ordination improvement.
5   Game skill techniques.

Kit

The pressures of commercialism cause some manufacturers of sports goods to pay a lot of attention to their logos and brand names and less to the quality of their product. Boots and track shoes are probably the most important item of equipment and should be carefully chosen. The current vogue for cutaway boots does much to increase the profit of the manufacturer (who uses less leather), but does little to protect the ankles of the players, thus increasing the possibility of ligament injury and long-term 'footballer's ankle', a type of degenerative joint disease.

Rugby players are notorious for failing to wash their training kit. This can lead to serious skin infections, interfering with the individual's availability for both work and competition.

Although initially viewed with suspicion, protective kit is now accepted by players and nowadays no player should neglect to wear appropriate protective wear. The gum-shield should be worn by all players who still possess teeth (see Chapter 13). Modified shoulder padding should be used by those players who have had recent or recurrent shoulder injuries. All forwards, and especially front-row players, should be encouraged to wear shin pads to prevent the common stud injuries to the slow-healing skin on the anterior aspect of the tibia. Protective knee and elbow braces are available but these should only be used after specialist opinion has been sought.

Diet and rest

Advice should be given to players on the need for proper sleep in the days before a major game. Changing the diet of the players is more difficult. It is advisable to eat sensibly before a big game but this must be coupled with timing of training. It is well known that a decreased glycogen storage and low blood-sugar levels impair the physical and mental performances of players and also increase their injury risk factor. Physiologically it takes about 36–48 hours to build up the glycogen stores by taking a diet high in carbohydrate content. Thus it is obvious that no hard training sessions should be held within 48 hours of a game or else the stores will be burnt up and none remain for the game. This often has been a reason for the lack-lustre performances of certain teams in the past. They have left their energy on the training ground due to poor management and have little to give in the big match.

Psychology

Sport is littered with psychosomatic cripples and rugby is no exception. The team doctor must play a firm and sympathetic role in preparing the player for the sport. The sportsman produces his best when top physical condition gels with the ideal psychological approach. The ability of a player to concentrate under extreme conditions is essential in sport. Too much or too little mental tension adversely affects concentration. In future seasons the doctor may be expected to help the player with this, and techniques such as biofeedback and meditation have been used with great success in golf and tennis.

Treatment of injuries

Effective sports medicine offers the injured player early assessment and prompt treatment. It is necessary to start evaluating the problem from the moment of the injury. If the accident is witnessed by the doctor who has a knowledge of the kinesiology of rugby, then establishing the diagnosis is made simpler. It is vital that after the injury the patient is not made worse by some well-intentioned but untrained person. It is all too easy for a simple fracture to be turned into a compound one, or for a fractured cervical vertebra without neurological problems to be converted by bad management into a neurological disaster. At all sports grounds where vigorous bodily contact sport takes place, suitable personnel and equipment should be available. These should include:

1 Trained personnel on duty, including doctor/physiotherapist.
2 Spinal stretcher and blankets.
3 Working telephone and list of emergency numbers.
4 Ice-packs.
5 First-aid kit, which should include:
(a) Brooke airway;
(b) tongue depressor;
(c) suture kit;
(d) slings;
(e) splints;
(f) disinfectant;
(g) bandages and cotton wool;
(h) analgesics;
(i) disposable gloves.
In 1981 a survey was done of Rugby clubs in Surrey and it was found that very few possessed these minimum requirements.[*]

---

[*] The responsibility for providing these items of equipment rests with the governing body of the home club. It would be prudent, however, for the team doctor to bring to the attention of the committee any perceived inadequacy in the first-aid equipment.

When assessing an injured player it is helpful for the doctor to have some guidelines to assist in making the decision as to whether he should leave the field of play. It is important that all concerned — coach, captain and player — know that the doctor is making the decision to safeguard both the player and his team-mates. Sometimes players unwisely stay on the pitch following injury and in so doing put themselves and others at further risk. The following injuries should be viewed as absolute indications to retire from the field of play:

1 Major laceration.
2 Severe muscle or tendon tear.
3 Dislocation of a major joint.
4 Head injury.
5 Spinal injury.

Major laceration

If a wound is deep, and especially if vital structures such as arteries or nerves are exposed, or if joints are involved, then, even if the function of the part is normal, the player should be advised to leave the pitch. Routine cleansing, antibiotics and antitetanus treatment should be effected as well as suturing the wound, although it is likely that a wound of such severity would require formal exploration and debridement under regional or general anaesthetic, to check the integrity of vital structures and to ensure complete removal of all foreign material. Under normal circumstances this of course means referral to hospital.

Muscle or tendon injury

If the tear is sufficient to limit function, then the player is at risk of further damage. If the muscle injury is associated with haematoma, then prompt initial treatment with compression and elevation of the injured part is likely to prevent troublesome sequelae. Unfortunately, as it is the lower limbs that are commonly injured in rugby football, this form of therapy makes it necessary for the injured player to adopt a recumbent position with leg elevated above the level of the head. Too frequently, social pressures cause such players to abandon therapeutic measures after cursory treatment and they are often to be found standing in the club bar with their team-mates after the game. The resultant oedema, however, will significantly lengthen recovery time.

Dislocation

Major joint dislocation normally gives extreme pain and loss of function and the player usually has no wish to continue. Dislocation of the interphalyngeal joints can often be reduced by experienced personnel and the player allowed to continue, though neighbour strapping and a follow-up X-ray are essential. Major dislocations, especially when complicated by fracture, should be referred immediately to hospital for treatment. Shoulder dislocation can be reduced immediately if a significant delay in hospital attention would otherwise occur; care, however, should be taken to assess the patient for fracture of the humerus, which may cause damage to the axillary nerve as a complication of the dislocation. In cases of doubt, treatment should be delayed until X-ray examination has taken place.

Fracture

The signs of fracture are: *Pain*

1 Deformity.
2 Abnormal mobility.
3 Crepitus heard and felt.
4 Local bone tenderness.
5 Loss of function.

In all cases of fracture the patient should be kept warm and moved as little as possible. The fracture should be splinted if possible before referring to the local hospital.

Head injuries

Any player who has had a loss of consciousness during play must take no further part in the game. This applies also to anyone who has suffered concussion. Concussion is a syndrome in which there is immediate impairment of neural function following a blow to the head. The player with the glazed look and rubbery legs is a danger to himself and others. Speed of reflex actions will become markedly reduced and he becomes prey to the 'sucker punch'.

In boxing now there is a statutory period of four weeks' enforced inactivity after a knock-out, and the same could be considered reasonable for all sports. Prior to playing again after head injury, the player should have a complete medical check-up.

Spinal injury

Amongst the most serious injuries in sport are the fracture, fracture–dislocation and dislocation of the cervical spine. These conditions are surgical emergencies and the risk of paraplegia is high if management is incorrect.

Horse-riding, rugby, rock-climbing and judo are the sports in which neck injuries are common. When faced with the problem of the player who falls awkwardly and stays down immobile, the doctor, the trainer and indeed anyone on the field of play should be aware of the physical signs which indicate serious injury to the cervical spine:

1 Loss of function in the limbs.
2 Deformity of the neck.
3 Unconsciousness.
4 Complaint of parasthesia in limb(s).

In the presence of these findings extreme care must be taken. An incomplete cord lesion can be converted into a complete one by improper handling.

Initial treatment

The first task is to ensure that the airway is patent and that normal breathing is occurring. The mouth must be examined immediately to remove the mouth-guards, chewing-gum and other foreign bodies such as broken teeth, and to ensure that the tongue is not obstructing the airway. These emergency measures having been taken, the injured player should not be moved until someone trained in moving a suspected cervical spine injury case is present. The patient should be kept warm by covering with blankets or coats.

Intermediate treatment

The patient should be transferred on to a special spinal stretcher. It is essential that the transfer of the patient from the ground to the stretcher is properly supervised, the aim being to support adequately the patient's neck. Three helpers on each side help lift the patient on to the stretcher, working in unison under the command of the trained person. Once the patient's condition has been stabilised, he should be transferred to a hospital for investigation and treatment.

Other injuries requiring hospital treatment

Trauma to the eye, genitals or serious intra-abdominal injury usually produce a shocked patient who should be treated for the shock along standard lines and referred to hospital as appropriate.

High-risk situations

When an analysis is made of the mechanism of Rugby injuries, certain factors stand out.

General

1 Mismatch (see p. 25). When opponents are roughly the same size and strength for their position, they are usually able to cope with the stresses of the game. When this is not the case, such as in schoolboys versus adults rugby matches, then the risks increase. This is especially pertinent to school rugby, where children should be matched by size and not age.

2 Incorrect equipment. No player should be allowed to take the field or to participate in opposed training in incorrect or inadequate kit, e.g. a forward using track shoes in a scrum instead of boots is 50% more at risk.

3 Unfit or inexperienced. Not infrequently a veteran, who may be unfit, is asked at the last minute to play or practise against strong opposition. Once, on an Irish tour in Australia an assistant manager, who was a past international forward, packed down in the front row without boots against the test side to illustrate a point. He emerged from the top of the scrum with two broken ribs — a sorry sight and a very chastened man.

4 Horseplay or foul tactics. There are still, unfortunately, individuals playing rugby who appear to derive pleasure from injuring their opponents. It is the duty of club members and selection committees to weed these people out as they have no place in the game.

Specific

1 Mistackle. Probably one of the commonest causes of serious injury. Serious neck injuries can occur if the tackler's head collides with the opponent's hips or thigh. This usually occurs when the tackler closes his eyes and/or does not position his head correctly to the side or behind the thigh of the oncoming opponent. The best prevention of this type of injury is thorough coaching and practice of correct technique.

2 Short-arm tackle. This occurs when the opponent changes direction at the last minute and goes inside the tackler, who throws up his extended arm, usually hitting the opponent across the throat or face, causing a whiplash type injury to the neck. The short-arm tackle is illegal within the laws of the game.

3 The pile-up. This describes a situation where a loose scrum evolves as forwards dive into it to win the ball. Those at the bottom may be injured by the force of the in-charging players. The rules regarding this have been recently improved and referees are recommended to stop play early if a collapsed scrum situation develops either in loose play or from a set piece.

4 The set scrum. Serious neck injuries can occur in association with the set scrummage. The front-row players are primarily at risk. In the set scrum the danger times are:

(a) impact. When the scrums pack down and the front rows collide shoulder-to-shoulder. Faulty timing of one player may cause his head to collide against his opponent's head or shoulder with obvious risk of injury;

(b) collapsing scrum. When the scrum has settled after the impact of the two sets of forwards, it may collapse unintentionally or be collapsed deliberately. There are many ways a scrum can be made to collapse which are not in this brief. The most obvious is the prop forward pulling down his opponent. With experienced players this is not usually dangerous as most competent front-row players have practised how to fall. It is usually when there is a mismatch in physique or experience between opposing front rows that injuries occur. The most dangerous part of a collapse situation occurs when the second and back rows continue to push whilst the heads and necks of the front-row players are trapped against the ground. This can be prevented by the education of players and the prompt whistle of the referee;

(c) aerial scrum. This is one of the most frightening and dangerous experiences for front-row players. It may happen when an entire front row is lifted off the ground by the superior technique of their opposition, whilst their own second row continue to push. The trapped players risk severe damage to their cervicothoracic spine, and any forward who has been in this situation speaks of his helplessness and fear. It is also the situation where 'sprung ribs' or fractures at the costochondral junction may occur.

Methods of reducing risks of injury

1 Players:
(a) must be fit;
(b) always wear correct equipment;
(c) do not play out of position;
(d) do not indulge in horseplay or foul play.
2 The coach:
(a) does not select unfit players;
(b) ensures that the skills of the game are learned and practised; this includes tackling, falling and scrummaging.
3 The referee.
(a) When a set scrum collapses, stop the play at once.
(b) If a loose scrum becomes a fight or collapses, stop the play at once.
(c) Repeat use of illegal techniques such as the short-arm tackle should be punished severely: sending off, followed by club disciplinary action.*
4 Administrators have a duty to keep the laws of the game under constant review with a view to improving safety for players and taking into account the evidence available from relevant research (see also Chapter 3).

---

* Intentional collapse of the scrum is of course illegal within the laws of the game. The difficulty for the referee arises in deciding which of the front rows was responsible for causing the collapse. The intricacies and tactics of front-row play are beyond the scope of this text. It seems clear, however, that the extremely serious form of injury resulting from this can be prevented most effectively by prompt action by the referee.

Conclusions

It is important that the doctor who undertakes the task of the team medical officer in rugby football should understand, enjoy and respect the sport which he or she serves. Likewise he or she should command the respect of the players and administrators whom he or she advises, so that unwelcome counsel is not ignored when it matters — e.g. advice to leave the pitch following injury. As long as Rugby Union remains amateur, the status of the club doctor will probably be honorary. He or she, like the coach, gives his or her time freely without tangible reward. The team doctor has an important role in rugby which can be enormously rewarding.

Recommendations

1 In England a restructuring of the game has seen the emergence of four divisional teams. It is suggested that centres of medical excellence should be set up for each of these where:
(a) injured players can be referred by club doctors and GPs to be seen by sports medicine specialists appointed by the Rugby Unions;
(b) a regular teaching commitment should be undertaken for team doctors, physiotherapists and first-aiders, etc.
2 The Rugby Football Union and other international unions give due attention to the issue of safety. It is suggested that, in addition to ongoing attention to the rules of the game, prescriptive requirements are made with respect to the adequacy and provision of first-aid personnel and equipment at the grounds of affiliated clubs.
3 It is suggested that any player who has received a serious injury (one that has necessitated him leaving the pitch) may only restart playing after he has had medical clearance to do so. The system employed in France could be adopted. Here all players of recognised clubs are issued with a 'licence' card. These record the personal disciplinary and injury record of each player. At the end of each season they are collected centrally for analysis and contribute greatly to a better understanding of the patterns of injury occurring within the game.
4 It is recommended that all players should be encouraged to take out adequate personal injury and disability insurance. In the UK affiliated clubs of the RFU may take advantage of corporate and individual policies offered.

25

The team doctor in international rugby

JOHN DAVIES

'A gentleman's sport played by ruffians'
Anon

As in all aspects of the profession, a doctor's prime function is advisory and nowhere is this more paramount than in the role of a medical officer to a national body, such as the Welsh Rugby Union. Besides advising on dope-testing, the role of the team doctor encompasses advice on vaccinations, medication and the general primary medical care of the squad.

The role of the team doctor

The medical needs of players in the national squad, whether at training sessions, at international weekends or on tour, are the responsibility of the team doctor. It is important to gain the players' confidence. The easiest way to do this is to involve oneself totally with the team's preparations, e.g. working closely with and assisting the physiotherapist in strapping techniques, and perhaps supervising the warm-up and pre-activity stretching exercises at training sessions. Familiarity, some people say, breeds contempt, but for rugby players, each with their own idiosyncrasies and superstitions, it is essential for them to have complete confidence in their team doctor, especially when playing conditions are adverse.

A prop forward, waking up on the morning of an international with a slightly wry neck following the previous day's scrummaging practice, or a wing threequarter, still troubled with a slight hamstring pull, must have the confidence to approach the doctor. In the case of the former, the author remembers a case where no approach was made to the doctor concerned and, as a result, the Wales scrummage had their worst performance in recent years. The prop eventually went off with cervical spasm, and Wales lost the match! As in any doctor/patient relationship, if there is a case for treatment, whether it be an infected ear, a swollen proximal-interphalangeal finger joint, a blister or just ligament or muscle problems, treatment must be instigated as early as possible. Drugs such as antibiotics or anti-inflammatory agents are occasionally supplied to players, or alternatively they may be advised after a training session, when indicated, to obtain a prescription or seek advice from their own general practitioners. Where physiotherapy is required, the patient's team physiotherapist will liaise with the physiotherapist of the player's own club.

During international matches, injuries do occur and players are occasionally substituted. One of the greatest concerns for the medical officer officiating in any collision/physical contact sport such as rugby is the occurrence of a serious spinal injury. The scoop stretcher has been designed with the spinal injury in mind and in order to produce the least possible chance of spinal damage. The ground staff should be trained to move a patient with suspected spinal injury: the player should be transferred to the stretcher by three on either side with the head being held in traction. At Wales National Stadium during international matches an ambulance is on standby, and there is a direct line available to the Cardiff Royal Infirmary for immediate admission if required. Other international rugby stadiums have similar equipment and emergency procedures available.

The team doctor must work very closely with the national team coach and his assistant, and also should liaise closely with the selectors, and must gain the confidence and respect of both parties. In the match situation the doctor can sometimes be of assistance to the coach and selectors by identifying subclinical injuries in players which may be apparent on close observation of their performance, e.g. a player favouring one leg. For each international, the doctor has to confirm that a player of his or her side is unable to continue the game, or that it would be inadvisable on medical grounds for that player to continue, before a substitution is allowed. Speed is of the essence in this situation, and occasionally before a player is substituted it has been known for the team doctor to advise the coach that a certain player has a problem, in order that the replacement can be adequately warmed up before going on to the pitch.

The laws of the game now state that treatment can be continued on the pitch whilst the game is in progress and this has certainly helped reduce the time for stoppages due to minor injuries. The team doctor is not allowed on to the pitch unless specifically signalled for by the referee. This may occur following a request by the trainer/physiotherapist who is already on the field, or the referee may make the decision himself if the injury obviously warrants a doctor's immediate attention.

The laws of the game at present state that no more than two players in each team may be replaced and a player who has been replaced may not resume playing in the match. In international matches, a player may be replaced only when, in the opinion of a medical practitioner, the player is so injured that he should not continue playing in the match.

If a referee is advised by a doctor or other medically trained person or if he for any other reason considers that a player is so injured that it would be harmful for him to continue playing, the referee shall require the player to leave the playing area.

The author recalls an incident in which a district club side which he was coaching was due to start a match against strong West Wales opposition without the benefit of their outside half, who had failed to turn up. The author was recruited to the team, but shortly after taking the field the missing player appeared on the touchline, having been delayed in traffic and hastily changed in his car on arrival. The delayed player signalled his wish to join the game but the author, although relieved, realised that such a substitution could not be automatic. A convenient minor injury occurred soon after this, and at the resulting stoppage in play the author declared himself unfit to continue. The referee, quite rightly at the time, informed the trainer and the author that no replacement would be allowed. The author duly informed the referee, to his total bewilderment and confusion, that he was a doctor, and limped off. The fly half ran on, but the matter did not end there. Two of the opponents' committee were unhappy and the author was followed to the changing-room. It was only the sight of a patellectomy scar which the author had fortunately acquired several years previously that appeased them, although not without a great deal of muttering and disbelief.

The law has subsequently been amended such that an injured player may be replaced:
1   at the advice of a medically trained person, or
2   if a medically trained person is not present, with the approval of the referee.

As physician to the Welsh Rugby Union one's advice is sometimes sought on medical and medico-legal matters.

The medical advisory capacity also includes lecturing to coaching conferences at a national level on medical matters such as conditioning, diet, body composition, effects of training and also injuries and their treatment. The WRU has nine districts, comprising in total 200 clubs, and in recent years each district has received lectures (with representatives from each club in attendance) on the necessity for and organisation of medical cover and the treatment of rugby injuries.

In the weeks preceding overseas tours, advice is usually also sought on the need for vaccinations if indicated. Together with the tour physiotherapist, lists of essentials are made bearing in mind the countries to be visited.

Psychological pressure at international level

Psychological pressures on players associated with an approaching rugby international are intense (and more so when playing in Wales). There is no escape from the media, well-meaning friends, ticket-seekers and critics. This overwhelming exposure must and does have an effect on the participants, in particular on newcomers to the international arena.

The Welsh team, replacements, coach, selectors and team doctor meet the day before a home international and stay overnight, all the training and technical work-outs having been completed. If any last-minute medical problems arise, they are dealt with and the evening is spent relaxing, usually watching a film on video. The players retire around 11 p.m. Over the years very few players have asked for hypnotics to help them sleep and, on the rare occasions that it was necessary, they have been given a shortacting benzodiazepine such as temazepam. This is very efficient and has little or no hangover effect so that the players feel fine the next morning. The players take a late breakfast between 10 a.m. and 11.30 a.m. and are allowed to take whatever they want or feel comfortable with. Most tend not to eat a great deal, preferring cereal, but it does differ widely. Some, usually prop forwards, have a voracious appetite, irrespective of the time of day or night.

Around 12.30 p.m. a team talk begins, with the coach going over a few last-minute details dealing with the game plan. Then it is time to assemble on the team coach to take us to the national stadium. Over the years it is our experience that the journey to the stadium produces the first significant increase in ~~adrenaline flow~~. *or excitement.* This continues until well after the match is over.

The team arrive at the dressing-rooms and make their own preparations for the game, aided by the physiotherapist and the team doctor in attendance. It is at this point that one becomes aware occasionally of the psychological pressures that may prey on individual players. Team motivation (particularly in a physical contact sport such as rugby) may be undertaken to its greatest effect at this particular moment. (I have taken my own pulse on several occasions whilst in the players dressing-room and ten minutes before the kick-off it has always been over 120 beats per minute — and I was not even playing!) The players, needless to say, are at a peak of arousal for psychological motivation. Some captains and coaches are tremendous motivators with their team talks. Whatever the approach, the players are very susceptible at this moment ~~in time~~ and those with motivational problems or perhaps excessive competitiveness can, on rare occasions, channel this into excessive aggression. This has led to ugly scenes in the first few minutes of a game on some occasions over the years.

The newcomer to the international scene, very often, is susceptible to an anxiety state which can impair performance. This is where communication through a personal introduction to the players in a sympathetic and welcoming tone can prove very beneficial in helping to put the newcomer at ease. Many players chosen to play for their country are found wanting at their début. It is often debatable whether they are physiologically and psychologically capable of moving into the 'overdrive' gear that separates the very good club player from the international. Physiologically they may or may not possess the additional qualities required at international level. Psychologically, if they are too anxious, then their output of energy may be misdirected, causing them to perform below their best.

Violence, foul play and the laws of the game

In considering psychological pressure at international level, the overspill effect of motivation in the extreme situation of the international stage has been discussed. Unfortunately, these social symptoms are manifest in a more florid form in certain types of personality. In physical contact team games they may move from team to team, usually because of their antisocial behaviour both on and off the field of play. Mercifully the game itself usually tends to weed these players out, and it is made known to them that they are unwelcome. The real danger lies in the psychopathic coach who will condone and even encourage such players, and will nurture unfair tactics and techniques involving intimidation of the opposition. This may result in aggressive and antisocial behaviour in the team as a whole. Thankfully this has not been the author's experience at international level. The persistent offender is normally penalised out of the game and punished accordingly. In 1978 a rugby injury survey published in the *British Medical Journal* (Davies & Gibson 1978) highlighted the incidence of Rugby injuries as a direct result of foul play. This was produced by personal interviewing of injured players partaking in the survey by the author. Almost 30% of the injuries were attributable to foul play, but the significant factor was that only a quarter of the injuries attributable to foul play were penalised by the referee. Some time following its publication, the four home unions introduced a new law whereby, at senior and international level, linesmen were allowed to adjudicate and bring to the attention of the referee any misdemeanour which the referee obviously had not seen.

This is perhaps a very good example of the way in which the medical profession may, through a scientifically performed survey, isolate risk factors in a sport and persuade the sports governing body to implement fundamental changes in the laws of the game to improve safety.

Since the 1970s several injury surveys in Rugby Union football have been undertaken, looking at injury trends in the game and in particular the incidence of serious cervical spine injuries. In January 1988 a paper in the *British Medical Journal* entitled 'The need to make Rugby safer' by Burry & Calcinoi from New Zealand showed that cervical cord damage is a known hazard of rugby, and that changes in the rules of the game have been accompanied by a dramatic fall in the number of such injuries in New Zealand. This paper met with much support but also a good deal of criticism.

There is no doubt, however, that the medical profession can contribute very considerably in assisting the organisers and administrators of the game of rugby football to make it safer and more pleasurable to play. Burry & Calcinoi state in their paper that a decision was made in April 1987 by an Australian court to award more than A $2 million damages to a youth who became tetraplegic after an injury sustained in a Rugby League scrum collapse. The judge castigated the State Government for failing to make known to the player and his coach the fact that players with long necks were much more vulnerable to cervical injury and should not be allowed to play in the front row of the scrum. Since the administration were known to be aware of this view, they were found to be negligent in not disseminating warnings.

Burry & Calcinoi conclude their paper by stating that a recent comprehensive study of cervical spinal cord injuries in various football codes in Australia found that in Rugby Union most injuries occurred in the 'collision phase' of scrum formation (Taylor & Collican 1987). As this danger can be eliminated be requiring the opposing front rows to engage and stablise themselves before the remainder of the players take up their positions, legal action could be taken against the administrators of Rugby Union by any player who damages his cervical spine during the formation or collision phase of a scrum. Failing to alter the rules of a game, despite the knowledge that existing practices were hazardous and that a safe alternative existed, could well be held by a court to constitute culpable negligence. The gauntlet has been taken up by the United States Rugby Football Union who in May 1988 held an International Injuries Conference in Boston, organised by the United States Rugby Football Union Foundation, a charitable trust. Speakers from as far afield as Wales, New Zealand, Canada, Japan and developing nations discussed injury problems. The main theme, however, which emanated from the conference was the very serious dilemma in which the USRFU could find themselves if they were held liable in a similar situation to that which had happened in Australia. Rugby Union is not played in schools in the USA, but is only taken up at the age of 18 or 19, on leaving high school. Previous playing experience for the vast majority is in American gridiron football, and players are therefore at risk when they encounter different tackling techniques, and especially through late introduction to scrummaging. With over 250000 players participating every weekend across America, the game is rising in popularity, but is in grave danger of being sued out of existence if every effort is not made to ensure that adequate safety factors are both acknowledged and implemented. The role of the doctor here is to promote information through research.

Random dope tests are held following each five-nations international rugby game and to date there have been no positive results.

Being an amateur sport, Rugby Union football players are perhaps far less likely to expose themselves to the risks of drug-taking than are their counterparts in the professional code of gridiron football, where in the USA cases of cocaine and marijuana abuse have been widespread.

Conclusions and recommendations

In concluding this chapter on the role of the team doctor in international rugby, the author hopes that most of the issues related, both in anecdotal terms and on the subject of scientific research, convey the fulfilment that can be obtained from this privileged post. It is obviously necessary to have a profound knowledge of the game to fully achieve the greatest satisfaction from what at times can be an exhausting but nevertheless enjoyable position.

The post demands the commitment of long hours throughout the season, attending squad training sessions in the worst of British winter. The returns, however, are great; the camaraderie of rugby folk results in many good and lasting friendships throughout the world with like-minded individuals who enjoy this, probably the best of all amateur team sports.

In considering recommendations, I have touched not only upon the drugs question, but also on the laws of the game, and how these have been altered and may be further amended to avoid or at least reduce serious injuries.

To avoid major litigation which could seriously harm the game internationally, the International Rugby Football Board should be kept appraised of developments, conferences and medical research that seek to identify the risks in order that hazards may be nullified. It is within the power of the governing body of the sport, by so doing, to make the game safer and more enjoyable for all.

References

Burry & Calcinoi (1988) The need to make Rugby safer. *British Medical Journal*
Davies & Gibson (1978) Rugby injuries survey. *British Medical Journal*
Taylor T. K. F. & Collican M. R. J. (1987) Spinal cord injuries in Australian footballers 1960–85. *Medical Journal of Australia* **147**, 112–8.

Association Football: the team doctor 26

J. CRANE

'All are fellows at football — on the playing field all are in equality'
Sixteenth century proverb

In the Football League, since 1981 it has been recognised that it is the responsibility of the home club to ensure that a qualified medical practitioner is in attendance throughout the match. Most clubs have been covered in this manner for many years. Dr Vernon Edwards at Watford, Dr Brian Curtin at Tottenham Hotspur and Dr Reid at Liverpool are all general practitioners who have been attending their clubs in excess of 25 years. The author has attended Arsenal for 17 years and, between us, Dr Leonard Sash and I have covered all games, i.e. first team, combination sides, youth teams and of course all cup matches. There is no formal contract of work between the clubs and their respective medical attendants and such club doctors are employed essentially in an honorary appointment. The club will, however, usually cover expenses and the doctor is often invited to accompany the team at the end-of-season tour, which may travel to any of the football-playing countries in the world, including Australia, Hong Kong and even America.

The role of team doctor has many facets. It is no longer appropriate for the sum total of the doctor's armoury and expertise to be restricted to use of 'the magic sponge'. A collection of medical and paramedical experts comprise the 'medical team' that provide advice and treatment to professionals of the present-day Football League. A doctor will supervise this medical team and may be an individual with training or an interest in orthopaedic or physical medicine. Most are general practitioners with an interest in sports medicine. It is also of practical importance that the medical officer should possess the capacity to mix well with all other dressing-room staff. As the GP gets to know his or her families in the general practice so he or she must get to know all the players in the squad — their problems, if any, and their likes and dislikes, especially about food. Minor anxieties such as 'team selection' and being on the substitutes bench should be discussed. Players being away from their families during a tour may also lead to reduced performance. The chronically injured player, who may have been out of the first team for anything up to three months, may need special attention.

For the team doctor the most important ally at the club is the trainer, who will be a physiotherapist permanently attached to the club and the man who organises the whole medical room. The trainer is with the players permanently and will also organise the regular weekly clinics. A list of injured players will attend and the trainer advises the doctor before the start of the clinic of his working diagnosis and prognosis. At the clinics all injuries are reassessed. Is progress normal for the injury? Have we made the right diagnosis? Do we need a second opinion? Most players like to know how long they are likely to be out of training. It is important that we can give them some idea. The manager will want to know so that he can change training schemes with a view to late team selection. Most joint injuries will have been X-rayed and these films will be very useful if we need to refer our player to an orthopaedic surgeon or other speciality. On match days a radiologist with equipment is in attendance and therefore acute joint injuries and suspected fractures can be X-rayed immediately. We make many referrals to ENT surgeons for management of fractures of the nose or facial bones. Clinical notes of each of the players seen at every clinic are kept under lock and key; the contents are private, known only to the patient and medical staff.* The medical officer at a club takes on a vital role when he is dealing with the examination of new apprentices to the club (at Arsenal this could be up to ten players per year). A medical assessment along the lines of an insurance medical is carried out. All joints are examined for mobility and possible deformity. This is important as so many young players are good athletes playing many other sports — they are generally speaking the élite sportsmen at their school and may represent the school or county in other disciplines. Several of the youngsters will have signs of overuse injury or stress injury, e.g. Osgood—Schlatter's disease of the knee, patellar tendinitis and chronic low back pain. They are not failed because of these findings but are offered specialist training programmes under the eye of the youth team coach. At the other end of the scale is the mid-season transfer of a player from another first-division club and possibly worth up to a million pounds. Medical examinations on such players often have to be on the day of transfer. Such medicals can be a headache especially if you find a blood pressure of 160/110 or that the player has a potentially serious condition, such as spondylolisthesis, but is asymptomatic. Maybe he has one leg shorter than the other by 2 cm because of an old fracture of the tibia and fibula. The player might be highly allergic to all antibiotics and drugs and has had very severe reactions in the past. All these signs have been found in players but in fact have not

---

*The same principles of medical confidentiality apply to this doctor/patient relationship as to the relationship between an occupational physician and an employee of a company. The physician may be employed by the company primarily to serve its interest. There may arise, therefore, a conflict of loyalties if the doctor were to detect a condition in a player which could preclude him from selection. The team doctor should also remember that GMC guidelines require that the patient's own GP should be kept informed of investigations and treatment supplied by the agents of the club.

stopped the transfer. In some cases of doubt we rely on specialist opinions. Even players with no medical history are fully X-rayed, including lumbosacral spine, hips, pelvis, knees and ankles. Urine analysis is performed, as well as tests for colour blindness and acuity of vision. The club doctors usually witness the next two home games with some degree of anxiety: is that super new player as fit as the doctor had declared?

Many young players experience a period in their career when they are over- or underweight. Even the manager may lightheartedly mention 'injections for that boy, doctor, he is skilful but does not have the weight'.* Most players are not underweight for their height. If there is a genuine problem, however, it may be useful to construct a week's calorie intake chart and calculate for an individual player how the deficiency may be rectified. For some players the problem is simply that they are away from home, and away from mum's cooking. These players are helped by counselling and guided in their dietary intake, and the problem is usually short-lived. Overweight players are easier to manage — the coaches see to that with more cross-country running! The doctor can help, however, by providing a suitable calorie chart. I will always remember the occasion when we took on a famous player who was about 12.5 kg overweight. He was sent to a special 'farm' which cost the club £500 for two weeks. He managed to put on 3 kg.

As the match approaches the players are under the trainer's control. A high-calorie carbohydrate diet is provided the night before the match and again at around 11.30 a.m. for a 3.00 p.m. kick-off. Cornflakes, tea, toast, butter, jam and honey are the norm.

Specific injuries on the field of play

The medical officer will rarely be called out to the field of play to treat injuries, this being the main province of the trainer. The doctor will, however, have to be available to advise on the more serious type of injury and in particular the unconscious player, and in incidents where there is injury to the cervical spine.

Contact sport by its very nature means soft tissue injuries occur during any match. Knocks and bruises are part of the game. Players will often ignore many of the minor injuries. For the more serious injuries, however, medical attention will usually be sought.

In football the most commonly injured joints are the knee (half of reported cases) and the ankle (one-third of reported cases). The most commonly injured muscle group is the quadriceps at the front

---

*Even if the manager's comments in this regard are not meant as a joke they should be treated as one. Performance-enhancing substances have no place in sport and the doctor should resist any pressure from management or players to provide non-therapeutic prescriptions in the form of anabolic steroids or banned stimulants (see Chapter 6).

of the thigh. 'Pulled' hamstrings and groin strains come an equal second. Lacerations which require suturing occur about every third game. Wounds are usually either facial or affecting the legs, below the knee. Following an injury during play the first man from the medical team on to the pitch to see the injury is the trainer. He must immediately assess the severity of the injury from two points of view — treatment required, and whether or not the player requires substitution. Fractures and severe sprains will require splinting and stretcher. At Arsenal the trainer and coach have the stretcher and are in charge of transport of the injured player. If the trainer wants the doctor on the field then a signal is given to the director's box. The 'doctor's bag' for use 'from the bench' should include an endotracheal tube and laryngoscope, an airway, a pneumatic splint, several triangular bandages, a hard cervical collar, stethoscope and ophthalmoscope. Also avaible should be a supply of antiseptic solution and sterile gauze. Any fracture, severe joint injury or muscle tear will necessarily mean the player coming off to the dressing-room. It is here that a final assessment is made.

If the player is unconscious an immediate testing of his vital function is made with observation of pulse rate and respirations. Resuscitation is carried out if necessary. If this is not necessary then the player is placed on his side and steps are taken to make sure that the airway is clear. The assessment of conscious level is made by testing the pupil reflex and response to pin-prick. If any spinal injury is suggested then the transport of the player to the ambulance and hospital must be under the supervision of the doctor.

Lacerations of the skin need careful examination to exclude any complicating factors, e.g. underlying fracture of a cheekbone, or deep tendon laceration around the ankle joint. The wound needs to be carefully cleaned and disinfected, using 1% lignocaine as local anaesthetic followed by a thorough cleaning with gauze or a sterile scrubbing brush. The wound is then sutured and the tetanus immunisation status of the player is checked. Lacerations around the ankle joint could be avoided if adequate protective pads were worn. In the author's view football shin pads commonly in use are not suitable and should be substituted for something more akin to hockey shin pads. The Swedes have a similar shin pad which offers all-round protection.

Muscle injuries are the most common soft tissue injury and are due to direct or indirect injury. The direct injury can cause immediate loss of function with associated haematoma formation. Such players may need substitution. The indirect injury is usually caused by the sudden 'pull' of a muscle working over two joints. The hamstrings are commonly involved in this way, and can cause symptoms of sudden pain and spasm from a tearing of fibres in the belly of the muscle. We recognise intra- and extramuscular injuries.

In the former, the tear is in the centre of the muscle bundle, causing much pain and spasm, and loss of function. Extramuscular injuries are bruises on the surface of the muscle groups. The bruise may be visible and can track down the fascia between the muscle bundles. The immediate treatment is the same for both types of injury, and can be remembered by the mnemonic 'ICE'. 'I' is for 'ice': a bagful wrapped in a towel and placed on the injured part for up to ten minutes. This controls further bleeding and exudation of fluid, thereby controlling the swelling. 'C' is for 'compression'. This also prevents further disruption of swollen tissues. 'E' is for elevation; the player is sent home and told to rest but keeping the injured area elevated to help absorption of exudate. Reassessment is made the following day. The intramuscular type of injury is usually a more severe form of injury than the extramuscular type.

Joint injuries must be diagnosed immediately and carefully. So-called sprains of the ankle joint may be classified as mild, moderate or severe. Mild sprains show tenderness and restricted range of movement and respond well to ice and compression; the player is, however, able to walk. The severe injury is self-evident and walking will be impossible. Usually the injury will need immobilisation in Plaster of Paris after an X-ray. We are fortunate at Arsenal in that we have an X-ray service available for every first-team game. The moderate sprain with capsular injury will be associated with fluid in the joint. This injury will need immobilisation for up to three days, then final assessment by an orthopaedic surgeon.

Knee joint injuries require careful examination. As a routine we test for effusion and instability in the collateral ligaments and cruciate ligaments. If there are any symptoms or signs of intra-articular instability, a meniscal tear is considered. Any player in whom this type of injury is suspected should see the orthopaedic surgeon within 24 hours of the injury.

It is inexcusable practice in the care of footballers to inject any sprained ligament with local anaesthetic and let him carry on playing. Such a practice will merely convert a minor injury into a potentially serious injury.

Dislocations of joints can be dealt with by the club doctor but only after X-rays have been taken. All fractures should be adequately splinted before the player leaves the field — a simple broad arm sling will suffice for upper limb fractures — as a temporary supportive measure pending definitive assessment and treatment, for which specialist help may be required.

Faciomaxillary injuries should be referred to special units. Depressed fractures of facial bone have been seen by the author on four occasions at Arsenal. Fractured nasal bones are not to be treated lightly. It is possible to have quite severe haemorrhage with these fractures. ENT opinion should be sought.

Prevention of injury

Managers, coaches and referees have an important part to play in the prevention of injuries. The manager must carefully consider a player's ability to play after injury. He must talk to the team doctor and physiotherapist. Risks are sometimes taken but it is only fair that the consequences should be known to all; the medical team and certainly the player should be consulted.

A recent survey carried out by the Football Trust found that there were as many injuries during training as during actual matches. It follows therefore that training methods should be scrutinised. The majority of injuries are from contact, and perhaps alteration in training methods may be able to reduce these. Other sources of training injury are stress fractures, from running on hard ground, and muscle strains. These are probably avoidable with better warm-up techniques. Clubs should aim to provide a full medical team and then should be prepared to follow its advice on the construction and requirements of the medical room. It would be prudent for professional clubs to ensure that their players are all covered by private medical insurance, to ensure early treatment of severe injuries.

Clubs should encourage the setting up of clinics devoted entirely to the treatment of sports injuries. Players with chronic injury or following a serious fracture may be assessed and rehabilitated away from the club in excellent surroundings and under excellent medical care, at the National Rehabilitation Centre at Lilleshall.

Legislation in the game is reviewed annually by the FIFA. The recent change of allowing two substitutes could mean that players with mild injuries could be substituted, thus avoiding the risk of making the injury worse by playing on. The substitution that is made is, however, in the hands of the manager. Unfortunately, at times tactical considerations will preclude the resting of an injured player.

There is still room for improvement in the medical care of footballers. Further training for the doctors involved is necessary for an increased awareness of the problems involved in treating footballers' injuries. It is the author's view that club doctors should have a formal contract with their clubs. Clubs in the lower parts of the Football League and those which are members of county associations should have trainers, at least to the standard of the FA five-years certificate. More courses are required to cater for club trainers.

International football: the team doctor[*]

Many of the problems which face the national team doctor are similar to those experienced at club level. There are, however, some important differences. For example, some of the players could be new caps, and therefore not seen by the doctor previously. It may be three months or more since the last international game. The first task for the doctor is to ensure that all the players are 100% fit. It is pointless asking players as soon as they arrive in the hotel about their fitness. They all answer 'very fit, Doc' because they want to stay! I usually make a point of paying an informal visit to each player. This is much more casual, and gives a chance to have a chat, talk about the last game, the result, etc., and discuss frankly any recent injury. The manager will want to know that evening. He will want to know the chances of the player competing. If there are any problems the manager will have little time to call a replacement if we are playing the following morning. During my round of assessing fitness to play I also ask about current medications, in particular to learn of any players taking non-steroidal anti-inflammatory drugs and any taking night sedation. I usually make a note of the player's last injury, as this is important from an insurance point of view. It is not uncommon for players to exacerbate a recent injury and on return to their club to find that they are unable to play. In this situation the medical insurance carried by the player's club may seek to recover monies from the insurers of the Football Association unless it can be shown that the injury predated the international match, and here the doctor's notes can be decisive.

The training programme at club and national level will be very similar, although some players complain of too little at national level. The training programme always includes at least half an hour of warm-ups: stretching muscles, co-ordination work, striking the ball. After these set pieces, movements and tactics are arranged. The ultimate is the so-called five-a-side — a short game on a small area. Players get to know their team mates, call names, etc.

When the national side travels abroad it is usual to make arrangements for a local orthopaedic surgeon to be available at the game, to help with the acute management of any severe injury during play. I usually contact the British Orthopaedic Association before leaving the UK to find an orthopaedic surgeon from the country to be visited. Immunisations to cover foreign travel is the responsibility of the team doctor. He must also attain up-to-date knowledge of the conditions of the environment with which the team might have to encounter. Altitude, high temperatures and humidity are such conditions. Acclimatisation is important.

[*] This post will be filled by only a privileged few in a professional lifetime. This account by the present incumbent to the English team is included as an interesting insight into an otherwise inaccessible magic garden in the realisation that most readers will not aspire to such dizzy heights.

27 Tennis injuries: avoidance and treatment

J. P. R. WILLIAMS

'Cannon in front of them Volley'd and thunder'd'
From *The Charge of the Light Brigade* by Tennyson

Lawn tennis has been played for several hundred years and derives from its predecessor 'real tennis', which was one of the favourite sports of Henry VIII. Tennis has progressed dramatically in recent years with markedly increased standards of performance and professionalism. Originally a game played on grass, many types of synthetic surfaces have now been introduced for most major championships.

It is hard to believe that tennis only became 'open' to professional players in 1968 and that the first Wimbledon Open Championships were the following year in 1969. Professional tennis-players are now highly paid and are subjected to tremendous pressure as they tour the professional circuit. Tournaments occur every week of the year and necessitate considerable world-wide travel. Such a physically demanding schedule predisposes not only to physical stress but also to mental stress and problems arising from repeated travel across time zones.

Types of injury

Joint problems

Elbow

Probably the best-known injury of all in tennis is that of 'tennis elbow'. This is a strain of the extensor origin in the forearm situated on the lateral aspect of the elbow. It is commonly caused by mistiming of the backhand stroke. This causes a strain in the extensor muscles and forces are transmitted to the extensor tendon origin on the lateral epicondyle, causing a partial tear. Correct stroke production is important in avoiding this injury and it is in fact a fairly rare condition amongst top players. Treatment of the established condition consists of rest, ice, compression and elevation. If this fails to be successful then properly monitored ultrasound treatment may be considered. Most cases of tennis elbow settle on this regime. However, a small percentage may require surgery. There are many different types of surgical procedure for this condition, but the simplest is that of a release of the extensor origin. This produces fibrous healing with cessation of pain.

Injury to the medial side of the elbow, the so-called 'golfer's elbow', is far less common in tennis-players. This condition involves injury of the flexor tendon and, as its name implies, is more common in the game of golf. Mistiming of the forearm tennis stroke could, however, result in this condition in tennis-players. Treatment is similar to that of extensor tendon injury.

Wrist

Injuries to the wrist joint involve sprains or partial tears of the dorsal and palmar capsule. As tennis is a 'stiff-wrist' game, relaxation of the wrist on impact of the ball can result in a sprain. Strapping or taping the wrist is effective, both as a prophylactic measure in cases of old injuries and to support a recent sprain.

Ankle

Ankle injuries are fairly common in tennis and most common amongst these are sprains of the lateral ligament. These are produced by an inversion injury to the ankle. It is, not surprisingly, more common on slippery surfaces. Although there is no bony injury involved, this soft tissue injury can lead to much pain, which can lead to a prolonged period of incapacity. Injuries to the medial side of the ankle are less common.

Shoulder

Soft tissue shoulder injuries are, not surprisingly, fairly common. These mainly involve rotator cuff problems, with inflammation of the four tendons comprising the rotator cuff as they travel over the shoulder joint. Rest, ice and compression are again important in treatment.

Back injuries

An incorrect service action may result in a chronic strain of the lumbar spine. Correct technique is important in avoiding this condition. The treatment is by physiotherapy. Back-strengthening exercises should be employed to relieve pain and to reduce the chance of further injuries.

Fractures

These in general are uncommon but, when they do occur, usually involve the ankle, through severe inversion injuries, or the upper limb following a heavy fall on to the arm. Assessment and treatment follow standard principles of traumatology with careful clinical assessment and radiological examination where necessary.

Treatment

Most soft tissue injuries can be treated non-surgically. It is only in chronic conditions which do not respond to conservative measures that surgery should be contemplated, for example in the case of chronic 'tennis elbow'.

Conclusions and recommendations

All tennis-players should attempt to reach a high level of fitness before participating in the sport. Prevention is better than cure, and the higher the level of fitness attained the less is the likelihood of injury. Attention to adequacy of playing surface is important as is a proper 'warm-up' prior to participation.

If injury does ensue, most are of the soft tissue variety and should be treated by rest, ice, compression and elevation for the first 48 hours. This reduces the bleeding of the soft tissues and facilitates active rehabilitation. Suspected fractures should be X-rayed in an accident and emergency department and the appropriate treatment given along standard lines. It is always better to err on the side of safety, from both the patient's and the doctor's point of view. Most soft tissue injuries will recover in time. In the competitive world of modern tennis, however, there is often not enough of this commodity available.

Medical care in cricket

F. T. HORAN

'The Ball no question makes of Ayes or Noes
But Right or Left as strikes the Player goes
And He that toss'd the down into the Field
He knows about it all, He knows He knows'
From the *Rubaiyat* by Omar Khayyam

Historical review

Until about 15 years ago the organisation of medical care in cricket was haphazard. Most counties had a doctor, usually a county member keen on the game, who made himself/herself available when required to a give advice on injuries to players. Not all counties had a physiotherapist, and some who did work within the game were not fully qualified. The provision of care at major matches tended therefore to be on an informal basis. Requests on the public address system for a doctor to attend the pavilion to treat an injured player during major matches were not uncommon. Changes in tactics in the deployment of fast bowling in the early 1970s led to an increase in injuries to batsmen. The England team who toured Australia in 1974–5 found Lillee and Thomson at their peak, and a number of batsmen sustained notable injuries. The West Indies toured England in 1976, and they again had a number of fine fast bowlers who did not hesitate to employ the short ball. The Test and County Cricket Board therefore decided that proper arrangements were required to deal with potential injury to players during major matches, and indicated that doctors should be available at all times in these fixtures. Since then far greater attention has been given to medical requirements in first-class cricket.

Present arrangements

The pattern of care now provided is similar in all first-class counties. A general practitioner is usually appointed as the honorary medical officer, and is responsible for the day-to-day health care of members of the county staff.

Most counties now have an honorary orthopaedic surgeon who

341

deals with injuries sustained during play. This individual is usually responsible for the recruitment of a suitable physiotherapist, who is contracted for the season. It is now mandatory to have a qualified physiotherapist available at the ground during all first-class games, and there is now a pool of qualified physiotherapists who are experienced in the requirements of first-class cricket.

Players who suffer more severe types of injuries which are not readily treated by the physiotherapist are referred to a specialist, who usually sees the patients on a private basis. Since most surgeons lead busy lives, few have time to watch much cricket, but those who undertake to look after players have a great interest in the game and are prepared to treat their cricketing duties as a priority. It is usual for the honorary surgeon to have the privileges of a committee member, and most become an integral part of the structure and organisation of their county club.

All the first-class counties carry insurance for the medical care of the players, which facilitates the speed and ease of treatment.

An important duty of the medical officer is to arrange (usually via the local hospital) for X-ray facilities to be readily available to injured players out of normal working hours, particularly since much first-class cricket is played at the weekends.

Apart from the management of acute injury or illness, team doctors are responsible for the routine medical examination of players who have been offered contracts, or whose contracts have come up for renewal. They may also be expected to give advice concerning the training and conditioning of players before and during the season. They must be able to advise the coaching staff on the likely recovery of players after injury, and must closely supervise the efforts of the physiotherapist in the rehabilitation of injured players. Liaison with doctors from other counties concerning injury to players from either of their teams is essential in order that continuity of care can be maintained.

Comprehensive records of the illness and injury of players are now kept, and it is necessary to ensure that these are up to date and properly stored.

Medical care at major games

For test matches, one-day internationals and major cup finals the responsibility for provision of medical care lies with the ground authority. It is customary to retain the services of suitable doctors on a fee basis. This guarantees a proper professional approach by the doctors concerned, who must ensure their easy availability before, during and after the game. These medical staff are there principally for the treatment of players, and are not available to treat spectators unless an extreme emergency arises.

Relationship with the players

Players must be treated as patients. The normal confidentiality of the doctor/patient relationship must be preserved, and disclosure of information concerning their health or physical fitness to the club officials needs the player's agreement. This, of course, is rarely refused, but it must be not be assumed, and the club should be aware that this is the case. It is in the interests of all concerned that information about injuries which might compromise a player's career is properly discussed with all interested parties. Similarly, if a player changes counties, exchange of medical information should be agreed before fresh contracts are signed.

Liaison with the Press is not a task for the doctor. Release of information to the Press depends on agreement between a player and the club. The Press are particularly persistent at times of injury to well-known players, and their requests for information need firm rebuttal.

A county cricket club is a close-knit organisation. Players become confidants and friends, and the doctor inevitably finds himself acting as an informal link between players, coach, captain and the cricket committee. Matters of family health or crisis may well be brought to the doctor, and the players must feel that he is reliable and discreet and has their interests at heart.

General responsibilities of the club medical officer

The responsibilities of the team doctor to the players have been discussed above, but on a wider basis the doctor may be called upon to advise the club in all medical matters. For example the doctor must ensure that the physiotherapist has proper facilities and working conditions. Until recently the overall level of resources available to physiotherapists in first-class cricket was poor, but in the last few years there has been considerable improvement. In 1989 the Test and County Cricket Board carried out an assessment of the arrangements in force in all of the first-class counties, and a report and recommendations will be issued which all counties will be expected to follow.

The club requires advice on proper insurance of the players, on the interpretation of regulations on the use of and testing for performance-enhancing drugs, and in the organisation of the medical care of spectators. Most grounds rely upon the cover provided by the St John's Ambulance Brigade or the Red Cross. However, in major games where large numbers of spectators are present, a more comprehensive service may be necessary. At Lord's the St John's

Ambulance Brigade have customarily provided spectator care. However, in recent years their numbers and back-up services have been considerably increased, and a Mobile Coronary Care Unit is present on big occasions.

The management of injuries

The aim of the treatment of injury is to return the player to maximum fitness in the minimal time. However, the interests of the club must not be allowed to override those of the player. Attempts at playing unfit players must be strongly resisted, and the doctor must have the final say. If his or her advice is overruled, he or she should make his or her position absolutely clear and be prepared to resign from the post if still ignored.

Treatment of minor injuries is undertaken principally by the physiotherapist. The player may be able to continue playing during treatment, and the experience and attitude of the players themselves are often a deciding factor.

Minor injuries require an early and precise diagnosis. A clear plan of treatment must be properly explained to all concerned, and a realistic programme of rehabilitation devised. Close liaison is necessary with the captain, the coach and the cricket committee.

In matches in which a doctor is not present the responsibility of the management of major injury falls upon the physiotherapist. He or she must be properly briefed and trained, and the arrangements for calling an ambulance and removal to hospital need to be rehearsed and understood by all concerned. Most counties now send their staff on first-aid courses. Many counties insist that their players understand the basic principles of first-aid, and before the start of last season all first-class umpires received instruction in basic resuscitation, including introduction of an airway, etc.

Training

The standard of physical fitness required in the professional game is a subject of controversy. Apocryphal tales of great players of former years who kept themselves at the peak of fitness by bowling twenty medium-paced overs per day are well known in the game. Cricket matches take a long time, and the effort and concentration required in varying phases of the game are plainly variable. However, the modern game, with emphasis on one-day matches requiring a high standard of fielding, demands a greater degree of physical fitness than was necessary in the past. In the view of the author, the level of true physical fitness in cricket could be greatly enhanced. The really fit players do perform at a consistently better level than those who take a more relaxed approach to training. Pre-season conditioning varies from county to county.

The availability of indoor nets now means that players may stay in reasonable cricket trim throughout the year, but bowling on the relatively unyielding surfaces found indoors does seem to promote injury in quicker bowlers.

Travelling

Modern county cricketers spend a considerable part of their lives travelling in cars on motorways. The arrangements of Sunday League fixtures have been criticised. Player fatigue is now a considerable problem. Men may be asked to play for 15 days in succession, with a considerable amount of travelling. This does not allow proper periods of rest and, particularly in bowlers, impairs adequate recovery from minor injuries, which may then progress to be more troublesome.

Drugs

The Test and County Cricket Board (TCCB) undertake a regular programme of random tests for performance-enhancing drugs. The Sports Council have instructed all governing bodies of sports to carry out such a programme, and, since the Cricket Council receives a grant from them, the TCCB are required to carry out a testing programme and have access to the appropriate laboratories.

The definition of a 'drug' in sport is that it be a performance-enhancing substance. The Medical Subcommittee of the International Olympic Committee have issued a comprehensive list of such drugs which is used as a yardstick for assessment. This list is heavily biased towards the athletic sports, but the Sports Council feel that it should be applied to all games, and it is therefore followed in cricket.

The TCCB have drawn up precise instructions concerning the use of drugs, which are circularised to all players each season. They are also sent a list of banned drugs, together with suggestions for permissible medicaments which can be bought over the counter in a chemist if necessary. It is a duty of the county medical staff to make sure that players are aware of the regulations and properly understand them.

The TCCB have introduced a clear protocol for the carrying out of tests. It is essential that such instructions be strictly followed and properly understood, so that in the event of a positive result being obtained no criticism of the conduct of the test can be made. If a positive test is obtained on a player, the matter is brought to the attention of the Disciplinary Committee of the TCCB and suitable action taken.

However, no evidence has emerged that so-called performance-enhancing drugs are used in first-class cricket, and indeed it is difficult to see that such substances would be of use in a game which may last for five days.

Overseas tours

A doctor does not customarily accompany the England team on overseas tours. An exception was made in the last World Cup in the Indian subcontinent, when a specialist in tropical medicine went with the team. The itinerary of cricket tours is long-established and local liaison with suitable doctors has been found to be satisfactory. If any doubts have emerged concerning the proper assessment of injured players, it has been customary to fly them home, so that they can be properly treated and a replacement sent if required.

Future prospects

Although there has been considerable improvement in the standards of medical care in first-class cricket we still require better facilities for physiotherapy and rehabilitation, a closer liaison between medical staff of the varying counties, and a better understanding of the standard of training and conditioning required for players in the first-class game.

Recent major disasters which have occurred at large sports grounds have emphasised the need for improvement in the medical facilities at the major games. The provision of adequate medical cover, coronary care facilities and improvements in stadium design are mandatory.

Motor sports injuries: the doctor's role in trackside management, and hospital care 29

P. G. RICHARDS

'Call the Doctor I think I'm going to crash
The Doctor said he's coming but you'll have to pay in cash'
From *Life in the Fast Lane* by The Eagles

Motor sport, which includes track racing, rallying, hill-climbs and sprints in both cars and motor-cycles, is steadily increasing in popularity among spectators and competitors alike. The combination of speed and competition means that accidents inevitably happen and injuries and fatalities are bound to occur. Fortunately they are relatively rare. A well-motivated medical presence is, however, essential to save life where this is possible, and to control unstable injuries so that secondary damage is prevented pending transfer for definitive treatment.

Medical examination

General practitioners are likely to have indirect contact with the sport if one of their patients needs a medical examination in order to obtain a licence. In order to compete, a valid licence and completed medical card have to be produced at each meeting. The basic requirements are that a competitor has to be fit enough to control his or her machine, have good vision and not suffer from any condition where a sudden loss of control may be a danger to himself/herself and others. Thus epilepsy, controlled or otherwise, is an absolute contraindication to holding a competition licence, as is a severe visual field defect. Diabetes may be acceptable, provided it is not unstable. Some disabilities which at first sight might seem a bar to competition may be acceptable, provided machine control is maintained, for example a number of motor-cycle side-cars are raced by one-legged riders! Some competitors may themselves suffer conditions which could be aggravated by further injury with serious consequences. This is not necessarily a bar to competition provided the competitor is made fully aware of the risk. The author gave an opinion on a professional racing motor-cyclist who in an earlier accident broke his neck, and sustained damage to a hip, necessitating prosthetic replacement. Further trauma could have been disastrous, but he knew and understood this and was prepared to take the risk. There was no contraindication to racing otherwise, so his licence was allowed to stand. If a doctor is not sure whether a competitor qualifies on medical grounds, then he or she should refuse to sign the licence, stating his or her reasons. If the competitor still wishes to carry on in the sport, then the problem will be referred to the medical committee of the appropriate sport, who will review the problem, taking appropriate specialist advice if necessary. Therefore if there is any doubt, it is safer not to sign the card.*

Accidents

Having received a licence and passed the medical, the competitor will then take up his or her chosen aspect of the sport. The vast majority belong to the breed of 'clubmen/clubwomen' racers, who take part in the sport for love, not money, and hold regular jobs during the week, racing only at weekends. A very small percentage enter the sport with a view to progressing to the highest ranks, and an even smaller percentage actually achieve this. However, most racers are very keen on their sport, and view injury as little more than a nuisance, preventing them from taking part in their next race. They are thus highly motivated to recover, and deserve and expect the highest standard of care at all levels. Types of injury vary with the sport involved. Accidents tend to be at a higher velocity than in road traffic accidents, but injury patterns vary for a number of reasons. First, competitors are invariably sober. They will realise when they have lost control of their machine and that an accident is imminent and will therefore brace themselves for impact. Secondly, all the vehicles are travelling in the same direction. Therefore head-on and side-on impacts rarely occur. Saloon cars have a tendency to roll, but drivers are usually well strapped in, and serious injuries rarely occur from rolling.

Protection

Motor sport competitors are invariably better equipped than the average driver on the road. Car-drivers are usually well strapped in with six-point seat-belts and correctly anchored seats. There is therefore a low incidence of seat-belt and steering-wheel injuries. Single-seated car chassis are much stronger, some of them now being made of carbon fibre and Kevlar which can withstand phenomenal impacts without transmitting the energy to the driver. In the motor-cycle field, all riders have to wear leathers and most choose the highest quality with additional padding in knees and elbows. Underneath leathers are worn polystyrene back protectors. Most

---

* Whatever decision is made by the doctor with regard to fitness to race it is of paramount importance that a note is made of the consultation, recording the clinical notes and indicating where appropriate that the risks to the prospective licence-holder have been discussed.

motor-cyclists who are experienced learn how to fall properly and slide, kicking the bike away from them if possible. Their major risk is that they will be run over by other machines, or that they will not get far enough away from their bike, and that it may strike them. A straightforward fall and slide rarely cause major damage other than the odd broken collar-bone or abrasion burns to the back or buttocks. More serious burns may be encountered in motor racing, where the driver may find himself trapped and surrounded by spilled petrol. For this reason it is mandatory to wear fireproof clothing. Fireproof socks, underwear, balaclavas, gloves and overalls made of several layers of flameproof material protect the driver so that the only exposed part of the skin is around the eyes. The best-quality fireproof clothing allows the driver between 30 seconds and one minute to escape in any major fire, which should allow ample time for fire marshalls, who usually wear similar protective clothes, either to get the fire under control or the driver out of the car, or preferably both.

Common to both car and motor-cycle racing is the essential need for good head protection, and it is mandatory to wear crash-helmets approved to appropriate standards. Two types of helmet are in common usage: the first is the open-face or 'jet'-type helmet, which is derived from the military aircraft pilot's helmet. This provides good protection for the cranial vault, but no protection for the eyes and face. In open-car racing or motor-cycle racing they must be used with a pair of good-quality goggles, but in saloon-car racing or rallying goggles are not absolutely necessary. They have the advantage of being relatively light, but give no protection to the facial bones. The more popular alternative is the full-face helmet which provides protection for the whole of the head. Part of the helmet is cut away at the front to facilitate adequate vision. Eye protection is provided by a hinged visor, which may be clear or tinted for use in sunny conditions. This helmet has the advantage of providing protection to the facial bones, but at the cost of increasing weight considerably. This in itself may put the wearer at increased risk of cervical spine injury in an accident, and also, depending on the size of the cut-away at the front, it may limit the visual field. For racing this is of limited importance. If used on the roads, however, a full-face helmet must allow adequate vision, particularly in the temporal fields. Several top-quality helmets, such as the American Simpson helmet, have been banned from road use, because of their restricted field of vision, even though they are widely used in motor sport.

Basic helmet construction is of a hard outer shell, usually made from polycarbonate, fibreglass or, more recently, Kevlar, with a polystyrene liner which absorbs a great deal of impact, and an inner comfort liner. It is held on the head by straps fixed to anchor points in the outer shell, although one type of helmet, the French GPA helmet, is held on the head by the whole of the base of the helmet unhinging. While this latter system makes it virtually impossible for the helmet to fly off in the course of an accident, it also makes it difficult to release and remove in the event of the wearer being rendered unconscious by the accident. This may make access to the airway difficult.

Helmets have been known to fly off and it is essential that the wearer gets a properly fitting helmet that cannot possibly slide off the back of the head in any way. In motor-cycle racing, following the deaths of two riders when their helmets came off, pre-race scrutineering now ensures that a rider must present his helmet to the scrutineers, who will test the fitness of the helmet and disallow its use if it is deemed to be too loose and therefore may be lost in the impact of a fall. Helmets for use in car racing are modified to take into account the risk of fire. They are coated with flame-resistant material and the best-quality helmets have inlets for piped oxygen which is carried in a separate bottle on the car to be released through the helmet, to give the wearer breathing space (literally) of 30 seconds to a minute in the event of him being trapped in a burning car.

Medical care

In the event of a rider suffering serious injury, there will be a medical presence rapidly available. In a local club event this may be an interested local general practitioner or junior hospital doctor recruited from the local hospital, while in the Formula 1 Car Grand Prix there may be as many as 50 doctors in attendance around the track, which works out at around two doctors for every driver. Such is the level of care in these circumstances that a few years ago at Brands Hatch, when a Formula 1 driver crashed in practice and was trapped in his car for a short period, he was attended while still in the car by a consultant anaesthetist, consultant general surgeon and two consultant orthopaedic surgeons! There is, however, always the possibility that, after this level of care has been shown at the track-side, when the patient finally reaches hospital the next doctor they see could be a casualty SHO. To prevent this happening, a little forward planning is required by the doctors attending the trackside.

In a local event early communication with the duty casualty consultant or a general surgeon a couple of days before the event will alert the department to the possibility of severely injured sports casualties arriving, who may require special care. For the larger events a great deal more planning is required. The international Grand Prix circus, both in car and motor-cycle racing, is a highly professional body, which expects and deserves top-quality care. Thus some thought ought to be given to the kind of injuries expected, and which local hospitals can handle them.

Major events usually have helicopters available, and this may increase the choice of hospitals to which casualties may be transported. Thus arrangements can be made to take multiple injuries to the nearest major trauma centre, severe head injuries to the regional neurosurgical unit and severe burns to the regional plastic surgery unit, but of course, for direct admission to these units, the co-operation of the duty consultants will be required. Contact should be made a couple of weeks in advance. It is of course pointless having helicopters to take injured people to hospitals if there are no landing facilities at the hospital, and that possibility must also be checked. The weather, particularly in Britain, must also be considered, and a number of alternative units approached if the main referring unit is closed down for helicopter access by the weather. When considering helicopter evacuation it should be remembered that severely injured patients do not travel well, particularly in a noisy vibrating helicopter, and that prior to setting out on the journey, the patient must be stable with all lines and tubes very firmly secured.

On arrival at the medical centre, further efforts must be made to stabilise the patient, and at this stage all available information concerning the nature of the accident should be assembled in order that the mechanism of injury may be understood. A great deal of misinformation may be offered by well-meaning helpers but usually the most reliable comes from the corner commander, who is a highly experienced marshal, or from the doctor on site, and attempts should therefore be made to obtain information from these individuals. In motor-cycle racing it is important to know whether the rider struck railings at the side, his own bike or another following bike, and an idea of the velocity of the accident is useful. In motor-car racing, a knowledge of whether the car rolled or was struck by another car or whether there was any fire involved is important. When examining the patient it is absolutely essential to remove all clothing. This may involve cutting off expensive leather or flameproof overalls, but that has to be done if it is the only means of undressing the patient. The level of consciousness should be assessed and any signs of chest or abdominal injury sought. The spine should be palpated for any evidence of spinal injury and the limbs closely inspected. Examination for signs of pneumothorax or haemothorax should be made. The pulse and blood pressure merits special attention. Most competitors will be young fit men and in these patients, therefore, a pulse of over 100 per minute (even though the patient may be warm and well-perfused with a normal blood-pressure) should alert the doctor to the possibility of occult blood loss through internal haemorrhage.

Good intravenous access is important: a small-bore cannula in a vein on the back of the hand is inadequate if there is intra-abdominal or intrathoracic bleeding. In a patient deeply shocked *in extremis*, a technique developed in the Vietnam war of cutting down to the saphenofemoral junction and putting in a giving-set directly may be necessary, although if such heroic measures are required at the site of the accident survival is unlikely. Blood is rarely available at the trackside, but plasma substitutes such as Haemocel and Gelfusion are normally carried along with normal saline.

The aim of treatment at the trackside is to stabilise the patient sufficiently well for transfer to hospital. The patient may die of overwhelming injury at the track or in the hospital, but should never die in transit. Having stabilised the patient and taken the decision to move him or her to hospital by the most appropriate mode of transport, be it ambulance or helicopter, the track doctor should then telephone the receiving hospital to give them as much warning as possible of the patient's arrival and condition. An assessment should be made of facilities required on arrival. This may include a general surgeon with an operating theatre standing by, or a functioning computerised tomography scanner, etc. For the severely ill patient, a doctor should accompany the patient to hospital even though this may necessitate suspension of the racing until he or she returns. It is essential, however, before the patient leaves that the history, examination and treatment thus far received are documented, both as an *aide-mémoire* for the track doctor, and for the subsequent investigation into the accident and its management. Thus, with the patient stable, the case documented and the doctor in attendance, the patient can be transferred to the receiving hospital where, hopefully, he or she will arrive in no worse a state than when he or she left the trackside.*

Patients who arrive at the receiving hospital following motor-racing accidents will usually have sustained serious injuries, the severity of which is usually greater than the majority of road traffic accidents. Thanks, however, to competent medical trackside attention the majority of racing injuries should arrive properly resuscitated. On arrival at hospital, therefore, they may appear deceptively well.

The principles of management of the severely ill patient will apply. Adequate oxygenation, adequate blood-pressure and administration of tetanus prophylaxis are immediate measures, followed by thorough examination of the patient and X-raying of all the clinically relevant parts. At that stage treatment priorities can be decided upon. Laparotomy, thoracotomy, closure and débridement of wounds, and setting fractures should be considered as indicated, as should transfer to regional neurosurgical or burns units. Specialist treatment usually follows the same lines as for any other road accident.

---

* There have to date been no recorded instances of a patient suing the doctor for negligent treatment at the trackside leading to damage or permanent disability. The fact remains, however, that the doctor's liability for providing negligent care in this situation is in principle no different from any other doctor–patient relationship. The notes may therefore assume an important medico-legal role in the event of a subsequent dispute over the standard of care delivered.

It should be recognised, however, that there may be pressure from the sports men and women themselves for treatment that will allow them early discharge, for the purpose of early return to racing. It may be acceptable to the individual concerned for a motor-cyclist injured in a 'highway accident' to wear a collar and cuff for a fractured clavicle or to stay in traction for three months for a fractured femur, but racing motor-cyclists, be it at club or international level, will often try and apply pressure on the surgeon to plate the clavicle or nail the femur, simply because it will allow them to get back to racing as soon as possible. Several international riders have broken collar-bones, had them plated and been racing within two weeks, and, however much they are advised about the risks of a further accident and breaking the plate, they would, in the author's experience, still rather run these risks.* This enthusiasm for the sport can lead to problems in the assessment of fitness to return to racing following injury. The rider may ask the advice of the doctor treating him at the hospital or the GP. If the leg or arm is too painful to control the machine because of a fracture, then they know they will not be able to race. If, however, they have suffered a head injury which has left them with no physical disability but some psycho-motor impairment, a dangerous situation can arise when the competitor appears to be functioning well, while in actual fact his or her driving or riding is unsafe. There may be difficulty in getting the rider to accept advice to stay off racing for three or six months. At present no guidelines from racing authorities exist to define when it may be safe for a competitor to return to racing after severe injury.†

Summary

In summary, severe injuries at the race-track are relatively rare. When a severe accident does occur, the initial aim of treatment at the trackside is to secure an airway, stop bleeding and obtain vascular access, and having done that the patient should be moved to the medical centre. In the medical centre, more thorough examination is possible, and the aim of treatment is to achieve a stabilised condition in order that the patient may be transferred to hospital. Following transfer to an appropriately equipped and forewarned hospital, treatment follows the lines of any other severely injured patient.

---

*The type of operation that a surgeon is prepared to perform in a given clinical situation will depend on numerous factors. The patient's wishes should naturally be taken into account. However, where the patient requests a treatment that the doctor considers to be potentially dangerous, the perceived dangers must be discussed with the patient before embarking on treatment. The ultimate decision on whether or not to employ the method requested rests with the doctor.

† The only safe course of action for the doctor who is consulted by a rider seeking certification of fitness is to apply a higher index of suspicion and to examine with care neurological and psychometric function, referring to specialist opinion where doubt exists.

30 Golf injuries: treatment and prevention

J. F. BUCHAN

'A good story at present is going round the clubs . . .'
From *The Right Stuff* by Ian Hay

Golf arouses increasing public interest. Television has shown it to be a well-organised enthralling game taking place in pleasant surroundings. Golf's top performers are seen as pleasing personalities and good sports men and women.

Historical background

The origins of golf are a matter of some debate. The Dutch believe it could have started in Holland. Old delft plates illustrate burghers whacking about a small object with carved sticks. Lema (1966) writes jokingly that the scene looks more like an American football scrimmage than a rehearsal for a Ryder Cup Match! Willhem Koolen (1608–66), the Dutch artist, also depicts a similar sort of game: four men playing on a frozen lake with clubs resembling old-fashioned woods. Was this a golf foursome of primitive ice hockey? It is anybody's guess.

The Scottish claim is based on sounder evidence. During the reign of James II (1437–60) the parliament prohibited the game because its popularity was jeopardising national defence by causing the young men to neglect their archery practice.

Mary, Queen of Scots, was rebuked for playing golf at Seaton House so soon after the murder of her second husband, Henry Darnley, in 1567. French-speaking, Mary had *'un cadet'* — a boy to carry her clubs, hence our term 'caddy'.

In 1592 the Burgh of Leith forbade golf 'during the course of the Sunday Sermons'. Golf's first club or society was formed there in 1744 and was at first entitled 'The Gentlemen Golfers of Leith', becoming subsequently 'The Honourable Company of Edinburgh Golfers'. Note the emphasis on 'gentleman's honour'. There is no game at which it is easier to cheat. Players are placed on their honour as in no other game. The Edinburgh golfers established a high code which still exists today and we owe them a debt of thanks. They were also responsible for drawing up the first set of rules.

The Society of St Andrews' Golfers, later dignified with the name 'The Royal and Ancient Golf Club', was founded ten years later, in 1754. It is now one of the senior decision-making bodies in the golfing world.

When the first Stuart king came to the English throne as James I, he and his courtiers used to go to Blackheath to play golf and it was there that England's first golf club was founded in 1766.

In the nineteenth century, with the spread of the British Empire throughout the world, golf spread with it. In 1971 the game took another giant leap forward when Captain Alan Shepard, Commander of the Apollo 14 spacecraft, hit two shots on the moon with a no. 6 iron. He was later reminded by telegram from the Royal and Ancient that 'before leaving a bunker a player should carefully fill up and smooth over any holes and footprints made by him. Failure to do so is in breach of the etiquette of the game'.

In the early days the number of holes constituting a round varied; Blackheath had five, Prestwick 12, St Andrews six, then 18 and later 22. However, in 1858, a new set of golf rules was issued, the first of which read 'a round of the links or 18 holes shall be reckoned a match unless otherwise stated'.

To start with, players made their own equipment but, with increasing refinement and standardisation, specialist club and ball makers arose. These professionals usually set up shop in a wooden hut beside the first tee, where they organised the caddies ('caddy-master') and made, hired out and sold golfing accoutrements.

For about 100 years the game was played with a ball called the 'feathery', which was made with 'a hatful' of boiled feathers stuffed into a small leather purse, which was then sewn up and hammered to make it more or less round.

The feathery was superseded in turn by the gutta-percha and 'gutty' balls. The first was made entirely of latex from Malayan gum trees, the latter of a composition of gutta-percha, powdered cork, leather particles and metal filings, all held together by an adhesive liquid.

Improvements in the golf ball necessitated changes in clubs. The feathery had many shortcomings: it tended to absorb moisture and hence became heavier if the ground was wet and it easily lost its shape, but it was very resilient and did not need particularly strong clubs to play with it. The harder gutty balls increased the wear and tear on clubs considerably. First the original face of the wood was inset with leather, later with bone and more recently with plastic. The type of wood constituting the head was changed from the original blackthorn, beech, apple or pear wood first to persimmon (the American date-plum), and then when this got scarce to laminated wood and now experimentally to metal 'woods' which consist of an aluminium shell filled with plastic.

Originally the golf club shaft was made of ash or hazel, and then, with the advent of the harder ball, hickory (a species of walnut) was used. Finally, today, the majority of players have stainless steel shafts although a few are trying carbon graphite.

Iron clubs, originally introduced as 'trouble shooters' to extricate the ball from bad lies, are now much used down the fairway, often off the tee and universally around the green.

In the 1890s an American dentist Coburn Heskell successfully completed his experiments with a ball consisting of a small central sac of gutta-percha which is encircled with rubber thread and the whole encased with gutta-percha. It was found that the Heskell ball flew further and it was soon adopted generally. In the last ten years a two-piece plastic ball has made its appearance. It is very tough but may lack the 'feel' of the rubber of the rubber-wound Heskell ball.

Injuries

Golf has, in addition to its 34 rules, a set of unofficial regulations to which all golfers are expected to adhere. These unofficial rules are called 'the etiquette of golf'. Despite the rules and etiquette, which exist to regulate both the nature of the game and the safety of its participants, there are a considerable number of injuries which occur on golf courses every year.

In chapter 5 of *Sport and the Law*, published by Butterworths, Edward Grayson cites two main sources of serious golf injuries:
1 Incorrect play.
2 Proximity of fairway to public access area.
Committee members should be aware of this second area and provide appropriate medical services and facilities accordingly. Some of the legal cases that record the type of injuries which occur and provide judicial precedent for the legal liabilities of the parties concerned are shown in Table 30.1. It is likely, however, that these records of novel legal principles represent only the tip of the iceberg of the real problem. They may realistically be multiplied in countless numbers in local newspaper reports and anecdotal archives.

Henry Cotton said that in his view golf is a game played predominantly with the hands, and, being closest to the point of contact, the hands and forearms are very liable to strain.

Blisters, cracks and callosities of the skin of the fingers and palms, 'golfer's' and 'tennis' elbows, sprains to the wrists and shoulders and back strains are the most frequently met with forms of local trauma. Lumbar disc lesions are not infrequent and tenosynovitis of the tendons of the thumbs and fingers occur but rarely.

Most medical men and women equate golf strains to 'golfer's elbow'! This condition, usually a strain of the common flexor tendon origin of the forearm flexors, is not confined to nor is it seen predominantly amongst golfers, yet it frequently occurs and is characterised by a pain on gripping, felt in the region of the elbow and down the forearm. Localised tenderness is present on the volar aspect of the forearm on its ulnar or medial side, over the common origin of the flexor muscles. It is usually caused by a 'jarring' injury — striking the rock-hard ground with a full shot.

'Tennis elbow' is likewise rather a misnomer. It is not confined to tennis players and is often met with in golfers. It is most frequently caused by a 'jarring' injury, like golfer's elbow, and the distribution of the pain is similar. The localised tenderness is situated in a small area on the volar aspect of the radial head or on its lateral aspect or over the lateral collateral ligament of the elbow joint.

In both these conditions the area of tenderness is very localised and requires careful palpation. The tenderness can also be very severe.

Back strain of the lower lumbar and sacroiliac regions arises as a result of restricted 'pivoting' (body rotation) during the swing. The weekend golfer is liable to 'forget' that the back and legs play an

Table 30.1 Legal cases involving golf injuries

	Decision	Principle
Golf ball played from 13th tee parallel with Sandwich Road, Kent, much frequented by motor-cars and taxicabs, into which road golf ball was hit. Windscreen of passing taxicab hit by ball and splintered glass, causing loss of driver's eye (*Castle* v. *St Austine's Links Ltd* [1922] TLR 615)	Golf club and player jointly liable for £450 damages and costs	Tee and hole were public nuisance from the conditions and in the place where they were situated. No precedent for different facts; but slicing of ball into roadway not only a public danger but was the probable consequence from time to time of people driving from the tee
Golfer not in course of play swings club during demonstration and injures person standing by. *Cleghorn* v. *Oldham* (1927)	Player liable	Not in course of play. Defence rejected of consent to negligent act, not unfair or vicious in recreation. Negligent misconduct actionable in recreation as in any other activity
Unreported pre-1962 decision of Sellers LJ on South Eastern Circuit (see [1963] 1 QB 43 at 55). Golfer in four-ball hit into rough, losing the ball. Said 'out of it' and encouraged better players to proceed. Resumed after finding ball, causing injury as victim turned round at defendant's cry of 'fore'	Player liable	Conduct outside the game; unnecessary for it; showed complete disregard for safety of those he knew were in line of danger from being hit from an unskilled instead of lofted shot over their heads
Pedestrian walking along narrow public lane injured on head by golf ball (*Lamond* v. *Glasgow Corporation* [1968] SLT 291)	Occupier liable for negligence	Although no previous history of any accident, 6000 shots a year played over fence should have created forecast of foreseeable happening
Lews Crown Court (unreported except newspapers), French J. Golfer in tournament injured by ball hit from fellow competitor without warning. *Bidwell* v. *Parks* (1982)	Fellow competitor golfer liable	Dangerous for 24 handicap golfer to take shot which could have gone anywhere without warning
High Court London (unreported except *Daily Telegraph* 24 January 1984). Awarded £10 000 damages when knocked unconscious on public footpath from golf ball knocking out five teeth and badly injuring nose, which required to be re-set *Smillie* v. *Woburn Golf and Country Club*	Golf club occupier of premises liable to pedestrian stroller	Golf club knew of risks of balls landing near pedestrian path. Neighbour as distinct from injured plaintiff had complained to club about golf balls landing in garden, 77 recorded between September 1979 and May 1981, and one had smashed conservatory window.

essential part but even professionals can strain their backs if for some reason their pivot is restricted (e.g. when playing from amongst trees).

An important point in avoiding back strain in the young is the development of a good orthodox golfing style. This is now being done at the various golfing schools. It is common experience that those with highly individual methods are very liable to back injuries.

Prevention

It was Gary Player who demonstrated the importance of physical fitness to the tournament. Player, not blessed with the same powerful physique as many of his top-class rivals, worked at physical exercises to such a degree that he has compensated for his lack of inches. He travels the world now with his own portable gymnasium.

Strength of the fingers and wrists is essential to good golf and is important in avoiding strains. Active exercises with spring grips and dumb-bells are valuable.

Jogging, press-ups, exercises on the static bicycle and with the rowing machine as well as back exercises form part of the professional's daily routine. Especially valuable are extension spinal exercises which can be carried out as follows:

1 Lie on the floor on the left side: with the legs fully extended and the arms down each side, the top leg (right) is carried straight back as far as possible by extending the hip and spine.
2 Turn on to the right side and similarly extend the spine and left hip.
3 Now turn face down, still lying on the floor. Extend the left hip and spine by lifting the thigh and leg straight up as far as possible.
4 Now do a similar exercise with the right hip.
5 Finally, still lying face downwards on the floor, raise the head and trunk upwards with the fingers of the hands interlocked at the back of the neck.

Warming up on the practice ground prior to play is valuable in relaxing stiff muscles and is conducive to a smooth unhurried swing. Warm muscles are less liable to be strained.

Drugs and the golfer

Delicate judgement and shrewdness are much needed on the golf course and any drug affecting the higher centres should not be prescribed during or immediately prior to play.

Stimulants, sedatives and analgesics are all best completely avoided. Even such comparatively innocuous substances as co-proxamal (distalgesic), co-codaprin (Codis) and solprin can adversely affect judgement.

Non-steroid anti-inflammatory drugs (NSAIDs) do not affect the higher centres and are permissible even during play. The most satisfactory are ibuprofen (Brufen), flurbiprofen (Froben) and indomethacin (indocid). All of these tend to produce gastric discomfort and should be taken ideally with food.

Early in 1987 Neil Foulds, a professional snooker player, informed the snooker board of control just before an important tournament that, on medical advice, he was taking beta-blockers. After much deliberation he was permitted to continue taking the drug and was also allowed to continue taking part in the tournament.

Where, it may be asked, is the line to be drawn in the Pharmacopoeia? Are we to permit any drugs to be taken by players if prescribed medically, despite the fact that they may also have performance-enhancing effects? The golfing world also will have to face this as yet unresolved dilemma. (See also Chapters 1 and 6.)

Conclusion

The golf 'tour' has spread world-wide and the participating tour professionals call for expert attention to their injuries and disabilities. It is hoped that these notes will be helpful to any one undertaking their care.

Reference

Lema T. (1966) *Champagne Golf*. London: Cassell.

31 The medical hazards of fencing

A. R. CRAWFURD

'I'll make thee glorious by my pen and famous by my sword'
J. G. Montrose

In one sense, fencing, the sport or pastime of swordplay, is as old in time and as widespread in distribution as the sword itself, and it is no more surprising that a fencing bout, complete with protective equipment, masks, judges and blunted swords, should appear in an Egyptian temple of 1190 BC (Arlott 1975) than that kendo should appear in Japan as a sport parallel to fencing in Europe. Man has ever shown himself able to sublimate his aggressive instincts and violent behaviour into ritualised forms of sport (as well as to do the reverse), so that swordplay as a recreation has always existed alongside that necessary practice with the sword which was required of the man whose life depended on his ability to use it effectively. The modern sport of fencing, however, has developed very largely from the swordplay of Western Europe, so it is particularly to France and Italy that one looks for the true origins of fencing.

Until the early sixteenth century, the European sword was a cutting weapon, principally used for hacking and hewing, but the development of the rapier, followed by the *flamberge* and then, a century or so later, the small-sword (Aylward 1960), changed the nature of swordplay into one that required skill, speed and dexterity far more than the brute strength required to cut one's opponent to pieces. This particular development, the use of the rapier, for which the Spanish and the Italians share the initial credit, rapidly became the expertise of the Italian fencing masters, and, among many famous names such as Manciolino of Modena and Marozza and Grassi of Venice, it was Camillo Agrippa of Milan, an amateur whose book *Trattato di Scientia d'Arme* was published in Rome in 1553, who 'first discerned the vast capacity for homicide which lay in the point of a sword, and how many souls could be rapidly released from the bondage of the flesh if puncturing, rather than slashing, was resorted to' (Pollock *et al.* 1889). This book marked the watershed between cut and thrust, even though it was to be a long time before England and even France recognised the new style as a legitimate means of swordplay. English monarchs have left

360

their mark on fencing in this country, as they have on many other sports, from Edward I, who, in 1285, banned fencing in the City of London, through Henry VIII, who, by granting a charter to the 'Corporation of Masters of Defence' sometime before 1540, established the first governing body of sport in England, to Edward VII, who, in 1906, granted the Tudor Rose as a badge to the Amateur Fencing Association (AFA) for use as its international colours.

About the middle of the eighteenth century, the fencing mask was reinvented (Pollock *et al.* 1889), traditionally by La Boëssière, though the macho rejection of an effective means of self-protection is by no means a modern phenomenon and it was many years before reputable fencers would wear them. France became the dominant influence, as Italian fencing became sidetracked into pedantry and absurdity, and it was masters such as Besnard, Labat, de Liancourt, Bertrand, Baron de Bazancourt, Cordelier, and the father and son Prévost who gradually changed the style of swordplay into the form recognisable today — developing the classic on-guard position as well as such basic moves as the lunge and the riposte.

The present century has seen many changes, but the most important milestone has been the introduction of the electrical recording apparatus, first for épée for the 1936 Olympics, shortly afterwards for foil, and now, at last, for sabre as well. The electrical apparatus not only reduced the inaccuracy and, dare one say it, the bias of judging hits by eye, but had a profound influence on the speed and style of fencing. A hit takes about 10–20 msec to be registered by the eye (Crawfurd 1989), so that, in the pre-electric era, a fencer had to let his point 'stay' on the target long enough for it to be seen by the corner judges, but any level of fencer can regularly make hits of 1 msec, and the present recording apparatus is permitted to register a hit of 1 msec (Paul 1985).

The effect has been that electric fencing allows the fencer to hit as fast (and therefore as hard) as he likes, safe in the knowledge that the hit will register. The great increase in speed of modern fencing has brought with it an increase in danger — the danger of penetrating injury from a broken blade — and, though much has been done to minimize that danger, fencing is not the only sport in which the perception of danger can add considerably to the excitement of competitor and spectator alike.

Fencing was one of the nine sports which made up the first Modern Olympiad in Athens in 1896 and it has remained an Olympic Sport ever since. The rules were first fully codified in 1914 and are now regulated by the Fédération Internationale d'Escrime (FIE), the international governing body of the sport, founded in 1913. The pressures and problems that beset sport today require considerable attention from governing bodies and the FIE's annual congress usually results in a dozen or more rule changes each year to try to keep abreast of the times.

Injuries and their prevention

Despite a few well-published fatalities, fencing is a very safe sport — there has been only one death in the history of British fencing — but there is no doubt that penetrating injuries due to broken blades attract attention, and, in both Italy and Germany, there was considerable pressure on governing bodies to be seen to be doing something in the wake of isolated fatal accidents. This illustrates the difficulty facing any sport trying to strike the right balance between making the sport as safe as possible and inhibiting its development through over-regulation. Defensive medicine has its parallel in sports legislation and, although nobody has yet suggested that we should have men and women in plate-armour fencing with rubber foils, the last ten years have seen more changes in that direction than the whole previous history of fencing. The 1985 recommendations of the FIE would, if implemented at all levels, have slightly more than doubled the cost of a beginner's equipment, and, in a low-budget sport such as fencing, this would have produced a very serious decline in the sport in this country. More resistant clothing is not only more expensive, it is heavier, more uncomfortable and restrictive to the fencer, and can produce problems in relation to heat regulation and fatigue. No serious fencers would put themselves at such a disadvantage unless their opponents were so constrained as well, so that any such regulations have to be made compulsory, not optional.

The pressure to be seen to be doing something has, in the view of many, produced a great deal of activity, sometimes in unprofitable directions. In the problem of protective clothing, for example, there has been little published work on the forces involved in lunging and the only unpublished experiments in this country were carried out with a female fencer using an intact foil against a stationary target. The flexibility of the intact blade reduces the force considerably, but, even so, the peak force reached was 190 newtons (Kerwin 1985). The force delivered by a fencer lunging behind a broken blade (particularly, as is commonly the case, when his opponent is lunging towards him) is massive, and of several orders of magnitude greater than a rifle bullet. Generally foil and épée blades break about 10–20 cm behind the tip, leaving a flat end approximately 4 mm × 4 mm for epee and 3 mm × 2 mm for foil. Top-class fencers are estimated to reach a speed of 10 m per second at the moment of impact. However, when a blade breaks, the potential energy stored in the blade, which is heavily bent just before it snaps, causes the blade to shoot out straight, reaching an estimated total speed of 22.15 m per second (Parfitt 1986a). The force of a 70 kg fencer travelling at 10 m per second would be 700 newtons, but the force behind the breaking blade would be of the order of 1550 newtons, and, if both fencers lunged at each other simultaneously, the force would be over 2000 newtons. The current FIE regulations require the 'vital parts' of the body to be protected with material resistant to 800 newtons (Crawfurd 1986), while the rest of the clothing should be resistant to 350 newtons. It is therefore perfectly clear that even the officially approved protective clothing would not be expected to stop a lunge with a broken blade and, indeed, that has been shown to be the case. The official apparatus for testing clothing involves measuring the forces as a conical plunger pierces the material, thus demonstrating that protection is only partial. The material which is in widespread use for fencing clothing up to FIE standards is Kevlar, but, unfortunately, this deteriorates both on exposure to sunlight and when washed with bleaching agents, thus reducing still further its protective value. New materials are now available with better characteristics, but a sport cannot survive frequent compulsory changes of expensive equipment. The AFA's Working Party on Equipment Standards, set up in 1983, as its title suggests, provides advice on the best steps to be taken within the UK to improve the safety of the equipment used, and has also produced, and regularly reviews, the AFA's published *Safety Guidelines*, and looks into all aspects of safety in fencing.

The common factor in almost all penetrating injuries is the broken blade. Injuries due to a blow with the intact point, although sometimes painful, are nearly always superficial. It follows that if blades could be manufactured which either did not break, broke less frequently, or broke more safely, then the danger of a penetrating injury could be much reduced. A great deal of ingenuity has gone into this search, and blades composed of fibreglass, plastic, spirally wound steel, and other materials, have been tried, but have all been found unsatisfactory. Blades with an integral weakness, or some form of joint at the base, have also been made and even blades incorporating an explosive charge which detonated when excess stress was put on the blade have been devised. So far, only one type of blade, made of maraging steel (B. Paul 1985), has received official approval. Maraging steel, which is specially heat-treated, has so far been shown to increase the life of foil blades by some two to three times, but has had, if anything, a negative effect on the life of épée blades, possibly because of the greater stresses involved in the manufacture of the unusual cross-section of an épée blade and possibly also because the amount of metal in the blade has been excessively reduced in order to reduce weight. On the other hand, it can reasonably be argued that if a blade lasts two to three times longer, there will be two to three times fewer broken blades and two to three times less chance of a penetrating foil injury over a given period of time. However, it is not fanciful to suggest that the tougher maraging blade might require greater force to break it and therefore the impact of the breaking blade would also be greater and therefore more dangerous (Fig. 31.1). A material with greater promise is Paul-Steel, a metal equivalent of glass fibre with long strands of hard metal fibres providing strength and springiness, held together by a tougher austenitic steel, which prevents crack propagation. Paul-Steel, like maraging, lasts longer but, more importantly, when the blade finally breaks, it breaks part through, rather

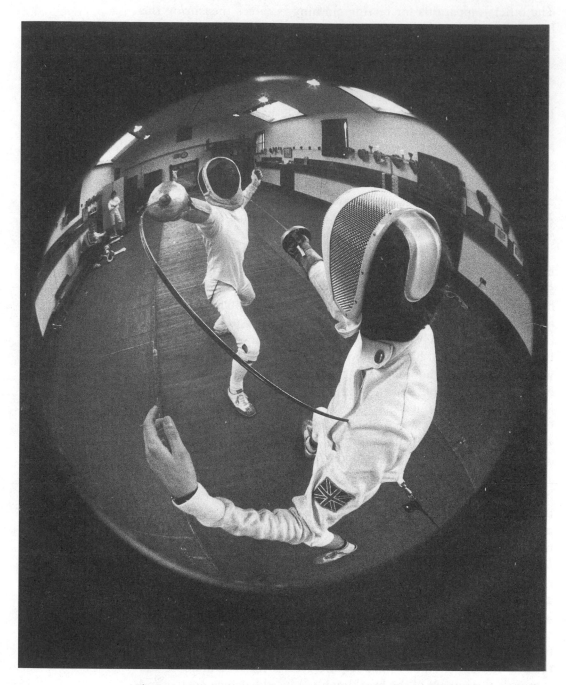

Fig. 31.1 Most penetrating fencing injuries are caused by broken blades, which often result from detective equipment.

like a greenstick fracture, so that the broken end, remaining attached to the blade, makes penetration much less likely. It is surely areas of research such as this that hold the greatest potential for greater safety.*

Some interest has been focused on subsidiary causes of accidents. The attack–counter-attack situation where both fencers lunge at each other almost simultaneously is a prominent feature of modern fencing and of serious accidents. It has been suggested that counter-attacks should be made illegal, but this would be almost impossible to implement. Penalties for uncontrolled fencing have been increased so that a hit scored by a fencer who is off balance is disallowed. Discipline amongst competitors and observance of a president's authority are, and have been for some time, at a low ebb, and attempts are being made to improve the situation, as some accidents have undoubtedly been caused by vicious hitting. A body of opinion blames the type of sword grip as a cause of accidents (Parfitt 1986b). A variety of grips exist but mainly they fall into two groups — the French grip with an almost straight handle, allowing greater flexibility, and the orthopaedic grip, giving greater strength at the expense of flexibility. Each grip has its devotees, though the orthopaedic grip is dominant in senior foil fencing and is the one that is most suspect because of the greater forces that can be exerted on the sword. In the absence of hard evidence, one must consider that the effect of the orthopaedic grip is likely to be small, and there are not, at present, sufficient grounds for banning it.

Accident statistics

Since April 1984, the Amateur Fencing Association has required the notification of all fencing accidents sufficient to cause a fencer to stop a bout. Over the four years since then, 24 accidents have been reported. It is very likely that injuries at the lower end of the scale have been unreported, but very unlikely that serious accidents, particularly broken blade accidents, will have gone unreported. A retrospective questionnaire carried out among Scottish university fencers (McKie 1987) revealed a small number of non-specific sporting injuries, and one cut from a very violent sabre attack. In other words, there is nothing to suggest that serious fencing accidents are being under-reported.

The accident statistics have been useful in highlighting some unexpected problems, dispelling a few myths and establishing some baselines. Among the conclusions were:

---

* It is perhaps for the legislators of the sport to draw the balance between rules which produce prohibitively expensive equipment changes whilst ensuring that measures are taken to safeguard the participants from possible injury, bearing in mind that fencing ranks fifth in the league table of incidence of sports injuries after Association Football, rugby football, women's hockey and men's hockey.

1   Serious accidents can happen to intermediate as well as top-class fencers.

2   The neck is a very vulnerable part of the body and attempts to increase protection to the fencer have not succeeded in protecting the neck adequately.

3   Aggressive fencing is not a constant feature of accidents.

4   Fencing pistes are commonly placed too close together, with resulting injuries to presidents and bystanders.

5   Particular care must be taken by presidents, when presiding over fights between children of very different height and physique, to control the weapon and style of fencing of the larger or stronger fencer.

Fatal accidents

There has been no systematic reporting of fatal accidents, but all those that are generally known about have been caused by broken blades. In the early years, there were occasions when penetrating injuries to the chest were associated with rotten or worn material in the jacket, particularly in the axilla, but this is rarely, if ever, a cause nowadays. In the 1982 World Championships, a former World Champion, Vladimir Smirnov of Russia, was killed when a broken blade penetrated his mask, passed through the orbit and caused a fatal brain injury. The mask was in good condition but the injury serves to illustrate further the force that can be generated in a broken blade accident. Attempts to improve the mask by replacing conventional tinned interannealed steel with stainless steel have been less than successful because stainless steel mesh cannot be welded, so that the wires can be forced apart. In the only fatal British accident, in 1983 (Crawfurd 1984), John Warburn, a member of the National Modern Pentathlon Squad, was killed when his opponent's épée blade broke on his chest, the broken end lifting the bottom edge of the bib of his mask and transfixing the trachea and left common carotid artery. It is true that this particular blade had been ground down to reduce the weight and stiffness, a practice that has now been made illegal, but the manner in which the blade broke was perfectly typical and very similar to injuries 2, 5 and 9 in Table 31.1. The problem of finding good protection for the neck has been a difficult one and, despite several new ideas, nothing has yet been found that gives good protection without seriously hampering the fencer's technique.

Other injuries

Fencing is a very asymmetric sport and élite fencers are commonly asymmetrically developed, but this does not apparently lead to any specific types of injury. There is the usual crop of sprains and strains,

Table 31.1 Fencing injuries

No.	Sex	Weapon	Level	Handle	L/R	Action	Aggression?	Injury
Broken blade injuries								
1.	M	Epee	Reg.	Ortho	R/R	Simultaneous attack	No	Blade transfixed left thigh
2.	M	Epee	Nat. U-18	Ortho	R/R	Attack/ counter-attack	No	Blade pierced bib and grazed neck
3.	M	Foil	Int.	?	L/?	Attack/ counter-attack	Yes	Blade transfixed non-Kevlar jacket and transfixed skin of chest wall
4.	M	Foil	Club	Ortho	L/R	Attack/ counter-attack	No	Superficial 5 cm cut on leg
5.	M	Foil	Club	Ortho	R/R	Attack	No	Pierced bib and grazed neck
Intact blade injuries								
6.	M	Foil	Reg	French	R/R	Attack/ counter-attack	No	Intact blade slid inside trousers and cut scrotum
7.	M	Sabre	Club	Sabre	?	Attack/ counter-attack	No	Intact blade slid inside trousers and transfixed base of penis
8.	M	Foil	Reg	Ortho	R/R	Attack/ parry	No	Intact point caused small puncture wound at base of thumb
9.	F	Foil	Nat.	Ortho	R/R	Attack/ riposte	No	Intact point slipped under bib and grazed neck
10.	F	Foil	Nat. U-16	Ortho	L/R	Attack at close quarters	Yes	Intact point slipped under bib and caused severe bruising to neck

Cuts and grazes, 4; sprained ankles, 4; pulled hamstrings, 1; other soft injuries, 6.
Level: Reg. = regional, including open competitions or others of approximately regional standard; Nat. = national; Int. = international.
Handle: orthopaedic or French grip as used by the fencer causing the injury.
L/R: left handers are common in fencing and it has been suggested that a left-hander fencing a right-hander is more dangerous than fencers of the same handedness fencing each other.
Aggression?: Whether the fencer causing the injury was, in the opinion of the injured fencer, unduly aggressive.

but, apart from a slight tendency to chronic knee injuries, there are no 'fencing-specific' injuries. Fencing is one of the few sports for women in which the bosom is an integral part of the target area, but the compulsory use of rigid breast protectors has meant that no significant breast injuries have been reported, although most protectors are made to a standard (and rather shallow) pattern which gives less than total protection to a well-developed woman. No specific studies on the incidence of breast cancer have been carried out, but there is no perception among women fencers that breast cancer might be a hazard of the sport.

The duties of an attending doctor

Only one set of rules for fencing exists (AFA 1986) and this sets the standards for fencing at Olympic and World Championship levels. For competitions at lower levels, organisers make *ad hoc* modifications as appropriate, but it is generally agreed that the presence of a doctor is only required at competitions of 'A' grade or above. At present, in this country, that includes the Commonwealth Championships, the Martini Epée Competition, the Eden Cup for U-20 Men's Foil and the Ipswich Ladies Epée Competition. At this level, the presence of a first-aid team and an ambulance are also required. At lower levels, access to some form of first-aid is advised.

The duty doctor, as well as being available to deal with injuries, may also be required under the 'ten-minutes rule'. This rule (no. 50) was introduced to try to put a stop to fencers feigning injury in order to take a break during a fight, and allows a maximum break of ten minutes, only if the duty doctor confirms the injury. In practice, it puts the doctor in a very difficult position. First, he or she has to be summoned from wherever he or she may be and has to arrive at the relevant piste. Probably without having witnessed the accident, he or she has to take the history (usually from a non-English speaker), make an examination on a fully clothed patient, reach a diagnosis, and pronounce whether the injury is genuine or not, all in a short enough space of time to deny the malingerer the advantage of taking a breather. If the fencer is injured, the doctor has to patch him/her up so that he/she can be back on the piste ready to fence within 10 minutes after the accident occurred. If this cannot be done, the fencer is automatically scratched.

A doctor in this position is well advised to take the following course of action. On arriving at the piste, ignore everyone except the president and enquire of him what actually happened. The rules specify that an accident in the course of fighting a bout must have occurred, so that cramp, injuries exacerbated by an awkward movement or obvious forms of time-wasting can be eliminated at the start. If no accident has taken place, inform the president that a medical opinion is not relevant and leave the rest to him. If an accident has definitely occurred, the president's account of what occurred is the only one worth relying on. The type of injury will dictate whether it is best treated at the side of the piste or in the first-aid room. Strapping to foot and ankle injuries has to be modified sufficiently to be applied with speed and for the fencer to be able to put on a sock and shoe over the dressing to continue fencing. Dressings which rely on adhesion to the skin frequently come adrift on sweaty skin, even when the skin has been thoroughly dried, but friar's balsam is usually effective in providing an anchorage for Steristrips or Elastoplast.

Where diagnosis or treatment has been, of necessity, perfunctory, it is important that the doctor instructs the fencer to return once there is sufficient time for the doctor to do the job properly. An even trickier situation faces the doctor when, surrounded by interested observers who know exactly whether the injury is genuine or not, he or she is asked to adjudicate on an alleged accident, with a histrionic fencer and with no hard physical signs for guidance. Once again, an experienced president is the best ally on such an occasion, but, if he or she is unable or unwilling to assist, then the doctor must either make a best guess, or fall back on low cunning. One strategy is to give the fencer a choice: either to continue fencing right away, or submit to a proper examination which will unfortunately take 15 to 20 minutes to carry out, so that, on return to the piste, he or she will, most regrettably, have been eliminated. Another alternative is for the doctor to take the view that, as he or she is unable to say categorically that the fencer is uninjured, the doctor should give the fencer the benefit of the doubt and recommend a break. However, Rule 50 states that 'the break should be strictly reserved for the treatment of the accident which brought it about'. It could be argued that simple rest is not 'treatment' and therefore the doctor can tell the president that, as no specific treatment is required, the bout may be restarted immediately. This may well be the signal for various coaches, physiotherapists and trainers to surround the fencer and start applying massage, sprays, liniments and bandages, while crying heaven's vengeance on the incompetent doctor who has failed to treat their injured lamb. The ball is now firmly back in the president's court, and it is up to him or her to make of the situation what he or she will. If the president is feeling brave, Rule 50 allows a penalty hit to be awarded for an unjustified request for a break in the fight. In any case, it is up to the president to restore order and restart the fight.

The doctor's official standing is, in the last resort, that of an adviser to the president, and he or she therefore does not have to make the decisions that are required, but merely advise the president of his or her opinion. The doctor's position is, or can be, ambiguous because, in the absence of the fencer's personal medical attendant, the doctor is also required to treat the fencer and do the best for him or her. To satisfy the fencer, president and spectators alike is a considerable test of a doctor's skill and personality.

The management of penetrating injuries

One anecdote exists of a sword entering the chest of an opponent and not being withdrawn, but, in all cases where details are known, the sword has been instinctively withdrawn from the wound, often without the fencer even realising he or she has caused an injury. The theory of first-aid treatment is straightforward in the sense that the bleeding must be stopped by direct pressure if possible, and urgent transport to hospital arranged. In practice the control of haemorrhage may be impossible and the British fatality occurred despite the fortuitous presence of a consultant surgeon in the *salle* at the time, and the location of the accident only a few hundred yards from a London teaching hospital. The FIE have called for the presence of a specialist in resuscitation to be present at any major competition, but, in the context of the British medical scene and in the light of the present experience of fencing injuries, such a requirement would be an unjustifiable waste of medical resources.

Doping and dope control

The aspect of competitive fencing which would most lend itself to doping is the necessity for a fencer to keep going against increasingly stiff opposition for one or two days. The normal pattern of major competitions is for the fencers to be seeded from the start and for those with poorer results to be progressively eliminated as the competition unwinds. It is not a straight knock-out competition because the first rounds are fought in pools, usually of six, in which each fencer fights every other fencer and those in each pool with the better results are promoted to the next round. This continues until an agreed number, usually 32, 24 or 16, are left. Then the formula changes to knock-out with *repêchage* until eight are left, when the formula changes again to direct knock-out. There are many variations on this theme, but the result is generally that a competition lasts between 12 and 20 hours. In pools, bouts last a maximum of six minutes' fencing time, being extended if the scores are then level, but, in knock-out, bouts last a maximum of eight minutes for women or ten minutes for men. Thus the winner of a major competition could expect to fight 15–20 short bouts and five–seven long bouts, although with considerable rest periods in between. This stop–start system, together with the fact that the fights become longer and harder as the competition goes on, puts a premium on mental and physical staying-power, and on the ability to reach a peak right at the end.

Apart from a brief flirtation with amphetamines, some 20 years ago when dope-testing was first appearing, fencers have not until recently shown themselves at all interested in doping, and the biggest problem for the authorities has been how to run a credible dope-testing programme when so many fencers casually dose themselves with cough mixtures and other medicines which may contain banned substances. This problem has been tackled in two quite different ways by the AFA and the FIE. The philosophy of the FIE appears to be that a positive dope test will lead to an automatic suspension, no matter how convincing the medical excuses and explanations given. To make up for the harshness of such a system, the penalties consist of only a six-month suspension on the first occasion, a two-year suspension on the second, and a life ban on the third. It is possible that such a system can be defended on the grounds that the medical profession, at least outside the UK, has shown itself to be quite unreliable and, indeed, sometimes frankly dishonest in the way that some doctors have attempted to promote and protect the doping of athletes.

Unfortunately, most of the victims of these sanctions so far have been household names in fencing who had inadvertently taken a catarrh remedy at the wrong time. Such results do little to promote the image and importance of dope-testing.

The AFA have adopted a different policy. When the Sports Council originally proposed random dope-testing in 1984, the AFA considered that there was insufficient distinction between bona fide medical treatment and *mala fide* doping, and declined to support the proposals. However, the Sports Council's revised proposals of 1985, allowing a flexible response to a positive dope test, have meant that the AFA could devise a scheme whereby innocent fencers could receive the benefit of an unrestricted Pharmacopoeia without fear of the consequences, while at the same time, genuine doping would be punished with far more realistic sanctions than those of the FIE. Under the AFA regulations, a positive test is followed by an inquiry, either formal or informal, and as a result of the inquiry the fencer may be found innocent or guilty, and the disciplinary committee can either impose no penalty at all, or anything up to a 5-year suspension on the first offence. Included within the ambit of disciplinary proceedings are not only the fencer concerned, but also any coaches, doctors or other fencers who may have been accessories. Even the withholding from the authorities of information concerning doping is considered a disciplinary offence. The disciplinary committee have it within their power to publicise their findings and even to inform the employers of the guilty party.

The validity of this approach has so far been demonstrated in that, in the two years of random dope-testing so far, no fencers have been found to be taking anything reprehensible, but, if FIE rules had been applied, perhaps as many as seven top British fencers might have found themselves in trouble for one reason or another. Even in such a short period of time a number of problems have emerged in what would appear to be a straightforward programme, though, of course, none of these problems are specific to fencing. Because of the considerable amount of perspiration involved in the sport, it is commonly the case that fencers cannot pass urine on demand, or even within two hours of a request. Unlike the AFA regulations, the FIE rules have now dropped the provision that a dope test can be called off after two hours if the fencer seems genuinely unable to urinate, and, in theory, fencer and doctor are doomed to sit and look at each other until nature calls, regardless of such mundane considerations as booked aeroplane flights or caretakers trying to lock up. If the fencer leaves first, he or she will almost certainly receive a six-month suspension, but, if the doctor leaves first, the fencer will be saved, although the doctor risks a ticking-off from the FIE, and in any case such a let-out would not be allowed by the independent sampling officers of the Sports Council.

The rules (608, article 2(n)) provide for a breathalyser type of test for alcohol, and set an upper limit for blood alcohol of 0.5%. This test is optional, but, if it is carried out and found to be positive, a quantitative test, using either a breathalyser or blood sample, is then mandatory, with sanctions for failing to comply. This rule is a curious measure on three counts. First, the alcohol test is very rarely used, unlike the ordinary urine test for dope. Secondly, alcohol is not likely to be a great help to a fencer, though it might just steady pre-final nerves. It is generally believed that the rule was introduced by the FIE in conjunction with the governing body of the modern pentathlon who found that alcohol was being used by pentathletes to steady them when a precision discipline followed immediately after an exertion discipline, even though such a consideration hardly applies to fencing on its own. Alcohol might almost be considered part of the staple diet of several of the top fencing nations, and the limit of 0.5% (as compared with the UK driving limit of 0.8%) corresponds approximately to 2 units of alcohol, and was introduced to allow for this national custom. However, if there is any benefit to be gained from alcohol in small quantities, it would almost certainly be abolished at levels higher than 0.5% so the rule would seem somewhat unnecessary. Thirdly, it introduces the principle of mandatory blood-testing while this is not allowed for in testing for other substances, even when the fencer is willing to submit to it. If the possibility existed of blood-testing, where the fencer agreed, it would make life a lot easier for the fencer and the doctor when the fencer is unable to pass urine.

Another problem concerns the dope-testing of minors. Random testing, to be an effective deterrent, must be carried out without warning, although it is common practice as a matter of convenience for it to be carried out at competitions or when fencers are training together in one place. It is probable that their parents will not be present when schoolchildren are being tested, and the teacher in charge may well consider that it would be inadequate for him or her to give personal permission for urine samples to be collected. Such an objection has indeed been raised. As a condition of holding an AFA licence, a fencer undertakes not to make use of drugs and to accept any form of test, and the holding of an AFA licence is obligatory for fencers over 14 entering section (regional) events or higher. It could be argued, therefore, that all minors, and, by implication, their parents, have been warned of the possibility of random testing and that consent can be inferred, although this is clearly less absolute than some form of written parental consent. Whatever the wisdom of this approach in today's world, it is in keeping with the attitude of fencing organisers at competitions in which children take part for which a disclaimer is signed in relation to accidental injury, but the signature is often that of the fencer or master in charge, and not that of the parent.

Fencing and the disabled

Fencing is a sport suitable for all ages and can be realistically enjoyed from nine to 90. It is a sport ideally suited to athletes who suffer from loss of full function of one arm; indeed, the last British World Youth Champion was so affected. With adaptation, fencing is also compatible with a wide range of disabilities. Wheelchair fencing is well established, with its own modified rules and its own section within the AFA. A wheelchair fencer can take on an able-bodied fencer sitting on a chair on equal terms. Although strictly speaking, fencing is a non-contact sport, the probability of knocks and grazes from the sword is too great to make it really suitable for an athlete with a haemorrhagic diathesis. A few blind fencers have managed to make a success of the sport, though this requires their opponent to maintain blade contact at least initially. For the supervisor, the most hair-raising of all disabilities to cope with is to try to control a pair of deaf fencers: shouting 'halt' achieves nothing, and it requires some courage to plunge repeatedly between the flying blades. Fencing has proved adaptable both to mental handicap and to mental illness, and, in the latter particularly, such aspects of the sport as the release of aggression and the anonymity of the fencer behind the mask have presented unusual and useful opportunities.

Summary and recommendations

Safety

Fencing is a very safe sport, and strenuous efforts are being made to minimise the danger of the only serious type of accident — the broken blade injury. The future lies in the perfection of specialised steel blades and their widespread adoption.

The doctor's role

The doctor attending a fencing competition has an important and unenviable task. As well as dealing with minor, major or even life-threatening injuries, he or she may be called upon to sort out malingerers from the genuinely injured, in the public gaze and against the clock.

Dope and dope-testing

Doping is not a serious problem so far in fencing. The development of an effective and credible dope-testing programme which does not penalise accidental or unintentional infringements has been achieved in the UK, but as yet not in the international arena.

Disabled fencers

Fencing is a sport suitable for people with many types of disability and for a wide age range.

References

AFA (1986) *Rules for Competition* (with amendments). Amateur Fencing Association.
Arlott J. (ed.) (1975) *The Oxford Companion to Sports and Games*. Oxford: Oxford University Press, pp. 301ff.
Aylward J. D. (1960) *The Small Sword in England*, 2nd edn. London: Hutchinson.
Crawfurd A. R. (1984) Death of a fencer. *British Journal of Sports Medicine* **18** (3), 220.
Crawfurd A. R (1986) Accident report for 1984–1985. *The Sword* (new series), no. 6, iv.
Crawfurd A. R (1989) Hits faster than the eye can see. *The Sword* (new series), no. 17.
Kerwin D. G. (1985) Amateur Fencing Association — fencing lunge study. Department of Physical Education and Sports Science, Loughborough University of Technology (unpublished).
McKie H. (1987) Thesis, Glasgow University (unpublished).
Parfitt R. (1986a) Report to the Fédération Internationale d'Escrime (unpublished).
Parfitt R. (1986b) Serious fencing accidents and their causes. *The Sword* (new series), no. 5, 4.
Paul B. (1985) The quest for the perfect blade. *The Sword* (new series), no. 4, 7.
Paul R. (1985) Report to the Amateur Fencing Association. Leon Paul Equipment (unpublished).
Pollock W. H., Grove F. C. & Prevost C. (1889) *The Badminton Library — Fencing, Boxing, Wrestling*. London: Longmans, Green, pp. 9ff.

Index